LATERALITY

Functional Asymmetry in the Intact Brain

This is a volume in

PERSPECTIVES IN
NEUROLINGUISTICS, NEUROPSYCHOLOGY, AND PSYCHO-
LINGUISTICS

A Series of Monographs and Treatises

A complete list of titles in this series appears at the end of this volume.

LATERALITY

Functional Asymmetry in the Intact Brain

M. P. Bryden

Department of Psychology
University of Waterloo
Waterloo, Ontario, Canada

1982 (AP)

ACADEMIC PRESS

A SUBSIDIARY OF HARCOURT BRACE JOVANOVICH, PUBLISHERS

New York   London
Paris   San Diego   San Francisco   São Paulo   Sydney   Tokyo   Toronto

ACADEMIC PRESS, INC.
111 Fifth Avenue, New York, New York 10003

United Kingdom Edition published by
ACADEMIC PRESS, INC. (LONDON) LTD.
24/28 Oval Road, London NW1 7DX

Library of Congress Cataloging in Publication Data

Bryden, M. P.
    Laterality : functional asymmetry in the intact brain.

    (Perspectives in neurolinguistics, neuropsychology,
and psycholinguistics)
    Includes bibliographical references and index.
    1. Cerebral dominance. 2. Laterality. I. Title.
II. Series. [DNLM: 1. Laterality. WL 335 B916L]
QP385.5.B79   612'.825   82-6692
ISBN 0-12-138180-3   AACR2

PRINTED IN THE UNITED STATES OF AMERICA

82 83 84 85   9 8 7 6 5 4 3 2 1

To my three P's
PAT, PENNY, AND PAM
who keep me going, each in her own way.

Contents

4 Visual Laterality Effects

5 Tactual Laterality Effects

6 Some General Considerations regarding Perceptual Laterality

7 Asymmetry of Motor Performance

8 Lateralization of Emotional Processes

9 Physiological Measures of Asymmetry

10 Handedness and Its Relation to Cerebral Function

11 Genetics of Laterality

12 The Development of Cerebral Lateralization

13 Introduction to Individual Differences in Cerebral Organization

14   Sex Differences in Laterality

15   Reading and Language-Related Deficits

16   Control of the Active Hemisphere

17   Some Final Words

Preface

This book grew from a concern with the sweeping generalizations about brain function and laterality that have become popular in recent years. When I first became interested in the possibility that behavioral techniques could be used to study the functional specialization of the brain in normal individuals, there were only a few relevant papers. Now, dozens of new articles appear each month, and an understanding of the differences between the two hemispheres is seen by some researchers as leading to the solution of almost all problems—from psychopathology and dyslexia, to stuttering and management effectiveness.

As I reviewed the literature, however, I found it important to adopt a more conservative stance. Cerebral lateralization is one factor affecting performance on a wide variety of behavioral tasks, but it is only one of many factors. Unless we understand the demands of the specific tasks chosen and the strategies subjects use to meet these demands, we risk the danger of overinterpreting the results of experiments on laterality. Thus, the central message of this book is that not all behavioral asymmetries are necessarily related to the differing functions of the two hemispheres.

A major goal of the book is to provide a single source that will introduce the reader to the various methods used to assess behavioral asymmetries. The initial chapters review the literature on perceptual-cognitive laterality effects in different sensory modalities, for it is research of this type that has generated much of the enthusiasm for laterality studies. These chapters indicate some of the problems with the existing research and offer suggestions about the direction of future research. Chapters 7–9 deal with the areas in which laterality research has become popular: lateralization of emotion and of motor behavior, and the electrophysiological evidence.

For many people, handedness is one of the most salient asymmetries.

General statements about brain organization and cerebral laterality are often prefaced by the statement that they do not apply to left-handers. Chapters 10 and 11 deal with the measurement and origins of handedness and indicate the extent to which handedness must be considered to be an important variable in laterality research.

In a broad sense, Chapters 12–16 are all concerned with problems of individual differences in laterality. First, I examine the question of whether laterality changes with age in young children. Second, I consider the data on laterality effects in special groups, especially those studies dealing with sex differences and with language-impaired subjects. Third, I consider the evidence for hemisphericity as a cognitive style. The concluding chapter summarizes the major points of the book and presents a general framework for laterality research in the normal subject.

This book is addressed primarily to neuropsychologists, experimental psychologists, neurologists, and educators. I am convinced that experimental psychology has a major contribution to make to the understanding of human brain function. Experimental psychologists can typically afford to test various hypotheses, develop precise methods, and rule out alternative explanations by careful experimentation. The practicing neuropsychologist can seldom afford such luxury: A patient with a particular type of brain damage may appear only rarely, and one cannot try a dozen alternatives before settling on an appropriate experimental procedure. In the domain of laterality research, this volume can direct the neuropsychologist toward those hypotheses that may be most fruitful and away from those that are less viable.

The book should also provide a similar function for the educator interested in special groups. Researchers in education often do not have access to the immense literature of experimental psychology, and yet a grasp of this literature is essential in planning good studies of dyslexia, language impairment, and related phenomena. By providing a general overview of laterality research, the book will give those researchers who wish to investigate particular types of laterality effects a view of how other researchers with different viewpoints have approached similar problems.

The book does not, however, provide a unified theory of lateralization of function. The more I read and wrote, the more convinced I became that there was as yet scant evidence to support any one general theory. There remain too many unanswered questions and too many unsolved problems to do any more than point in the direction of an integration of the laterality data. That will have to wait for more experimentation. In the meantime, this book may suggest fruitful lines of research.

Acknowledgments

In the preparation of this book, the contributions of two individuals stand out. Frances Allard started this project as a collaborator, but found it necessary to withdraw from active participation because of other demands on her time. Fran wrote the initial draft of the chapter on motor asymmetries and commented critically, often caustically, and always helpfully, on the entire manuscript. Marion Tapley, my research technician and colleague, worked above and beyond the call of duty to supervise the typing of the manuscript, organize and check references, and prepare the figures. She made my task vastly easier and prevented innumerable disasters with her planning and organization.

I must also acknowledge the support of Harry Whitaker, the series editor. Whit encouraged the project from the beginning, reassured me when I was most pessimistic, tolerated the lengthy time it took to complete even the first draft, and made wise suggestions about all parts of the manuscript. I looked forward with some trepidation to the pages of single-space commentary he sent me on each chapter. Derek Besner, Ernie MacKinnon, Janice Murray, and Sid Segalowitz also read and commented on my penultimate draft, and their advice has colored the final project. Many thanks are also due to Bonnie Lee Bender, Laurie Westlake Bruin, Bev Dakins, Diane Hagan, Paula Kovacs, and Lyn Spaetzel who did an outstanding job of typing page upon page of manuscript. Finally, my own contribution was aided by a grant from the Natural Sciences and Engineering Research Council of Canada and by the willingness of the Department of Psychology at the University of Waterloo to assist with both typing services and computer facilities.

Introduction

The notion that the two cerebral hemispheres have different functions and that this is important in our daily lives has become very popular in the past few years. Such ideas have a long history (Wigan, 1844) but were given new impetus by the exciting work of Sperry and his colleagues on the behavior of patients following section of the corpus callosum and anterior commissure (e.g., Gazzaniga, Bogen, & Sperry, 1962, 1963, 1965). This work revealed that the isolated left hemisphere perceived, remembered, and responded in a fashion quite different from the isolated right hemisphere (see Bogen, 1969a, 1969b; Gazzaniga, 1970 for reviews). At about the same time, work by Doreen Kimura (1961a, 1961b, 1967) in auditory perception provided some suggestion that the different functions of the two hemispheres could be measured in the normal, intact brain.

The popular appeal of this work has been such that it has led to a vast number of speculations. Cerebral asymmetries are now taken as givens, and ideas derived from the study of cerebral asymmetry are used to explain almost every imaginable kind of behavior, from reading disability to schizophrenia, from stuttering to the gender-related difference in spatial ability, from infantile autism to the generation gap.

The objective of the present book is to review the evidence pertaining to cerebral asymmetries in the intact human brain. We shall be concerned primarily with two issues. First, can one reliably assess the different function of the two cerebral hemispheres with noninvasive techniques? Second, do the patterns of cerebral asymmetry relate in any consistent way to meaningful behavior? One of the viewpoints developed in this book is that many of the studies supposedly dealing with cerebral asymmetries do not in fact do so. Nevertheless, sufficient consistencies do exist for one to believe that functional cerebral asymmetries can be measured and that they do have some meaningful consequences for normal behavior. The aim of the succeeding pages is to provide a realistic assessment of the current state of the art.

A Simplistic View of Cerebral Asymmetry

Ever since the work of Dax (1865) and Broca (1861) in the mid-nineteenth century, it has been known that damage to certain portions of the left hemisphere results in disturbances of language (*aphasias*) that do not occur following damage to the right hemisphere. Thus, in some fashion the left hemisphere is functionally specialized for at least some language processes. In the late nineteenth and early twentieth century, there were a number of reports of aphasias following right-hemispheric damage, often in individuals who were left-handed or had some familial history of left-handedness. It was an easy step from these observations to the notion that left-handers were the reverse of right-handers, using the right hemisphere rather than the left for speech and language processes. While current evidence indicates that this is an oversimplification, it is generally agreed that the incidence of right-hemispheric speech is higher in left-handers than in right-handers (Herron, 1980).

Perhaps because disturbances of speech and language are relatively obvious and important in one's daily life, much of the early clinical neuropsychological work concentrated on the aphasias and on the functions of the left hemisphere. Only in the past 30 years has much attention been paid to the right hemisphere and to nonverbal skills. Although the deficits may not be as striking or as clear-cut, recent evidence has suggested that the right hemisphere plays an important role in a variety of nonverbal activities, including music (Gates & Bradshaw, 1977b), spatial abilities (Benton, 1979), face recognition (Geffen, Bradshaw, & Wallace, 1971), and emotional expression (Ley & Bryden, 1981). At a simple level, then, the left hemisphere can be viewed as concerned with speech and language, whereas the right hemisphere is concerned with nonverbal skills. In the search for a better distinction, the left hemisphere is often described as analytic or concerned with sequential processing, whereas the right is considered to be concerned with the integration of information over space and time, a holistic or gestalt processor (cf. Bradshaw & Nettleton, 1981).

It is only a small step from this elementary description of functional asymmetry to the view that those people who excel in verbal skills are using their left hemispheres in preference to their right and, conversely, that those who excel in spatial skills use their right hemispheres. One might even hope that if we can find out which hemisphere people use, then we ought to be able to say something about what kind of people they are, and therefore some assessment of functional specialization should be useful in the study of individual differences.

Similarly, one can argue that if an individual is poor at verbal skills, there must be something wrong with his or her left hemisphere. If, for example, language functions fail to lateralize clearly in one hemisphere, then an individual might be expected to show some form of language disturbance. Such an argument has been used to suggest that poor readers, stutterers, the congenitally deaf, and many other special groups suffer from a disturbance of functional lateralization. In many of these cases, the argument also implies that functional lateralization develops and that the particular group in question suffers from a "developmental lag."

Not all individuals are left-hemispheric for speech and language (Hécaen, DeAgostini, & Monzon-Montes, 1981; Satz, 1980), and likewise, it is presumed that not everyone is right-hemispheric for nonverbal processes. We have known for a long time that left-handers are somewhat more likely to have right-hemispheric speech, and, certainly, we have often considered left-handers to be peculiar (Hardyck & Petrinovitch, 1977; L. J. Harris, 1980). Perhaps, then, there is something peculiar about those individuals who have speech and language functionally represented in the right hemisphere. This logic leads one to argue that the particular pattern of functional organization is important and that at least some left-handers are qualitatively different from the "normal" right-handers.

Finally, one might argue that we do not use our brain as well as we might. Most particularly, since the majority of us are left-hemispheric for speech and since our culture seems to depend very heavily on speech and language, perhaps we are missing a facet of our education. There are other cultures less dependent on language, and we may very well be missing something important by ignoring this aspect of our experience. With training, we might give significance to integrative, intuitive (right-hemispheric) behaviors. By implication, our training and experience can dictate the way in which we use the two hemispheres of our brain, and we would perhaps be better persons if we made full use of the potential of our right hemispheres.

The preceding paragraphs should not be construed as a statement of the position to be espoused in this book, but rather as a resumé of contemporary views concerning the relevance of lateral specialization. It is intended to give an overview against which the remainder of this book can be evaluated. From this beginning, the relevant issues can be addressed.

What Is Lateralized?

It is very easy to argue that if one hemisphere acts in a particular way, the other hemisphere must do the opposite. The notion of a balanced or dual asymmetry has been very popular, and it most certainly has led to such distinctions as verbal–nonverbal or analytic–integrative. Bogen (1969a, 1969b) and Corballis and Beale (1976) have tabled various views as to the functional differences between the hemispheres. These tables make it clear that there is no general agreement as to what it is that differentiates the functions of the left hemisphere from those of the right. Certainly, one can search for some dichotomous relationship: At the same time, one should recognize that a dichotomy is not necessary. If a particular region of left frontal cortex is important in the expression of language, it does not imply that the homologous region in the right hemisphere is important for the "opposite" function, whatever that might be.

Issues of reliability and validity become an essential part of any discussion of cerebral laterality. In the middle 1960s, any argument that a behaviorally measured laterality measure such as those offered by Kimura (1961a, 1961b) or Bryden (1965) might actually be related to cerebral asymmetry was greeted with a certain amount of derision (e.g., Harcum & Filion, 1963; Inglis, 1965). More recently, however, the pendulum has swung the other way, and virtually any observed lateral asymmetry is interpreted as being necessarily related to cerebral asymmetry and virtually any deficit in spatial or verbal function is interpreted as indicating some malfunction of one or the other cerebral hemispheres.

One of the basic concerns of this book is that many of the tasks employed to assess lateral specialization actually measure a diversity of things (Bryden, 1978). Although a simple behavioral task, such as the auditory dichotic listening procedure employed by Kimura (1961a), may very well be related to the lateralization of language, other factors—attentional biases, strategies of encoding or remembering the stimuli, and the like—may influence the magnitude of the laterality effect observed and may even reverse the effect under some conditions or for some people. Without understanding and controlling these extraneous factors, we run the danger of grossly overinterpreting our results.

Despite these cautions, both the clinical and the experimental literature point toward the conclusion that the two cerebral hemispheres have
very different functions. One of the objectives of this book will be to
consider the evidence about what it is that is lateralized and to see
whether or not there are any general principles that can be enumerated.

What Are the Mechanisms of Lateralization?

A second issue concerns the mechanisms of lateralization. In many
ways, such a question is the domain of the neurophysiologist rather
than the behavioral scientist, but the existing behavioral evidence can
serve to point us in the proper direction.

There are at least two general theories to consider. One may be
termed a structural theory: It is the view that different functions are
lateralized to different hemispheres because of the underlying structure
of the nervous system. Such a view places emphasis on the neuroanatomical differences between the hemispheres that have been
found to exist even at birth and sees the functional differences as being
derived from these structural differences. An alternative approach considers the cerebral cortex to be a much more dynamic system and views
lateral asymmetries as emerging dynamic factors that change the overall
level of activity in one hemisphere or the other. Such an approach em-
phasizes the spread of neural excitation from one portion of the cerebral
cortex to adjacent areas. There may be other alternatives as well: One
might argue, for example, that there are different optimal levels of activation for the two hemispheres and that the observed differences between the two hemispheres are somehow related to optimizing the conditions under which each hemisphere can function most efficiently.

What Are the Origins of Lateralization?

When one asks what the origins of lateralization are, one is essentially
asking two distinct questions—one ontogenetic and one phylogenetic.
The human brain shows lateral specialization to a far greater degree than
is manifested in subhuman species: In some way, evolution has led to
the development of a human brain exhibiting lateral specialization. The
fact that lateralization is the result of evolutionary processes does not,
however, mean that lateralization must change in the developing organism. This issue of the ontogeny of lateralization is a separate question.

Lenneberg (1967) popularized the idea that speech and language functions gradually become more and more lateralized in the developing child, reaching full lateralization at about the age of puberty. This notion has led to many speculations that particular special groups of children, such as the reading disabled, stutterers, or the deaf, manifest incomplete lateralization and thus exhibit a "developmental lag." More recent evidence (e.g., Witelson & Pallie, 1973) indicates that there may be anatomical asymmetries observable even at birth. Such a finding suggests that lateralization does not develop in any true sense but is determined by the anatomical and physiological properties of the individual at birth (or even at conception). Of course, lateralization of cognitive functions *does* change with age, in some trite sense, for the language capabilities of the adult are certainly different from those of the child and the spatial abilities of the adolescent different from those of the infant. The question that we must be concerned with is whether or not there is any developmental change in functional lateralization over and above changes in the capacity to perform certain tasks. The way in which this question is answered has implications for many assertions that have been made about the significance of lateralization in children.

At the same time, it becomes germane to at least speculate about the evolutionary origins of lateralization. To some extent, this question can only be dealt with at a speculative level, because evidence about lateralization of behaviors are not preserved in the fossil record. Although it will not be discussed here, the nature of lateral specialization in subhuman species is certainly relevant to the topic of human brain function. The data concerning the possibility of a genetic basis for lateralization are also important. While in many instances, this topic turns us away from cerebral lateralization to manual specialization, we must examine the evidence concerning the evolutionary development of lateralization.

Does It Make Any Difference How the Brain Is Organized?

In the preceding sections, the important questions of what is lateralized, how it is lateralized, and when it is lateralized have been raised. At least provisionally, it is clear that one cerebral hemisphere functions in one way, while the other functions in a different way. At the same time, there are both clinical and experimental data to suggest that not all people have the same functional organization. Left-handers as a group, for example, have long been suspect: the incidence of aphasic disturbances following left-hemispheric damage is not nearly so great in left-handers as it is in right-handers, and concomitantly the incidence of aphasia following right-hemispheric damage is much greater (Hécaen *et al.*, 1981; Satz, 1980). As a result, it has often been thought that left-handers, or some particular subgroup of left-handers, have a functional organization that is the reverse of that usually observed. Other investigators have raised the possibility that women are less clearly lateralized than men and have sought to explain some of the sex-related differences in cognitive functioning in terms of different patterns of lateralization (Bryden, 1979a; Levy, 1974; Ounsted & Taylor, 1972).

The possibility that different people have different patterns of organization raises some interesting problems for research in human lateralization. Much effort has been devoted to determining the characteristics of individuals who have reversed lateralization (e.g., Levy & Reid, 1978) or who have bilateral representation for certain functions. If the end result of this work is simply to provide a better description of the cerebral organization of the individual, our efforts become largely academic. The end result will be only that we can better predict the consequences of unilateral brain damage. The immediate benefits of such knowledge are not clearly evident, unless one proposes to produce a lot of people with unilateral brain damage.

If knowledge of cerebral organization is to be of use, we need to demonstrate that different patterns of cerebral organization have different consequences. Two general hypotheses come to mind. One is that "reversed" organization is somehow deleterious: Left-handers have long been maligned. They are accused of being odd, eccentric, devious, and even stupid (L. J. Harris, 1980). Perhaps this arises from those left-handers who show a pattern of lateralization reversed from the normal. Admittedly, it is not self-evident why a reversed pattern of lateralization per se should be deleterious, but certainly enough questions have been raised about the idiosyncracies of left-handers to warrant investigation of the question.

A second and somewhat more plausible hypothesis is that those individuals with bilateral or diffuse representation of function are different from those with unilateral or focal representation of function. If the same cortical tissue is involved in both spatial and linguistic functions in one individual and not in another, one might expect to find differences between the two individuals. Diffuse or bilateral representation could lead to interference in some conditions and to mutual facilitation in others. The notion of investigating the relation between patterns of cerebral organization and behavior, then, is one deserving continued investigation. If it can be demonstrated that there are meaningful differences in intellectual abilities, cognitive styles, or personality variables that are related to the pattern of cerebral organization, then the investigations of cerebral laterality in the intact brain emerge from the academic ivory tower and become pertinent to our general understanding of behavior.

Do People Habitually Use One Hemisphere?

It is currently popular to invoke hemispheric asymmetries to "explain" individual differences in behavior. In our enthusiasm for dichotomous classifications, people are seen as being fundamentally either verbal or nonverbal in their behavior. Certainly it is true that some people are verbally fluent and relatively inept at, say, spatial tasks, whereas others show the reverse pattern. It would be easy to assume that the verbal individual is one who habitually makes use of his or her left hemisphere, whereas the nonverbal or spatial person makes use of his or her right hemisphere.

In one sense, this linkage of brain and behavior is trivial. If a particular individual habitually approaches all problems in a verbal fashion, and if the left hemisphere is peculiarly specialized for the processing of verbal material, then the activity of the left hemisphere will be different than that of the right, and very possibly greater than that of the right. To consider this an "explanation," however, is quite another matter. Do we become verbal (or nonverbal) because we learn that verbal strategies are the most successful for us, or because we learn to use one hemisphere in preference to the other? If the person who uses visual imagery is truly using his or her right hemisphere selectively over the left, this should have other implications: For instance, other processes that are dependent on the right hemisphere should be facilitated in such individuals.

We do not doubt that there are individual differences in verbal ability, in the use of imagery, and in spatial ability. The basic question is whether attributing such individual differences to some underlying concept of "hemisphericity" adds anything to our knowledge. Is the left (language) hemisphere of the highly verbal individual any different from the left hemisphere of the verbally deficient person? Is language lateralized more strongly, or less strongly, or in some different way in the verbal person? Or, alternatively, are we dealing with a person who has learned to employ some constant substrate in an efficient way?

Because our educational system prizes verbal skills, it has often been argued that we selectively educate the left hemisphere. Techniques have been developed that purportedly train people to use the right hemisphere and are claimed to have wondrous consequences in education, interpersonal relations, management, and so on. What do these procedures do? Do they really train the right hemisphere in any legitimate sense, or do they simply emphasize the use of nonverbal problem-solving strategies, imagery, and the like? The essential question is whether it is necessary to invoke any concept of hemisphericity to deal with such ventures, or whether they are best described as techniques for altering one's strategy of problem solving.

The preceding pages provide a very brief introduction to the basic concepts in the study of human lateralization and to the issues that seem to be important. Most simply, the issues of what, how, when, and so what are the critical ones. In the following pages, these questions will receive continued emphasis as the present state of various approaches to lateralization in the normal brain are considered.

Methods and Measurement in Laterality Studies

In this chapter, we shall provide a general introduction to some of the behavioral techniques that have been developed to measure hemispheric asymmetry in the normal brain. We shall examine in some detail the procedures and findings of some of the early experiments in each sensory modality. As work on lateralization has progressed, the techniques have improved and the specific hypotheses being tested have become more sophisticated. However, at the beginning it is illustrative to examine some of the earliest experiments, so that the basic issues in the measurement of hemispheric asymmetry can be brought out more clearly. This chapter, then, is concerned not only with familiarizing the reader with the basic findings but also with raising a number of questions about procedural detail to be kept in mind as we progress to a more detailed consideration of current experimentation.

The initial indication of the possibility of a behavioral assessment of cerebral specialization in the intact brain came, oddly enough, from the study of brain-damaged individuals. In 1961, Doreen Kimura published two papers that showed a clear relationship between speech lateralization and patient's performance on an auditory task called dichotic listening. The dichotic procedure involved the presentation of short lists of numbers, arranged in such a way that some came to the left ear while others arrived simultaneously at the right ear. Thus, a patient might hear the list "7–9–1" at the left ear and "8–3–4" at the right ear. Kimura found that temporal lobe excision resulted in a considerable drop in performance on the ear contralateral to the removal. More interestingly, her patients showed consistent and marked asymmetries in recall performance even preoperatively, finding the items from one ear typically easier to recall than those from the other.

Fortunately, Kimura had available knowledge of the speech lateralization of her patients, obtained through sodium amytal testing (Wada & Rasmussen, 1960). In this procedure, sodium amytal is injected unilaterally into the carotid artery: It produces a transient hemiplegia on the side contralateral to the injection. If the speech-dominant hemisphere is injected, the drug also produces an aphasia that outlasts the hemiplegia. In the past two decades, the Wada test has become a fairly common clinical procedure for assessing speech lateralization prior to surgery, although the side effects and potential risks preclude its use with normal populations. The availability of sodium amytal data made it possible for Kimura to test both left- and right-handed patients of known speech lateralization on the dichotic task. Her data indicated that those patients with speech in the left hemisphere recalled more items from the right ear, whereas those with speech in the right hemisphere recalled more items from the left ear. There were also small differences between handedness groups such that right-handed left hemispherics showed a bigger right-ear effect than left-handers and right-handed right hemispherics showed a smaller left-ear effect than left-handers. These differences, however, were not statistically significant, according to the analyses Kimura performed.

In her second study, Kimura tested a group of normal young adult females on the dichotic listing task and found that normal subjects showed a significant right-ear superiority in recall accuracy. Since one would expect the vast majority of normal adults to be left-hemispheric for speech, the obvious conclusion is that one performs better in the dichotic listening task on the ear opposite to the speech hemisphere. Although there are both crossed and uncrossed pathways from the ear to the cortex, Kimura cited evidence to indicate that the crossed pathways were dominant over the uncrossed ones and that information passing along the contralateral pathways would block or occlude information ascending the ipsilateral paths. Thus, right-ear information would have direct access to the left auditory cortex, whereas left-ear information would be forced to the right hemisphere and then have to be passed transcallosally before it could be analyzed by the speech centers of the left hemisphere. Left-ear information would therefore take longer to reach the speech centers and/or be degraded by the longer transmission route. Kimura's model is shown in Figure 2.1.

Since reasonably adequate dichotic tapes could be prepared by anyone with a little patience and a stereophonic tape recorder, Kimura's findings offered the very exciting possibility that experimental psychologists could assess hemispheric specialization for speech in healthy normals. So much of our data on functional localization have come from studies of people with head injury, stroke, and brain tumor that the

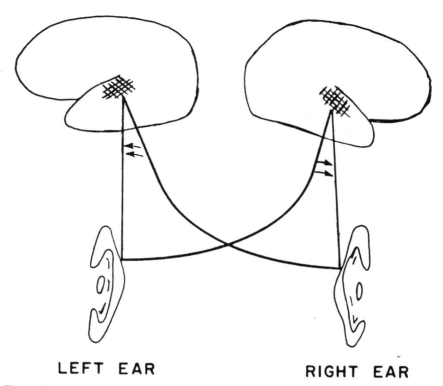

LEFT EAR   **RIGHT EAR**

Figure 2.1. Kimura's model for asymmetries in dichotic listening. With speech input, the stronger pathway from the right ear to the left hemisphere occludes the weaker ipsilateral pathway from the left ear. With music or environmental sounds, the primary analysis is in the right hemisphere, and information coming from the left ear occludes that from the right. (From Kimura, D. Functional asymmetry of the brain in dichotic listening. *Cortex*, 1967, *3*, 163–178. Reprinted with permission.)

discovery of the relationship between right-ear superiority in dichotic listening and speech lateralization represented a very significant breakthrough.

A number of experiments provided support for Kimura's model. If the right-ear effect is due to an access advantage for right-ear information to the speech center, then dichotic nonverbal material should not show a right-ear superiority. In fact, nonverbal dichotic material might well be expected to show a significant left-ear superiority if the right hemisphere has developed its own set of specializations. In support of her model, Kimura (1964) demonstrated a significant left-ear advantage for the recognition of dichotically presented musical passages. The ear advantage observed under dichotic presentation, then, changes as a function of the nature of the auditory material being presented.

If Kimura's notion of the contralateral auditory path occluding the ipsilateral path is correct, an ear superiority should only be observed with dichotic presentation. In general, this has also proven to be true (Bryden, 1969), although monaural effects have been reported (Henry, 1979).

Although the general form of Kimura's model has been supported, it has become popular to assume than one can administer any dichotic listening test to any subgroup of individuals, adult or child, and make precise inferences about the functional organization of the individual's brain. As the dichotic listening literature has amassed, major problems with the dichotic paradigm have become evident. Many researchers seem to have forgotten that they are dealing with active, scheming human beings. A subject enters the laboratory and is faced with the task of identifying or otherwise responding to a particular set of stimuli presented in a unique fashion. Because most dichotic listening experiments are very difficult, the subject is going to do those kinds of things that maximize performance, or seem to please the experimenter, or get the subject out of the situation. As argued elsewhere (Bryden, 1978), the whole structure of the experimental situation permits the subject to adopt idiosyncratic strategies that help him or her cope with the demands of the task. To the extent that these strategies influence performance, they may dictate the magnitude and even the direction of the behavioral laterality effect. Unless we become aware of these problems and develop procedures to control the strategies that subjects adopt, we run the danger of building complex theories on shaky grounds. We may discover, for example, that poor readers have a smaller right-ear advantage for verbal dichotic material than do good readers. It is easy to make the inference that language is less lateralized in poor readers than in good readers. In fact, we may be making two errors. It is very possible that good readers do the dichotic task in a different way than do poor readers, since good readers may have more systematic strategies in dealing with perceptual information. We have to be very sensitive to the demands of the task to be sure that this is not the case. Second, Kimura's original (1961b) study showed only that people with left-hemispheric speech showed a right-ear advantage for verbal material presented dichotically. Her data did not address the issue of individual differences in the *magnitude* of the observed effect; there is little evidence to indicate that a person who exhibits a big right-ear effect is any more dependent on the left hemisphere for speech processing than the individual who manifests a small right-ear effect. Yet it has become commonplace to interpret differences in the magnitude of laterality effects as indicative of differences in the relative involvement of the two hemispheres; this may turn out to be a totally unjustified assumption.

The Kimura Study

To illustrate the problems we have just described, we will now consider Kimura's initial experiment in some detail. This will allow us to raise issues dealing both with inferences that can be made from dichotic listening studies and with the measurement of laterality effects.

Because Kimura's work was essentially an exploratory application of Broadbent's (1954) dichotic listening technique to the study of temporal lobe patients, her selection of stimulus material included a variety of different types of lists. In all cases, subjects heard 6 numbers, apparently selected from the set 1–10. On most of the trials, these were arranged as three dichotic pairs, with 3 numbers arriving at the left ear and 3 arriving at the right, and with a presentation interval of .5 sec between pairs. However, some lists were presented at slower rates (1961b, p. 159), and in some trials, the numbers alternated between the two ears with a .5-sec interval between succeeding numbers. In most of the analyses, the data from all 32 trials, regardless of the specific stimulus parameters, are pooled. Only once are the conditions separated, when we see that the postoperative loss on the ear contralateral to temporal lobe excision is confined to the dichotic condition (1961b, pp. 161–162). Normal subjects heard the same test materials as did the temporal lobe patients (1961b). Presumably, 6 different numbers were heard on any one trial, so that one could determine which number was being recalled. With a pool of only 10 numbers, subjects who bothered to report (or guess) 6 numbers on each trial would average 60% accuracy on each ear purely by chance.

By current standards, Kimura's recording technique was highly primitive. She practiced reading numbers at a set rate, much in the way an accomplished IQ tester does, marked the starting position of her tape with a grease pencil, and then recorded on one channel. Next, the tape was rewound to the original starting point, and the remaining three digits recorded on the other channel. Binaural monitoring of the result served as a check on whether the numbers were appropriately synchronized. This technique provides only gross checks on the timing of the individual numbers, the synchrony of the dichotic pairs, and the relative loudness of the paired inputs.

Finally, it is important to note the instructions that were given to the subjects. Effectively, they were told only that they would hear lists of numbers arriving at both ears and that they were to "recall as many of them as they could, in any order they chose." It is not clear whether subjects were told that there would be six numbers on each trial or that numbers would not be repeated within a trial, but a reasonably alert subject could be expected to learn this within the 32-trial test session.

A dichotic listening task, such as the experiment by Kimura we have just described, does result in a significant superiority in accuracy of report for material presented to the right ear. Knowing what we do about how Kimura's experiment was actually performed, we would now like to discuss what might be the cause of such a right-ear superiority. Kimura attributed right-ear superiority to the more direct access of right-ear material to the left-hemispheric speech processor. But what does this direct access model mean in terms of the psychological advantage enjoyed by right-ear material?

There have been many ideas about the nature of the right-ear advantage for dichotic listening. Different experimenters have attributed the right-ear effect to report order bias, attentional biases, perceptual differences, and memory trace differences. It is important to consider each source of the right-ear advantage in order to evaluate the dichotic listening task as an assessment tool.

An early notion of the nature of the right-ear advantage was that the direct access of the right-ear material translated into a tendency for subjects to start their reports with right-ear information. The right-ear material in memory would thus be fresher in memory than the later reported left-ear material, resulting in more accurate right-ear report (Inglis, 1962). Note that the "starting-ear theory" makes an interesting prediction about the ear advantage seen for a dichotic task—it claims that the greatest accuracy will be seen for the ear with which subjects initiate their reports. It should be possible to reverse the normally observed right-ear effect by simply instructing subjects to start their reports with left-ear material. Experiments showed that subjects, when instructed which ear to report first, continued to show greater accuracy of report for right-ear material whether it was reported first or second (Bryden, 1963).

A second possible source of the right-ear effect is through attentional bias. By the simplest form of an attentional bias theory, it is easier for subjects to focus their attention on information coming to the right ear. In fact, a frequent observation in studies designed to probe the nature of selective attention has been that subjects are more accurate when shadowing right-ear material (e.g., Treisman & Geffen, 1968). As will be seen later, the attentional factor in dichotic listening is an important element in a subject's performance, an element we are still not certain how to evaluate.

A more complex version of the attentional bias argument has been proposed by Kinsbourne (1972). According to Kinsbourne, activity going on within a hemisphere will bias a subject's attention to one side of space or the other. Ongoing activity in the left hemisphere, such as verbal thought, will bias a subject's attention to the right side of space. Ongoing right-hemispheric activity, such as involved in humming a tune, will bias a subject's attention to the left side of space. In a dichotic listening experiment involving report of verbal material, a subject must gear up the left hemisphere in order to respond. This left-hemispheric priming will result in an attentional bias to the right side of space, and hence a right-ear advantage. Although there is some experimental support for Kinsbourne's theory (Spellacy & Blumstein, 1970), more systematic attempts to influence the direction of the ear advantage in dichotic listening by hemispheric priming have had little success (Allard & Bryden, 1979).

The third possible factor to which a right-ear advantage could be attributed is a perceptual advantage. By this argument, the more direct link between the right ear and the left hemisphere results in a stronger sensory signal from the right ear. Such a view would suggest that the signal-to-noise ratio of the right ear is the larger than that of the left ear. A perceptual locus of the right-ear superiority makes good common sense and adequately describes a large body of experimental data, although it may not be possible to assign a perceptual locus to all dichotic laterality effects.

The fourth potential locus of the right-ear advantage lies in memory. By this theory, right-ear material is encoded into memory in a more permanent fashion, making right-ear information more resistant to decay or output interference.

In any dichotic listening task, the trick is to control or eliminate as many as possible of those factors that influence the direction or magnitude of the observed ear advantage but are not related to the underlying hemispheric asymmetry. Early experiments, such as Kimura's, used lists of dichotic digits as stimuli, confounding such influences on the observed ear advantage as starting ear, attention, and memory. More recent studies avoid these confounds by presenting a subject with a single pair of dichotic stimuli for report. Even this procedure raises problems of interpretation. A more thorough discussion of the dichotic procedure must wait until the next chapter. First, it is important to examine other ways of approaching questions of lateralization.

Approaches through the Visual System

The intrinsic appeal of Kimura's (1961a, 1961b) work with a verbal dichotic listening task made it inevitable that there would be attempts to extend her logic to visual paradigms. The anatomy and functioning of the visual system are sufficiently different from that of the auditory system to make a wholly analogous procedure impossible to achieve. Over the years, two procedures for assessing laterality by visual means have become relatively popular—one that will be called *unilateral* presentation, and another that will be called *bilateral* presentation.

In the visual system, it is not the case that the left eye sends fibers to the right hemisphere and vice versa. Rather, the left half of each retina sends its ascending fibers to the left visual cortex, and the right half of each retina sends its fibers to the right visual cortex. Because of the optical reversal of the lens, this means that the image of objects lying to the right of the line of sight for either eye are transmitted to the left cortex, while those lying to the left of the line of sight pass to the right visual cortex (see Figure 2.2).

In order to ensure anything even remotely analogous to the dichotic listening situation, then, we must present material lateralized to one visual field or the other, not to one eye or the other. If we do this, verbal material presented to the right visual field will be transmitted directly to the left visual cortex and can obtain access to the language processing centers of the left hemisphere via intrahemispheric connections. In contrast, material presented to the left visual field will be transmitted first to the right visual cortex, and an extra interhemispheric connection will be required before it can gain access to the same language processing centers. Thus, one might expect to find a right-visual-field advantage for verbal material.

Lateralizing stimuli to one visual field or the other is not simply a matter of presenting them to one side or the other of the line of sight. The eyes are constantly in motion, glancing from one location to another, and some control must be exerted over this. One approach is to fix the image of the target on the retina so that when the eyes move, the target moves with it. This can be accomplished either through the use of a tight-fitting contact lens system (Pritchard, Heron, & Hebb, 1960) or through the use of a prolonged after image (MacKinnon, Forde, & Piggins, 1969). Because of the technical problems involved with these approaches, they have rarely been employed systematically for the study of perceptual asymmetries (but see Zaidel, 1976).

The more common approach is to present the stimuli so briefly that the eyes do not have the time to move from one location to another

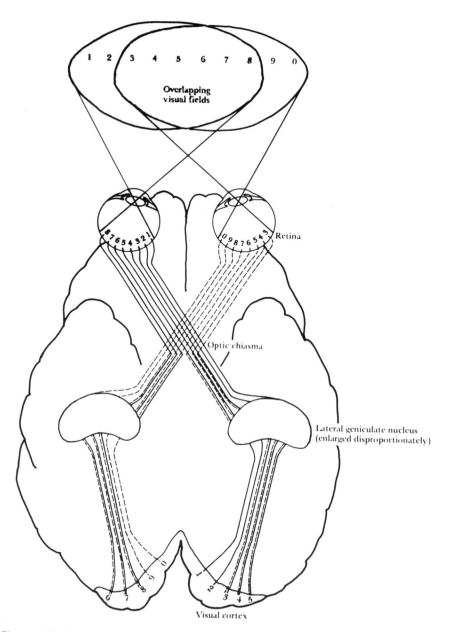

Figure 2.2. The anatomical arrangement of the visual system. Note that information from the left visual field of either eye (1–5) is projected to the right hemisphere and that from the right visual field (6–10) is projected to the left hemisphere. (From Lindsay, P. H., & Norman, D. A. *Human information processing: An introduction to psychology.* New York: Academic Press, 1977. Second edition.)

during the exposure. Woodworth (1938) is usually cited as evidence that it takes some 180 msec to initiate a saccadic eye movement to transport the eyes to a new fixation point. More recent evidence suggests that it may take up to 300 msec to initiate an eye movement when the subject does not know which of two locations will be stimulated (Hulme, 1979). Certainly, exposure durations of 100 msec or less make the likelihood of an eye movement during exposure negligible. Thus, the vast majority of visual laterality experiments have employed a tachistoscope—a device to permit rapid, controlled, visual exposures. Subjects are initially requested to fixate a central fixation point or cross, and then lateralized stimuli are presented. Of course, the success of the procedure depends on the subject following the instructions to fixate the central point. Furthermore, one should note that the stimuli used in dichotic experiments are perfectly intelligible when played monaurally: Errors in perception are achieved through the competition of two simultaneous signals. In contrast, tachistoscopic experiments degrade the stimulus by exposing it briefly in an area of reduced visual acuity.

Even prior to Kimura's (1961b) work, there was a history of studies of perceptual asymmetry in vision, although these studies were not related to concepts of hemispheric asymmetry. In 1952, Mishkin and Forgays had reported that English-reading subjects identified English words more accurately when they were presented in the right visual field, whereas Yiddish-reading subjects identified Yiddish words better in the left visual field. They related their findings to directional processes acquired in learning to read, Yiddish being read from right to left. Shortly afterward, Heron (1957) undertook a systematic study of this phenomenon. He employed single letters and groups of letters rather than words. He found that accuracy was much better on the left for a row of letters centered at fixation and spreading into both visual fields. In contrast, single letters or groups of letters exposed in only one visual field were more accurately identified when they appeared in the right visual field. Heron developed a theory of the serial processing of alphabetic material to account for these effects.

Because of the influence of Heron's (1957) work, most of the early attempts to measure a visual hemispheric asymmetry employed a unilateral presentation procedure (e.g., Bryden, 1965; Kimura, 1967) (see Figure 2.3). Stimuli were presented in only one visual field at a time, randomly appearing to the left or right of fixation. Because of the fact that scanning processes of the sort postulated by Heron (1957) might affect words or letter rows, Bryden (1965) chose to use single letters. He found a right-visual-field superiority for the identification of briefly exposed single letters in right-handers, but not in left-handers, who would

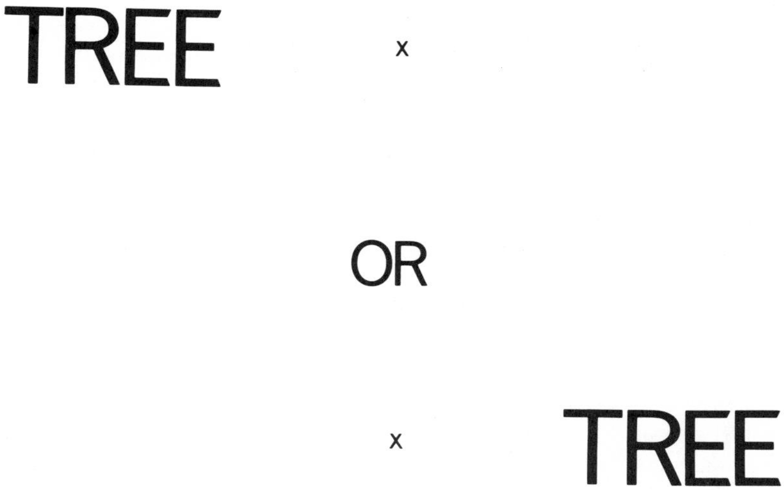

TREE   x

OR

x   # TREE

Figure 2.3. The arrangement of stimuli for unilateral tachistoscopic presentation. On any one trial, a stimulus appears in only one visual field.

more often be expected to have right-hemispheric speech lateralization. Other workers have extended the approach to words, either ignoring Heron's work and presenting the words in horizontal orientation, or showing them vertically (e.g., Barton, Goodglass, & Shai, 1965). Even vertical presentation may not solve the problem, because one must wonder whether words have the same properties when shown in an unfamiliar orientation as they do when shown horizontally (Bryden, 1970).

The adequacy of any tachistoscopic presentation procedure is dependent on its success in controlling fixation. Most people have assumed that subjects follow instructions and that unilateral presentation gives no special advantage to biasing fixation to one side or the other, since it is unpredictable where any given stimulus will appear. However, unilateral presentation does not have the competitive property of dichotic listening, since there is but a single stimulus to identify.

Others have been impressed with the success of the dichotic listening task and have attempted to construct an analogous visual procedure. Thus, for example, Zurif and Bryden (1969) and Hines, Satz, Schell, and Schmidlin (1969) have presented a series of pairs of numbers, with one number of each pair appearing in each visual field. Such a procedure not only is technically difficult but also introduces all the order-of-report and attentional complexities of the dichotic list procedure. A more common approach has been to present a single pair of stimuli on each trial, with one item in each visual field. This is usually referred to as bilateral presentation (see Figure 2.4). Since the subject knows where the stimuli will appear on every trial, fixation control is considerably weakened. Subjects also find it tempting to report the items in a left-to-right order, thus generating a left-visual-field advantage (Heron, 1957). McKeever and Huling (1971) have attempted to control for this by introducing a small number at fixation. Subjects are required to demonstrate that they are fixating by reporting this number correctly before the trial is scored. Right-visual-field effects with this form of bilateral presentation are unusually large and robust.

The fixation digit control may not solve all the problems, however. By directing attention to the fixation digit, one may lead the subject to continue a serial scan to the right, as one does in reading English, and thus to process the right-visual-field item next. The robust right-visual-field effect may then arise because of a primacy given to the processing of the right-visual-field item. (See the debate between M. J. White, 1973, and McKeever, 1974.) In fact, Hirata and Bryden (1976) have shown that simply introducing a gap between items in the left visual field and those in the right leads subjects to first process the items to the immediate right of fixation. It may very well be, then, that the bilateral presentation procedure enhances the right-visual-field effect by introducing factors quite unrelated to cerebral lateralization.

The right-visual-field superiority for bilaterally presented words is certainly far more robust than that obtained with typical unilateral presentation procedures. For instance, both Kershner and Jeng (1972) and Hines (1976) found larger and more statistically significant effects with bilateral presentation than with unilateral presentation. Furthermore, the right-visual-field superiority is impervious to a number of manipulations that would be expected to influence scanning strategies. McKeever (1971) showed that a robust right-visual-field effect persisted when the subjects were instructed to report the items from left to right, or when the left-visual-field word was presented 20 msec in advance of the right-visual-field word. In McKeever's study, however, the unilateral effect was also very large and more significant than some of the bilateral conditions.

TREE   8   BARN

Figure 2.4. The arrangement of stimuli for a bilateral tachistoscopic presentation. In this illustration, the digit 8 appears at the fixation point; subjects would be expected to identify this correctly for the trial to be counted. The use of such a fixation digit is optional.

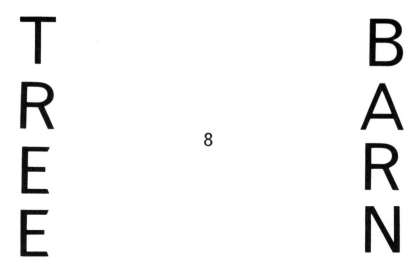

Figure 2.5. A bilateral stimulus arrangement with a vertically aligned word.

McKeever and Gill (1972) employed the bilateral presentation procedure, coupled with a fixation digit, with both vertically displayed words and single letters (see Figure 2.5). In both cases, clear right-field effects were obtained, though they were smaller than those obtained with horizontal words, thus suggesting that some property of horizontally aligned words enhances the effect. Very similar results were obtained by Mackavey, Curcio, and Rosen (1975), who investigated the effects both of vertical presentation and of eliminating the fixation digit. Virtually all subjects showed right-visual-field effects in all conditions, though the absolute magnitude of the right-field effect was not so large with vertical presentation as with horizontal presentation. Eliminating the fixation digit served primarily to increase accuracy and did not change the laterality effect.

To complicate the picture further, Kershner, Thomae, and Callaway (1977) report that the laterality effect with digits depends on the nature of the fixation item. In a study with children, they found a left-visual-field effect when a geometric form was used as a fixation control, but a right-field effect when a letter was employed. If this finding holds for adults, it would suggest that the use of a central fixation digit also serves to prime the linguistic capacities of the right hemisphere.

Thus, although the bilateral procedures give robust effects to which there is little doubt that cerebral lateralization contributes (McKeever, 1974), a number of problems remain. Presentation at known retinal loci make it crucial that proper fixation be maintained, and the idea of a fixation control item is an appealing one. Further, the presentation of two items per trial means that the subject must select the order in which they are to be reported, and this can lead to contaminating influences of short-term memory. Finally, Kershner *et al.*'s (1977) data raise the possibility that the fixation item itself may have an effect. A potential solution to these problems has been employed by Piazza (1980). She used a small arrowhead, pointing to the left or right, as a fixation control item: The arrowhead also cued which visual field was to be reported. By this technique, one can improve the likelihood of proper fixation and at the same time eliminate order-of-report effects by using partial report. In addition, the depth of processing involved in dealing with an arrowhead may well be insufficient to produce selective priming of one hemisphere.

This is not to argue that unilateral presentation procedures are inappropriate. Many of the more convincing visual laterality studies have employed unilateral procedures, and the results obtained with such procedures are at least as convincing as those found with bilateral presentation. Hines (1975), however, has argued that unilateral presentation provides a situation in which the more specialized hemisphere will always carry out the task. In his view, unilateral procedures are appropriate for assessing the efficiency of interhemispheric communication or interhemispheric transmission time. In contrast, he argues that the presence of items in both visual fields inhibits interhemispheric communication. Thus, bilateral presentation provides a better means of assessing the capacity of each hemisphere to deal with the task.

Hines's (1975) argument is based on the notion that bilateral stimulation activates both hemispheres. One must certainly consider the nature of competition in visual studies. In dichotic listening, not only are there two events competing for cerebral space, but there is a true attentional competition. Subjectively, one of the problems comes from disentangling the two stimuli, and blends of the two are common (Studdert-Kennedy & Shankweiler, 1970). With bilateral visual presentation, there may be competition for cerebral space, but there is certainly no perceptual confusion. Subjects do not make visual confusions and blends between the left and right stimuli, as they do in dichotic listening. If it is this perceptual confusion that is a critical aspect of dichotic competition, we are perhaps constructing the wrong visual analog to the dichotic situation. One alternative would be to use unilateral presentation and binocular rivalry. Thus, one could present different stimuli to the left (or right) visual fields of each eye. This would produce the perceptual competition that is lacking in current procedures.

A final problem concerns the choice of dependent measures. Virtually all the early experiments required a verbal identification of the stimulus and compared accuracy in the two visual fields. With the advent of modern mini- and microprocessors, recording and analyzing response times became much more feasible, and such research as that of Posner (e.g., Posner & Mitchell, 1967) has popularized the reaction time approach to information processing. Not surprisingly, many investigators applied reaction time measurement to questions of laterality (e.g., Cohen, 1973; Klatzky, 1970; Moscovitch, 1979). Both approaches have their benefits and their dangers: It is unlikely that there is any one "correct" approach. Verbal responses, whether timed or simply used to indicate accuracy, involve left-hemispheric speech output mechanisms, and somehow the information must reach these systems. There is thus an intrinsic left-hemisphere bias in verbal response procedures. While this may simply enhance right-field effects with verbal material, it may counteract any evidence for a nonverbal right-hemisphere superiority. Further, accuracy measures are relatively insensitive to small effects, since a given trial or item can yield only a binary (correct–incorrect) response. On the other hand, response time measures with manual responses introduce questions of stimulus–response compatibility and interactions of hand and visual field (Berlucchi, Crea, DiStefano, & Tassinari, 1977). One partial solution to these problems has been to use a bimanual response, in which the hand responding fastest stops the timer (Geffen, Bradshaw, & Nettleton, 1972). In addition, response time experiments lead to questions about what to do with extremely long or extremely short latency responses, and how to treat data that may very well not fit the normal distribution. Most investigators choose to set some upper cutoff on response time and to work with the median or geometric mean of the response times for each subject. Finally, response time paradigms have been developed to assess the resource limitations of subjects (Norman & Bobrow, 1975). As such, they have investigated how fast a person can perform a particular task, given a clearly visible stimulus. Laterality experiments involve brief exposures to control eye fixation and therefore put a considerable data limitation on the task. It may not always be appropriate to apply resource-oriented measures to data-limited situations.

We cannot provide a prescription as to the appropriate way to carry out a visual laterality experiment. A variety of different approaches have been employed, and all lead to the general observation of a right-visual-field superiority for verbal material and a left-field superiority for at least some types of nonverbal material. All have their problems, and the specific procedure may introduce components that enhance or reduce the laterality effect in various ways. Just considering the bilateral presentation procedure as an example, both McKeever (1974) and M. J. White (1973) have their points: Neither cerebral lateralization nor directional scanning is a *sufficient* explanation for the right-visual-field superiority, but both may be necessary. If one wants to use such data to make inferences about cerebral lateralization, it is necessary to understand how other factors, such as directional scanning, can influence the results.

Somatosensory Studies

In contrast to the multitude of studies that have been reported using dichotic and tachistoscopic procedures, relatively few experiments have employed somatosensory procedures to investigate hemispheric specialization. Whereas the anatomical situation is relatively simple, in that the left half of the body projects to the right hemisphere and vice versa, somatosensory stimuli are notoriously difficult to construct and control, and this is certainly one of the reasons why there are so few investigations in the area.

Although there are some early studies of somatosensory laterality involving unilateral presentation procedures (e.g., S. Weinstein & Sersen, 1961), most recent studies have tried to construct a parallel to the dichotic listening situation—a dichhaptic stimulation test.

Witelson (1974), for example, had subjects feel raised block letters for 2 sec with their fingertips. In strict adherence to the dichotic test situation, she presented different letters to each hand for 2 sec and then, 1 sec later, followed this with two additional letters for 2 sec. Her subjects were then asked to name the four letters they had felt. In this particular study, the subjects (young boys) showed only an insignificant right-hand superiority on this task, but they also showed a highly significant left-hand superiority on a similar nonsense shapes task. This nonverbal task differed from the letter task in that subjects were given 10 sec to feel two simultaneously presented figures, only a single pair was presented, and a pointing response rather than a verbal response was required.

As suggested earlier, dichotic list procedures such as those employed by Kimura (1961b) introduce many experimental effects influencing the observed laterality. These include starting position, attentional bias, differential memory loss, and the like. These same experimental effects are even more likely to influence the results in Witelson's (1974) letter procedure, which employs a list approach with much longer stimulus durations and intertrial intervals than are encountered in dichotic listening. The single-pair procedure used for the nonsense shapes eliminates some of the problems, but the subject is still left free to determine how to divide attention between the left and right stimuli. Particularly with a 10-sec palpation time, it would seem likely that the patterns of fingering the two stimuli would be quite different.

Oscar-Berman, Rehbein, Porfert, and Goodglass (1978) tried a slightly different dichhaptic procedure in an attempt to control for some of these problems. They had two experimenters draw figures on the palms of the hand simultaneously. Thus, subjects did not actively palpate the stimuli, and exposure time was under 2 sec. Furthermore, they instructed subjects to report either the right hand first or the left hand first. Most of their significant effects were found for the hand reported second. Letters were better identified on the right hand, line orientations on the left. The authors suggest that laterality differences in tactile perception are more evident after a delay than directly following stimulation.

The study of Oscar-Berman *et al.* (1978) controls some of the problems that we might have raised with respect to Witelson's (1974) study but leaves the question of attentional bias unsettled. It remains possible, even with the ordered report studies, for a subject to devote more attention to one side than to the other. Perhaps solutions such as those we have proposed for the dichotic listening situation could be fruitfully applied to somatosensory tasks.

Summary of Studies

The preceding pages have provided a review of some of the more common experimental procedures that have been employed to investigate perceptual laterality and cerebral specialization. If this section has seemed critical, it is because of the conviction that there are many potential sources of variation in lateral asymmetry and that only some of these are directly indicative of the differing activities of the two cerebral hemispheres. If we continue to use procedures without understanding them, we are only building our theories on shaky foundations.

The review has also tended to concentrate on verbal studies; those showing a right-side, or left-hemispheric, advantage. To some extent, this is because they provide better examples for a critical commentary. At the same time, the left-hemispheric specialization for language is so well established that it is clearer what should happen if we had a successful behavioral technique for measuring cerebral organization. However, one should realize that there are many nonlinguistic tasks for which a left-side (right-hemispheric) superiority has been reported, in all three of the sensory modalities that we have reviewed. Fundamentally the same issue of separating experimental effects from true hemispheric effects exists for these studies. A detailed consideration of them must wait for the ensuing chapters.

Laterality Measures and Cerebral Function

In introducing some of the techniques that have been employed to assess lateralization, a variety of procedural factors that could influence the magnitude of any observed laterality effect have been pointed out. So long as there are alternative explanations for a laterality effect, one should not assume that the effect is due to the functional asymmetry of the brain. Simply showing a right-ear effect or a right-visual-field effect is not enough to justify the claim that one has discovered some process that is dependent on the activity of the left hemisphere.

How, then, can we make the case for a relation between behavior and functional cerebral lateralization more convincing? Certainly, some of the strongest evidence will come from studies of individuals with brain damage. If we have available to us individuals who have had their cerebral commissures sectioned, and the isolated left hemisphere can perform a task while the isolated right hemisphere cannot, then we have good evidence that the left hemisphere is important for performance on the task (cf. Gazzaniga, 1970; Gazzaniga & LeDoux, 1978). Similarly, studies of unilateral brain damage can be useful: If damage to the left hemisphere produces a different effect than damage to the right hemisphere, then one can relate the behavior to functional cerebral asymmetry.

This is not to argue that studies of clinical populations following commissurotomy or unilateral brain damage are the only approach to linking behavior to brain function, or even the most desirable approach. In dealing with neurological populations, we cannot pretend that we are dealing with normal brains, and what holds true for the brain-injured population may not be true for the general population. Often there has been brain dysfunction of long standing that may have led to the involvement of different structures or pathways in a particular behavior. Further, it is often not possible to obtain both preoperative and postoperative measures of performance, so one cannot be certain just what the effects of a particular surgery are. One must also recognize that the brain-injured patient may use quite a different strategy for carrying out a task than does a normal subject. To the extent that the choice of strategy determines the data obtained, such an effect could lead to false conclusions. Finally, one must use the same task with brain-injured subjects and with normals. The fact that damage to the right parietal area leads to deficits in face recognition (Meadows, 1974a) does *not* demonstrate that the left-visual-field superiority often obtained in studies of face recognition in normals with unilateral tachistoscopic presentation (e.g., Ley & Bryden, 1979a) is a reflection of this right-hemispheric superiority. While such data may make the argument for a brain–behavior correlation in the normal studies, they do not close the door on alternative explanations: The procedures used in the clinical studies are quite different from those used in the studies of normal adults.

Not only are suitably brain-damaged patients hard to come by, but they may not provide unequivocal evidence that a particular pattern of behavior in normals is related to a functional cerebral asymmetry. What other approaches are there? One approach, rather too often ignored, is to compare samples of left- and right-handed subjects. We are reasonably confident that the incidence of right-hemispheric or bilateral speech is much higher in left-handers than in right-handers (Rasmussen & Milner, 1977; Satz, 1980). If the laterality effect under study is really related to cerebral asymmetry, the effect should be attenuated or reversed in left-handers (Bryden, 1965; Piazza, 1980; Zurif & Bryden, 1969). As will be seen in the discussion of Kimura's (1961a, 1961b) work in the next chapter, there is some possibility that handedness could have an effect on laterality measures independent of its relation to speech lateralization. Further, it would be a major step forward if there was an objective and reliable means of determining which left-handers had right-hemispheric speech representation (see Chapter 10). Despite such problems, however, handedness does provide one means of defining groups with predictable differences in cerebral organization, and any behavioral measure of lateralization that is in fact related to cerebral asymmetry should manifest predictable differences between handedness groups. In examining the studies of perceptual laterality, such handedness differences are one of the things to be noted.

Another approach is to dissociate verbal and nonverbal laterality effects. If we find a left-visual-field superiority for some nonverbal task, such as face recognition, we do not have very strong evidence for the effect being due to right-hemispheric function. However, if we find that the same subjects also show a right-visual-field effect for verbal material, the argument for relating the behavior to cerebral asymmetry is bolstered. This is particularly true if the two effects can be obtained simultaneously, with trials of different types being intermingled, because such a procedure ensures more satisfactorily that similar attentional and fixation strategies are being used for both types of material. Statistically, one is looking for a side by type of material interaction. Thus, a further type of evidence to be noted is an indication of this dissociation of verbal and nonverbal effects.

In many studies, the experimenter wishes to make statements about the relative magnitude of the laterality effect in different groups, in different individuals, or for different types of material. Any developmental study of laterality, for example, takes this form. Groups of subjects of different ages are tested and then compared as to the magnitude of the laterality effect. Studies of sex differences and differences between pathology groups, and even reliability studies of laterality, require some way of quantifying the degree of lateralization shown on a particular task. Over the years, a number of suggestions have been made as to appropriate ways of carrying out this measurement. At this point, it is appropriate to examine some of these measures of lateralization and to comment on their merits and demerits.

Perhaps the best way to grasp the various measures of laterality that have been employed is to work through some examples based on actual data. Let us begin with the data presented by Kimura (1963) in her developmental study of dichotic listening. In this experiment, children listened to lists of numbers presented dichotically. The lists varied in length from a single item at each ear to three items per ear. Subjects were instructed to recall as many of the items as possible, in any order they chose. Scoring was based on the number of items reported correctly from each ear. Since there were 10 trials at each list length, the maximum score for each ear was 60. Mean accuracy scores for each age–sex combination are shown in Table 2.1: These data are reproduced from Kimura's article.

The most common approach to these data would be to employ the analysis of variance on the left- and right-ear scores. In effect, such an analysis determines whether the mean score for the right ear is significantly different from the mean score for the left ear. It is equivalent to determining whether the difference score $(R-L)$ is significantly different from zero. In fact, Kimura (1963) carried out 12 separate t tests rather than an analysis of variance, but the principle is the same. The difference score is treated as a measure of laterality. These scores are shown in the third column of Table 2.1.

An examination of these difference scores indicates that they have a

Table 2.1
Development of the Right-Ear Advantage in Dichotic Listening

Age/Sex		Left ear	Right ear	Difference	Total correct	Total errors	POC[a]	POE[b]	e[c]
4	F	23.2	35.8	12.6	59.0	61.0	.214	.207	.214
	M	16.0	30.0	14.0	46.0	74.0	.304	.189	.304
5	F	32.9	44.1	11.2	77.0	43.0	.145	.260	.260
	M	25.6	38.6	13.0	64.2	55.8	.202	.233	.233
6	F	39.3	53.3	14.0	92.6	27.4	.151	.511	.511
	M	35.7	44.9	9.2	80.6	39.4	.114	.234	.234
7	F	45.8	50.0	4.2	95.8	24.2	.044	.173	.173
	M	44.1	49.9	5.8	94.0	26.0	.062	.223	.223
8	F	48.9	54.7	5.8	103.6	16.4	.056	.354	.354
	M	50.2	55.0	4.8	105.2	14.8	.046	.324	.324
9	F	52.4	55.1	2.7	107.5	12.5	.025	.216	.216
	M	52.9	55.5	2.6	108.4	11.6	.024	.224	.224
rho	F			−.771			−.943	+.086	+.086
	M			−1.000			−1.000	+.371	−.229

Note. Data from Kimura (1963).
[a] Percentage of correct items.
[b] Percentage of errors.
[c] Laterality index.

rather curious property: They tend to decrease with age. If one simply interpreted the difference scores, one would say that the magnitude of the laterality effect decreased with age—that cerebral lateralization lessened as one grew older. There is no theory that would predict such an effect, and to most researchers, it would seem nonsensical. (Kimura, 1964, was far too wise to fall into this trap.) The declining trend is clearly demonstrated by the negative rank-order correlations with age shown at the bottom of the column.

A little thought will make it clear why this relationship holds. Young children find the task relatively difficult. Four year olds identify less than half the numbers correctly. With three pairs of digits, a young child might remember only two or three of the items. Knowing what we do about order of report in dichotic listening (Bryden, 1962; Witelson & Rabinovitch, 1971), it would not be at all surprising if all the items came from one ear. It would thus be easy for a child to accumulate over trials quite a large right-ear advantage. The oldest children, in contrast, identify about 90% of the items correctly. Even on the three-pair lists, they remember items from both ears and identify, say, three from one ear and two from the other. Difference scores in the older groups are small because they do the task well, and there is little room for a large absolute difference to emerge.

What we need, then, is some correction for overall accuracy. One common approach has been to use the score $(R-L)/(R+L)$. This is equivalent to calculating the percentage of correct items (POC) that were on the right ear, $(R)/(L+R)$, since:

$$1 + \frac{R-L}{R+L} = \frac{R+L+R-L}{R+L} = \frac{2(R)}{R+L}$$

This computation involves determining the ratio of the difference score to the total number of items identified correctly; it is shown in column 6 of Table 2.1. As can be seen from the rank-order correlations given at the bottom of that column, this manipulation does little to change the negative relation between age and the measure of laterality. Despite the popularity of POC, it does not succeed in correcting for overall differences in accuracy level.

A third alternative is to compute a score that might be called POE, or percentage of errors. This would involve dividing the difference score by the total number of errors, rather than the total number correct, or equivalently, by computing L_e/L_e+R_e. Such a measure has been advocated by Krashen (1973), on the empirical basis that it tends to be uncorrelated with overall accuracy in a number of dichotic listening studies. Values of POE for the Kimura data are shown in column 7 of Table 2.1. The rank-order correlations with age indicate that POE has eliminated the age trend and has largely solved our problem of interpretation. We would now argue that there is no systematic change in degree of lateralization with age.

Halwes (1968) has recommended yet another approach. He has derived a laterality index (e) that expresses the observed lateral difference as a proportion of the maximum possible difference that could occur at that level of accuracy. For instance, if subjects make only 12 errors, as do the 9 year olds, the most extreme distribution would assign all 12 errors to one ear and yield accuracy levels of 48 items at one ear and 60 at the other. Thus, the index of laterality should be $(L_e-R_e)/12$. On the other hand, if the subjects get only 46 items right and make 7 errors, as do the 4-year-old boys, then the maximum laterality effect would be obtained by assigning all 46 correct responses to one ear, and the index of laterality should be $(R-L)/46$. This procedure is equivalent to using POC when overall accuracy is less than 50% and POE when overall accuracy is greater than 50%. It also solves the problem of the relation between age and laterality. Marshall, Caplan, and Holmes (1975) and Repp (1977) have also argued in favor of this index.

A more general argument in favor of the laterality index can be seen if we examine plots of left-side accuracy against right-side accuracy (see Figure 2.6). In Figure 2.6, we have plotted what might be termed *iso-laterality curves* for various measures of laterality: These curves represent constant values of the measure of laterality at different levels of accuracy. Thus, the isolaterality curves for the difference measure $(R-L)$ are straight lines parallel to the major diagonal. Not every difference score can be obtained at all levels of accuracy: A difference of 20, for instance, can be obtained only if the subject makes 20 or more errors and also gets at least 20 items correct. Thus, the magnitude of the difference score is constrained by the overall performance level.

Isolaterality curves for POC are straight lines emanating from the lower left corner of the diagram. Up to an accuracy of 50%, the limits of POC are +1 and −1, but the measure is constrained above that. At 75% accuracy, the maximum value is .33 $[(100-50)/(100+50)]$, since the most extreme distribution possible would assign a 50% score to the poorer side. POE is simply the mirror image of POC: It is constrained below 50$% rather than above.

The laterality index (e) combines the useful features of POE and POC. It has limits of +1 and −1 at all levels of accuracy. In fact, the figure for e begins to approximate the familiar ROC curve from signal detection theory. The one awkward point about e is the inflection along the minor diagonal, at the point where the overall accuracy is 50% and the measure calls for a shift from POC and POE.

Bryden and Sprott (1981) have proposed a new measure of lateralization (λ) based on the log odds ratio. λ has certain advantages over other measures in that it provides a significance test for each individual as well as for the group data. Let us imagine a simple experiment in which we have run 20 independent trials for each side, as in a unilateral tachistoscopic experiment. Suppose our subject has identified 14 items on the right and 8 on the left. The odds of identifying the item on the right are 14/6, while the odds of identifying the item on the left are only 8/12. One of the merits of treating these values as odds rather than as probabilities is that odds ratios have some very interesting properties. The natural logarithm of the odds ratio has an approximately normal distribution and a variance that is equal to the sum of the reciprocals of the component frequencies. What we really want to know in a laterality experiment is whether the odds ratio for identifying something on the right exceeds that for identifying something on the left, that is, whether $\lambda_R - \lambda_L > 0$. Thus,

$$\lambda_R = \ln \left(\frac{\text{correct } R}{\text{misses } R} \right) = \ln \frac{14}{6} = 0.847$$

$$\sigma^2_{\lambda_R} = \frac{1}{\text{correct } R} + \frac{1}{\text{misses } R} = \frac{1}{14} + \frac{1}{6} = .238$$

$$\lambda_L = \ln \left(\frac{\text{correct } L}{\text{misses } L} \right) = \ln \frac{8}{12} = -.405$$

$$\sigma^2_{\lambda_L} = \frac{1}{\text{correct } L} + \frac{1}{\text{misses } L} = \frac{1}{8} + \frac{1}{12} = .208$$

$$\lambda = \lambda_R - \lambda_L$$

$$= \ln \left(\frac{\text{correct } R}{\text{misses } R} \right) - \ln \left(\frac{\text{correct } L}{\text{misses } L} \right)$$

$$= \ln \left(\frac{\text{correct } R \times \text{misses } L}{\text{misses } R \times \text{correct } L} \right)$$

$$= \ln \left(\frac{14 \times 12}{6 \times 8} \right) = 1.252$$

$$\sigma^2_\lambda = \sigma^2_{\lambda_R} + \sigma^2_{\lambda_L} = \frac{1}{14} + \frac{1}{6} + \frac{1}{8} + \frac{1}{12} = .446$$

The fact that there is a known variance for this expression makes it possible to test each individual subject. In the example, $z = 1.252/\sqrt{.466} = 1.87$, a figure significant at the .05 level by a one-tail test.

Table 2.2 shows data from a unilateral tachistoscopic study. In this experiment, subjects were given 24 trials in each visual field with vertically displayed consonant–vowel–consonant (CV) nonsense syllables. Subjects were scored as either wholly correct or incorrect, with no partial credit being given. In Table 2.2, we have shown the difference measure (d) for each subject, the laterality index (e) computed by Halwes's (1969) method, and the λ value. If we test each subject by dividing the individual by the standard deviation, we can see that Subjects 4, 5, and 14 have significant right-visual-field superiorities, and Subject 12 has a significant left-field effect.

Rather than being a two-branched function, like e, λ is a continuous function for all values of P_L and P_R (see Figure 2.6). Otherwise, λ and e

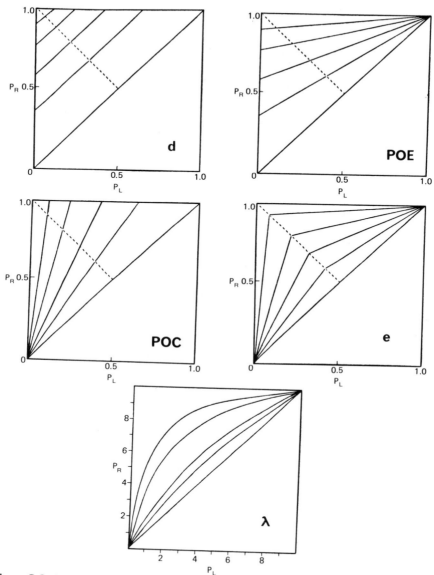

Figure 2.6. Isolaterality curves for various measures of laterality. Points on a given line represent a constant value of the laterality index. Left-side accuracy is plotted along the abscissa, and right-side accuracy along the ordinate; thus, all the curves drawn show right-side superiorities. Top row: the difference score and percentage of error score. Middle row: percentage of correct score and Repp's (1977) *e* score. Bottom: Bryden and Sprott (1981) lambda values.

Table 2.2
Computation of Laterality Measures for Individual Data

Subject	Left	Right	Difference	Laterality index (e)	λ_L	λ_R	λ	σ_κ^2	Z
1	6	8	2	2/14 .143	ln(6/18) −1.099	ln(8/16) −.693	.406	.410	.634
2	9	13	4	4/22 .182	ln(9/15) −.511	ln(13/11) .167	.678	.346	1.153
3	9	5	−4	−4/14 −.286	ln(9/15) −.511	ln(5/19) −1.335	−.824	.430	1.256
4	6	13	7	7/19 .368	ln(6/18) −1.099	ln(13/11) .167	1.266	.390	2.027
5	11	18	7	7/19 .368	ln(11/13) −.167	ln(18/6) 1.099	1.266	.390	2.027
6	10	5	−5	−5/15 −.333	ln(10/14) −.336	ln(5/19) −1.335	−.999	.424	1.534
7	18	14	−4	−4/16 −.250	ln(18/6) 1.099	ln(14/10) .336	−.762	.394	1.214
8	18	19	1	1/11 .091	ln(18/6) 1.099	ln(19/5) 1.336	.236	.475	.342
9	18	13	−5	−5/17 −.294	ln(18/6) 1.099	ln(13/11) .167	−.932	.390	1.492
10	14	18	4	4/16 .250	ln(14/10) .336	ln(18/6) 1.099	.762	.394	1.214
11	11	17	6	6/20 .300	ln(11/13) −.167	ln(17/7) .887	1.054	.370	1.733
12	21	13	−8	−8/14 −.571	ln(21/3) 1.946	ln(13/11) .167	−1.779	.549	2.401
13	11	16	5	5/21 .238	ln(11/13) −.167	ln(16/8) .693	.860	.355	1.443
14	6	15	9	9/21 .429	ln(6/18) −1.099	ln(15/9) .511	1.609	.400	2.544
15	10	12	2	2/22 .091	ln(10/14) −.336	ln(12/12) 0	.337	.338	.580
16	13	19	6	6/16 .375	ln(13/11) .167	ln(19/5) 1.335	1.168	.421	1.800
Mean	11.94	13.63	1.69	.069			.272		

have very similar properties: The rank-order correlation between the two for the data of Table 2.2 is .99. The advantages of λ are that it makes use of all the data by treating each trial as a separate event and that it is possible to test each individual as well as the group mean. However, it should be noted that the particular method of calculating λ will depend on the design of the experiment. Here the computations have been illustrated with data from a unilateral tachistoscopic experiment. Other procedures call for testing somewhat different hypotheses. For instance, the typical dichotic listening experiment calls for the presentation of a pair of items, followed by the identification of these items. Only trials on which a single item is identified provide any information about laterality, and the appropriate question is whether single-correct trials are more likely to involve the right-ear item or the left-ear item. Thus, the correct calculation of λ is given by ln (single correct on R/single correct on L). Given other approaches, other procedures may be appropriate. These procedures are discussed in further detail by Bryden and Sprott (1981) and by Sprott and Bryden (forthcoming).

In the foregoing section, we have considered various approaches to measuring laterality in experiments in which the dependent measure is number correct. In such experiments, λ is clearly the most sensitive measure, although e is a reasonably adequate approximation. What about reaction time experiments? They have become increasingly popular, yet there is no formal literature on the measurement problems associated with such experiments. Most experimenters have been satisfied to determine the mean or median reaction time for each subject in each cell and apply the analysis of variance. Yet some of the same problems that plague accuracy experiments also appear in reaction time studies. Can, for instance, a difference in reaction time of 10 msec be considered the same when it reflects a difference between 340 and 350 msec as when it reflects a difference between 1140 and 1150 msec? Further, lateral differences are stable for some subjects and not for others. Present methods of analysis throw away information about individual subject distributions. An approach based on the same logic as used in developing λ would clearly have advantages. In effect, one should test the significance of the lateral difference for each subject, using the data from each trial, and then combine these probabilities across all subjects. To date, however, no detailed treatment of such an approach has been provided.

3

Dichotic Listening and Auditory Lateralization

Of all the procedures for investigating cerebral function in normal individuals, the dichotic listening technique is certainly the best known. In dichotic listening, a subject is presented with two different signals at the same time, one arriving at each ear, and is required to make some identifying response. In general, accuracy for speech-related material is better on the right ear than on the left, whereas accuracy is better on the left ear for nonspeech material. The preceding chapter provided a brief introduction to dichotic procedures and to some of the problems associated with their use. The present chapter provides a more detailed examination of the results of dichotic listening experiments.

The ascending auditory pathways are relatively complex (see Figure 3.1), and information is transmitted from each ear to both ipsilateral and contralateral auditory cortices. However, there is some evidence that the crossed pathways have a greater number of fibers and faster transmission speed than do the ipsilateral connections (Majkowski, Bochenck, Bochenck, Knapik-Fijalkowska, & Kopec, 1971; Rosenzweig, 1951). Ferraro and Minckler (1977), on the other hand, have noted gross individual differences in the asymmetry of the lemniscal pathways. If these individual differences are carried into higher levels of the auditory system, there could be major individual differences in the relative dominance of the contralateral pathways. If there is an asymmetry in the auditory pathways, information from the right ear would reach the left hemisphere first, whereas the reverse would be true for left-ear input. Kimura (1967) has proposed that the laterality effects in dichotic listening depend on such an asymmetry of the ascending auditory pathways.

Kimura's initial discovery was that normal adult subjects were more accurate in identifying verbal material presented to the right ear than that presented to the left ear under conditions of dichotic competition.

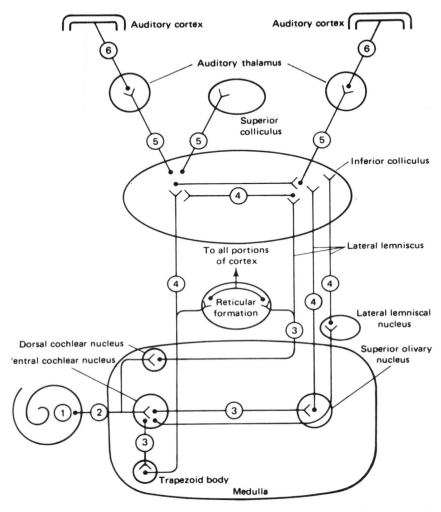

Figure 3.1. Schematic diagram of the ascending auditory pathways. Note that information from each ear reaches both hemispheres. (Figure 3.26, p. 123, from *The psychobiology of sensory coding* by William R. Uttal. Copyright © 1973 by William R. Uttal. Reprinted by permission of Harper & Row, Publishers, Inc.)

She also found that neurological patients with known left-hemispheric speech representation showed a right-ear superiority, whereas those with right-hemispheric speech representation exhibited a left-ear superiority, regardless of handedness (Kimura, 1961a, 1961b). The dichotic listening technique thus held promise for providing a means of assessing speech lateralization in the neurologically intact subject and for studying the cerebral organization of the normal brain.

Kimura's pioneering work has generated a vast body of experimental literature. The technique has been refined and polished by procedural alterations, employed with specific classes of speech sounds, and revised to make it appropriate for use with nonspeech material. It is now commonplace to find studies with normal subjects in which dichotic listening performance is used as a criterion of speech lateralization and from which sweeping conclusions about the organization of the normal brain are drawn.

There are difficulties with such a strong interpretation of the dichotic listening procedure as providing a measure of speech lateralization. The clinical literature on aphasia (e.g., Penfield & Roberts, 1959; Roberts, 1968) and studies of speech lateralization involving unilateral cortical suppression through sodium amytal (e.g., Milner, Branch, & Rasmussen, 1964; Rossi & Rosadini, 1967) indicate that the incidence of left-hemispheric speech in right-handers is on the order of 97–99%, yet the incidence of right-ear superiority in dichotic listening tasks in normal right-handers tends to be in the range of 75–85%. Some of this discrepancy is undoubtedly due to a lack of reliability in the dichotic listening procedures. Although few workers report reliability measures, Bryden (1975) gives values of .61 and .66 for two different dichotic tests, Shankweiler and Studdert-Kennedy (1975) a value of .70, and Blumstein, Goodglass, and Tartter (1975) a value of .74 for verbal material. These values are not impressively high if one wants to use the dichotic task as a diagnostic tool.

One must remember that many different factors affect performance on dichotic listening tasks (cf. Bryden, 1978). Despite the multitude of different procedures that have been employed, none have fully succeeded in controlling the situation so that only cerebral lateralization is pertinent. To properly understand the factors influencing dichotic listening performance, and auditory asymmetries in general, it will be necessary to take a detailed look at the results obtained with different procedures and with different types of stimulus material. To make this clearer, the best place to start is with a further examination of Kimura's original studies (Kimura, 1961a, 1961b).

The Kimura Experiments

The original report on dichotic listening performance and hemispheric asymmetry appears in two separate papers. The first (Kimura,

1961b) deals with the effects of temporal lobe excision on performance in patients with focal epilepsy. Both pre- and postoperatively, left temporal subjects were found to be less accurate than right temporals, frontals, or subcorticals. Furthermore, left temporal lobe excision resulted in a greater postoperative deficit than other removals. Temporal lobe excision, regardless of side, produced a sharp drop in performance on the ear contralateral to the removal. Thus, the importance of the temporal lobes in dichotic performance was established. The second paper (Kimura, 1961a) deals with the relation of performance to speech lateralization. Here data are reported from 13 normal controls, who show a significant right-ear effect. In addition, 120 patients with epileptogenic lesions and known speech lateralization, as determined by the sodium amytal procedure (Wada & Rasmussen, 1960), were also tested. Subjects with left-hemispheric speech were more accurate on the right ear, whereas those with right-hemispheric speech were more accurate on the left ear (see Table 3.1).

An examination of this table is rather revealing. Because of fluctuations in accuracy between groups, ear differences have been expressed in terms of a laterality coefficient (Halwes, 1969; Chapter 2) that is independent of overall accuracy. While Kimura (1961a) states unequivocally that handedness is not a factor in producing laterality differences, she never reports a full analysis of her data, and Table 3.1 does not entirely support her contention. In terms of the laterality coefficient, handedness has an effect about half the magnitude of that produced by speech lateralization. Although one cannot assess the significance of this effect from the data given, it is possible that the dichotic laterality effect is influenced by handedness independently of speech lateralization. If this

Table 3.1
Summary of Data Relating Dichotic Performance to Speech Lateralization

Group	N	Left ear	Right ear	Laterality coefficient (e)
Left-hemisphere speech	107	76.64	83.01	.197
Right-handers	93	77.03	83.73	.214
Left-handers	10	72.50	77.00	.106
Right-hemisphere speech	13	85.00	74.85	−.316
Right-handers	3	83.67	81.67	−.075
Left-handers	9	85.00	71.44	−.298
Normal controls (right-handers)	13	90.25	92.25	.211

Note. From Kimura (1961a).

is true, it would weaken our earlier argument that comparisons between handedness groups provide a way of bolstering the argument that a particular laterality effect is related to cerebral asymmetry.

When we consider the original Kimura experiments, perhaps three major questions come to mind. Let us consider each of these in turn. First, the free recall of lists of numbers or words gives the subject a great deal of freedom in what he or she chooses to do. To what extent does the use of lists of material introduce spurious factors unrelated to cerebral lateralization? Second, what laterality effects are obtained with other types of material? Third, is it necessary to have dichotic competition for laterality effects to be observed?

Word List Experiments

When a subject is faced with the task of identifying the items in a list presented dichotically, he or she has many alternative ways of accomplishing the task successfully. When the pairs of items are presented fairly rapidly, most subjects spontaneously report all the items that arrive at one ear before giving any that come to the other ear (Bryden, 1962). This strategy of report implies that items from the second ear will be at a distinct disadvantage: Not only will they be reported later in time, but they will also be subject to more output interference than items from the other ear. As one slows the rate of presentation, it becomes more commonplace for subjects to report the items in a pair-by-pair fashion, in their order of arrival. Even at fast rates of presentation, however, there are many exceptions to the neat ear-by-ear report strategy. The particular sequence in which the items are reported will influence which ones are correctly identified and will thereby influence not only the magnitude but also the direction of any left–right difference that is observed. Further, with the general instruction to "report all you can remember," subjects may choose to deploy their attention in a variety of different ways. Some will divide attention between the two ears; others will focus on one ear. The manner in which attention is deployed will have an effect on the observed laterality effect.

These considerations would suggest that the dichotic free-recall task employed by Kimura (1961a, 1961b) can be influenced by a variety of factors that need have little to do with cerebral lateralization. Despite this caution, the observation of a general right-ear superiority has proven to be one of the most robust phenomena of contemporary experimental psychology, and it has been replicated literally hundreds of times. Nevertheless, procedural variations do have an effect, and it is totally unjustified to assume that *any* right-ear effect observed with verbal material is necessarily related to some lateralized cerebral process.

It is an easy job for most normal adults to remember three pairs of numbers, even in the novelty of the dichotic situation. One obtains no information about lateralized processes if the subject identifies everything correctly. Early dichotic experiments increased the difficulty of the task for normal subjects by increasing the amount of material to be recalled or by employing other types of verbal material to increase the size of the stimulus set. Thus, Bryden (1967a) used up to five pairs of numbers, and Satz, Achenbach, and Fennell (1967) as many as six pairs of words. In right-handed samples, strong right-ear effects were consistently observed and did not seem to bear any systematic relation to the amount of material presented. The right-ear advantage was also observed with various types of material, from nonsense syllables (Curry & Rutherford, 1967) through meaningful words (Satz *et al.*, 1967). There have been occasional reports of such factors as imagery value affecting the magnitude of the right-ear effect (e.g., Kelly & Orton, 1979), but these data may be wholly interpretable in terms of recall strategy. The free recall of dichotic lists does not provide a convenient way of assessing laterality effects for different types of stimuli.

In free recall, many subjects choose to report the items from the right ear before giving those from the left ear. In fact, the magnitude of the right-ear effect correlates with the frequency of starting from the right ear (Bryden, 1963). This, of course, raises the question as to whether the right-ear effect is simply an order-of-report effect. A variety of solutions to this question have been proposed. Bryden (1963) instructed subjects to report first the items from one ear and then those from the other. On half the trials, the subject gave the left-ear items first, and on half the right-ear items. While items from the first ear were recalled much more accurately than those from the second, an overall right-ear superiority emerged when the data were collapsed across the two orders of report. Similar results have been reported by many others (e.g., Satz, Achenbach, Pattishall, & Fennell, 1965; Wilson, Dirks, & Carterette, 1968; Zurif & Bryden, 1969), although there have been a few failures to obtain a right-ear effect with ordered recall (e.g., Inglis, 1968; Oxbury, Oxbury, & Gardiner, 1967). In general, the right-ear effect obtained with ordered recall is of much less magnitude than that seen with free recall, although the proportion of subjects showing the effect is roughly the same. This would indicate that starting-ear bias cannot be considered as an *explana-*

tion of the right-ear superiority, although it contributes to the magnitude of the effect.

Even with ordered recall, subjects are asked to attend to both ears, and they may well vary in their success in dividing attention. M. Schwartz (1970) attempted to control this problem by using a dichotic monitoring procedure. He presented lists of six pairs of words and required subjects to attend to one ear and report items only from that ear. Again, a robust right-ear superiority was observed. In fact, Schwartz found rather larger right-ear effects than are seen in most ordered-recall experiments. By avoiding the attentional strategies of the ordered-recall task, Schwartz may have eliminated some of the extraneous variance. As we shall see, monitoring tasks have more recently been used with some success in single-pair dichotic studies.

Even with a monitoring task, however, it still may be easier for subjects to attend to the right ear than to the left. In fact, many subjects spontaneously report such a feeling, despite careful equating of intensity at the two ears. Bryden (1967a) has developed very complex scoring procedures to correct for some of these biases that can be applied to free-recall data. He first eliminated all trials on which an "ear order" of report was not used—that is, only those trials on which items reported from one ear preceded items reported from the other ear were scored. Such trials were then separated into those on which the right ear was given first and those on which the left ear was given first, and separate means for each ear and each report order were computed. The scores for left ear given first and left ear given second were then averaged, as were the comparable scores for the right ear. In effect, this procedure gives a measure of how a subject would have performed had he or she always used an ear order of report and given the left ear first half the time and the right ear first half the time. It eliminates the components of the right-ear effect due to memory and to starting bias. In addition, it may be the only procedure that also compensates for attentional biases, leaving us with a pure measure of perceptual laterality. This, of course, depends on the assumption that the subjects are paying as much attention to the left ear when they spontaneously choose to start with a left-ear item as they are to the right ear when they start on that side. Such an assumption may not be fully justified, but the procedure may very well correct for attentional biases better than instructing subjects to monitor one ear. The difficulty is that with long lists the scoring is cumbersome and results in a loss of much of the data. Finally, one should note that the right-ear effect can be reduced or eliminated by making the left-ear signal louder, by increasing the overall signal intensity, or by cutting out the high frequencies (Cullen, Thompson, Hughes, Berlin, & Samson, 1974).

The considerations raised in the preceding paragraphs indicate that the right-ear effect observed in early dichotic list experiments is influenced by a variety of factors, many of which may be quite unrelated to cerebral asymmetries. It is quite inappropriate, then, to argue that a reduced laterality effect in some pathological group is evidence for an abnormality of cerebral representation. Rather, one must consider the alternative explanations for the altered laterality effect.

This is not to argue that one of the bases for the right-ear effect does not lie in cerebral asymmetry. Since Kimura's studies, a number of investigators have found that the laterality effect is reduced in left-handers as opposed to right-handers (Satz et al., 1967; Satz et al., 1965; Zurif & Bryden, 1969), although ambidexters seem to show as large an effect as right-handers (Pizzamiglio, 1974). Since right-hemispheric speech representation is more prevalent in left-handers than in right-handers, this reduction of the right-ear effect should be expected. As Zurif and Bryden (1969) have shown, it exists with ordered-recall procedures as well as with free-recall ones.

Further, the sensitivity of dichotic word lists to lateralized cerebral damage has also been verified (e.g., Mazzucchi & Parma, 1978; Schulhoff & Goodglass, 1969), and Milner, Taylor, and Sperry (1968) have reported an almost complete suppression of left-ear input in individuals with surgical disconnection of the two hemispheres. There can be little doubt that the dichotic listening procedure taps some lateralized function of the speech-dominant hemisphere. The problem arises in using it as a diagnostic tool. So many other factors interact to determine the specific level of performance on tasks involving dichotic lists that data from such tasks become very difficult to interpret.

Single-Pair Studies

In 1970, a major paper by Studdert-Kennedy and Shankweiler popularized a new approach to dichotic studies. In their procedure, only a single pair of CVC nonsense syllables was presented on each trial. By carefully aligning the onset of the two simuli, and by using a stimulus set that was very highly confusable, they generated single-pair material that was sufficiently difficult for subjects to make errors. The use of single pairs reduces the memory load on the subject (but see Darwin & Baddeley, 1974) and eliminates many of the response organization factors that complicate the interpretation of list data. The subject is still free to deploy attention in a variety of ways, and even two items must be reported in some order, but the complexities of interpretation are greatly reduced.

Each of the CVC syllables employed by Studdert-Kennedy and Shankweiler (1970) consisted of an initial and terminal consonant, and a medial vowel. The consonants were the six stop consonants /b, d, g, p, t, k/, while the vowels were /i, ɛ, æ, a, ɔ, u/. To investigate the effect of the initial consonant, they used 90 different stimulus pairings: each of the 15 possible pairings of two different stop consonants, followed by each of the six vowels and the terminal consonant /p/. Thus, the subject might hear /bap/–/dap/ or /dip/–/kip/. A similar approach was used to investigate terminal consonants, while vowels were presented in two separate environments, one in which the initial stop varied and one in which the final stop varied. Subjects were instructed to attend to both ears and to report both consonants (or vowels) in their order of confidence.

The results of this study are quite compelling. All subjects showed a right-ear advantage for initial stops. For terminal consonants, the right-ear effect was still present, but to a lesser degree. In contrast, vowels were inconsistent in their lateralization, although there was a trend toward a right-ear effect. Further, the voiced consonants /b, g, d/ always showed a greater right-ear effect than the unvoiced consonants with the same place of articulation /p, k, t/. Many of the errors that occurred were the result of combining or blending the voicing feature from one consonant with the place feature from the other.

The very robust right-ear effects found by Studdert-Kennedy and Shankweiler (1970) for initial stops led most investigators to abandon list experiments and adopt stop consonant sets. Since the terminal consonant seemed to have a weaker effect, CV stimulus sets with the six stop consonants in a common vowel environment have been the most popular.

A number of procedural improvements have been suggested. A number of investigators have been concerned with the fact that the typical instructions do not specify how one is to deploy attention, and even a single pair provides some freedom in which item to report first. One solution is to have subjects attend to one ear for a block of trials and report only the item from that ear (Haggard & Parkinson, 1971; Hayden, Kirstein, & Singh, 1979). There is some evidence that such a procedure leads to less variability in the right-ear effect than does a more open-ended instruction (Bryden, Munhall, & Allard, 1980). Another approach is to make the two members of the dichotic pair so similar that they fuse, and only a single sound, usually the right-ear stimulus, is heard on any given trial. Repp (1977, 1978) has used this procedure very successfully with synthetic speech stimuli, where it is possible to manipulate the acoustic parameters of the signal very precisely. He finds very large and robust right-ear effects with this fusional approach and reports that the way in which attention is distributed does not affect the stimulus that is heard. Unfortunately, Repp's approach does require the use of synthetic speech.

A slightly different procedure has also been given the name dichotic monitoring by Geffen and her colleagues (Geffen & Caudrey, 1981; Geffen & Traub, 1980; Geffen, Traub, & Stierman, 1978). These researchers present a long list of word pairs in which a particular target word appears randomly at one ear or the other. The subject is required to initiate a button-press whenever he or she detects the target word. The procedure permits determination of both hit rates and response times for each ear, and normal subjects are both faster and more accurate on the right ear (Geffen et al., 1978). Further, the task has been shown to classify subjects of known language lateralization reliably (Geffen & Caudrey, 1981). Thus, this particular task does seem to provide good classification of language lateralization even though subjects have some freedom as to how to deploy attention.

Yet another approach is to concentrate on reaction time measures. Springer (1973), for instance, had subjects monitor one ear and indicate whenever a particular target syllable appeared. Even though the speech material was paired with white-noise bursts on the other ear, and not competing syllables, reaction items were 13.6 msec faster to right-ear targets than to left-ear targets. The reaction time procedure eliminates the necessity of a verbal response, and the fact that a right-ear advantage still exists indicates that it does not have its origin in very late stages of accessing the speech system. However, Sidtis and Bryden (1978) found that a right-ear reaction time advantage for dichotic words emerged only after practice on the task.

There is little more than argument to indicate that one procedure is better than another for measuring cerebral organization uncontaminated by other effects. However, much support can be mustered for the attentional monitoring procedure. In this procedure, subjects are required to attend to one prespecified ear and to identify or respond to only the items arriving at that ear. In counterbalanced blocks, subjects are tested while attending to the left ear and while attending to the right ear. Because of practice effects, the use of several blocks for each ear is desirable. This procedure, coupled with the use of single-pair stimulus material, overcomes most of the problems we have raised in the preceding pages. Memory factors are reduced to a minimum, and the manner of deploying attention is experimenter determined rather than subject determined. Bryden *et al.* (1980) have employed this procedure and found less variability in the right-ear effect with monitoring instructions than when the subject was asked to divide attention between the two ears. This result would suggest that strategy effects had a greater effect on the magnitude of the right-ear effect under divided attention instructions. In addition, Piazza (1980) has reported that familial left-handers show a very reduced right-ear effect with monitoring instructions, a pattern that would be expected from our knowledge of the relation between handedness and speech lateralization.

What about different speech sounds? The stop consonants are convenient material to use because they begin rapidly, and temporal alignment is much easier to accomplish. Nevertheless, there have been studies with other classes of speech sounds. Thus, right-ear effects have been reported for fricatives (Allard & Scott, 1975; Darwin, 1971) and for liquids and semivowels (Haggard, 1971), although the effects are not as large as those observed with stops. Hayden *et al.* (1979) investigated performance on 21 different consonants, using a monitoring procedure. They found large right-ear effects for both stops and nasals, much smaller ones for liquids and affricates, and virtually none for continuants (/f, v, s, z/). Most curiously, the continuant–affricate and nasal–liquid pairings led to much larger right-ear effects than would be predicted from effects observed with the constituents. However, Hayden *et al.* do not provide a breakdown of their data, and one cannot determine, for example, whether the very large right-ear effect for nasal–liquid pairings comes from the nasals or the liquids. Further, by pairing 21 different syllables with one another in all possible combinations, they were left with only a single presentation of each pairing for each subject. However, the large right-ear effect for nasals has been replicated by Murray, Brown, Saxby, Tapley, and Bryden (1981). Despite the problems of pairing consonants of differing durations, there still remain some interesting questions concerning the magnitude of the right-ear effect for different classes of phonemes.

Although most researchers have agreed with Studdert-Kennedy and Shankweiler (1970) in finding that vowels produce only a small right-ear effect, Godfrey (1974) and Weiss and House (1973) have indicated that vowels show a significant right-ear effect when the task is made difficult. Almost in contrast, Haggard (1971) found a right-ear effect for vowels when they occurred in different voices, produced either by changing the fundamental or the formant frequencies. Spellacy and Blumstein (1970) found a right-ear effect for vowels when they appeared in the context of other word pairings, but a left-ear effect for the same material in the context of nonverbal material. Thus, the particular ear advantage depends in part on the nature of the task the subject is performing.

Given that stop consonants produce the largest and most robust right-ear effect, what is it about these consonants that produces the effect? The important features for the identification of a stop consonant are the initial burst of energy and the change in frequency from the onset of the sound to the steady state of the following vowel (A. M. Liberman, Cooper, Shankweiler, & Studdert-Kennedy, 1967). By editing real speech sounds, Allard and Scott (1975) attempted to remove the transitional cues or the burst cues from stop consonants. They found a larger laterality effect when only the bursts were present than when only the transitions were present. Cutting (1974), using synthetic speech material, found as big a right-ear effect with stops having no first formant transition (but a second formant transition) as with normal sounds. Repp (1978) has found very robust right-ear effects by manipulating voice onset time. Others have found bigger effects for unvoiced than for voiced syllables (e.g., Lowe, Cullen, Berlin, Thompson, & Willett, 1970). These results would all suggest that timing information is very critical in determining the right-ear effect and raise the possibility that the left hemisphere is specialized for detecting very fine temporal differences or executing fine frequency analyses.

Not only is there a large and robust right-ear superiority for dichotically presented stop consonants, but performance on the stop consonant material is selectively influenced by unilateral brain injury. For example, Oscar-Berman, Zurif, and Blumstein (1975) found that left-hemispheric damage led to a complete reversal of laterality, with accuracy being better on the left ear than on the right. They found that left-hemispheric subjects made relatively little use of feature sharing, not showing improved accuracy when the two dichotic consonants shared a common feature.

In summary, there is fairly convincing evidence that the right-ear effect obtained with carefully paired phoneme contrasts is related to the left-hemispheric specialization for language. Further, single-pair techniques are far less contaminated by subject strategies than are list procedures. In particular, the attentional monitoring (Hayden et al., 1979) and fusional (Repp, 1978) procedures may provide a good metric for assessing individual laterality effects. We do not know, however, that phonetic processing is the only language function that shows a perceptual laterality effect. The concentration on phonetic distinctions has turned research away from the use of more meaningful material.

A third procedure that holds promise, and may be very useful in the investigation of laterality effects for more meaningful material, is the list monitoring procedure of Geffen et al. (1978). Although this procedure does involve lists of words, the target monitoring task eliminates most of the problems associated with list studies, and it would be easily possible to manipulate the semantic characteristics of the target or the context.

Is Dichotic Stimulation Necessary?

Kimura's (1967) early model of dichotic performance proposed that information ascending to the brain along the ipsilateral auditory pathways was blocked or occluded by competing information (see Figure 2.1). Because of this occlusion, information from one ear would reach only the contralateral auditory cortex. Thus, speech information would be at an advantage when it was presented to the right ear because it would be transmitted directly to the hemisphere specialized for speech and language. Left-ear input, on the other hand, would travel to the right hemisphere and then have to be transmitted callosally to the left hemisphere. This model suggests that dichotic competition is necessary for an auditory perceptual laterality effect.

However, if the crossed auditory pathways are in fact more efficient than the uncrossed ones (Majkowski et al., 1971), dichotic competition may not be necessary for a right-ear effect. Rather, dichotic competition may simply serve to make the task sufficiently difficult for one to observe a right-ear advantage. Remembering a CV syllable or a list of three numbers is not hard when the material is presented monaurally; it only becomes a challenge when there is competing material present. Thus, one might expect to find laterality effects with monaural stimulation under the appropriate conditions.

In a bibliography of published research, Henry (1979) found 74 studies that reported significant laterality effects employing monaural presentation procedures. Unfortunately, Henry does not enumerate the studies that failed to find any monaural asymmetry (e.g., Bryden, 1969), nor does he comment on how fragile some of the effects seem to be (e.g., Bakker, 1967). Nevertheless, there does seem to be a large body of evidence indicating that auditory laterality effects can be obtained in the absence of dichotic competition.

As one example, Catlin and Neville (1976) found a right-ear advantage in voice reaction time to spoken letters of the alphabet. This difference was the same order of magnitude as that observed when competing white noise was presented to the other ear. Very similar results were obtained for manual reaction time by Catlin, VanderVeer, and Teicher (1976). Although Springer (1973) did find a right-ear effect for speech material with competing white noise, it may not be the ideal way of producing a dichotic effect (Corsi, 1972). If there exists a subcortical occlusion mechanism such as that postulated by Kimura (1967), it might well depend on the spectral characteristics of the competing material. We still do not have strong evidence that any monaural laterality effect is of the same magnitude or due to the same mechanisms as the dichotic effect. It might be interesting to use the target search task ("respond when you hear /ba/") employed by Springer (1973) and by Catlin *et al.* (1976) under conditions of dichotic competition, where other speech signals were arriving on the unattended channel.

In fact, there is some evidence that monaural laterality effects are qualitatively different from dichotic ones. Lowe *et al.* (1970) not only found no monaural laterality effects but also found that the types of errors made in monaural presentation were different from those observed with dichotic material. For instance, unvoiced consonants are more accurately perceived in a dichotic situation, but this difference is reduced or reversed with monaural stimulation. Similarly, Bryden (1969) found no signs of a monaural laterality effect even under conditions in which there was uncertainty as to which ear would receive the stimulus.

Furthermore, there is strong evidence that monaural and dichotic masking effects are quite different. For instance, the effects of a second stimulus, lagging in time slightly behind the first, are quite different monaurally and dichotically (Studdert-Kennedy, Shankweiler, & Schulman, 1970). Dichotic masking effects depend on the acoustic similarity of the masking signal to the target, but do not require that the masking signal be identifiable as speech. Differences can be seen between monaural and dichotic effects using only the second formant of the signal as a mask—a "bleat" that is not recognized as speech (Berlin & McNeal, 1976; Porter & Whittaker, 1980).

One is tempted to argue that the monaural laterality effects observed with manual response time measures are a reflection of the contralateral control of hand movement, rather than being an indication of any left-hemispheric superiority in processing auditory material (cf. Klisz & Parsons, 1975; Provins & Jeeves, 1975). There remain, however, some monaural effects that cannot easily be explained on this basis. For instance, Frankfurter and Honeck (1973) and Turvey, Pisoni, and Croog (1972) have reported monaural right-ear effects for the recall of syntactically complex verbal material. Safer and Leventhal (1977) found a dissociation between the recall of content and emotional tone of sentences heard monaurally, with subjects listening to the left ear being guided more by the emotional tone and those listening to the right ear being guided by the semantic content. Finally, in a difficult music discrimination task, Bever and Chiarello (1974) found a left-ear advantage in unskilled musicians, but a right-ear advantage in skilled musicians. Data such as these would lead one to accept the notion of monaural laterality effects, though it remains unclear as to how they relate to the more common dichotic ones.

A second attack on the question of competition has come from Morais and his colleagues (Hublet, Morais, & Bertelson, 1976; Morais & Bertelson, 1973, 1975). These investigators have found that true dichotic stimulation is not necessary for the right-ear effect but that it can be obtained by presenting the two messages in free field, through loudspeakers. In this case, both messages are heard at both ears, although the timing and intensity parameters differ for the two signals. Morais and Bertelson (1973), using lists of CV syllables, found a right-speaker advantage when the speakers were placed to the left and right of the subject, but an advantage for the voice in front of the subject when it was compared to a voice to one side or the other. They argue that the right-ear effect arises, not from competition, but from a tendency to attend to particular parts of space, with the front dominating the sides and the right dominating the left. In fact, they may very well have identified one of the extraneous components that contributes to the right-ear effect with lists of material, but Kimura's (1961b) original data (see Table 2.1) make it very clear that there must be some component directly related to speech lateralization.

Nonverbal Studies

Having found a right-ear advantage for the perception of dichotically presented speech stimuli, it was an obvious next step to search for tasks that led to a left-ear superiority. In 1964, Kimura reported just such an effect in the perception of melodies. She paired 4-sec excerpts from instrumental chamber music. After each pair, four melodies, including the two that had been played dichotically, were presented in succession binaurally (using the general procedure illustrated in Figure 3.2). The subject's task was to indicate which two of the four binaural melodies had been presented earlier. In selecting the melodies to be played, sets of four were chosen in which the instruments were the same and the pitch range and tempo very similar, so that melodic pattern was the primary cue. Kimura found a left-ear advantage for normal subjects on this task.

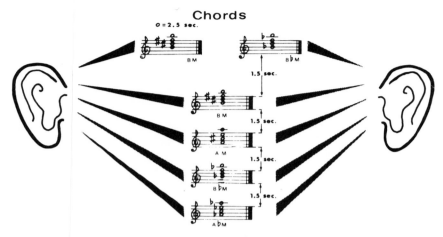

Figure 3.2. Paradigm for dichotic presentation of chords. A single pair of chords presented one to each ear, followed by four multiple choices presented binaurally. In this example, the first and third choices are correct. [From Gordon, H. W. Degree of ear asymmetries for perception of dichotic chords and for illusory chord localization in musicians of different levels of competence. *Journal of Experimental Psychology: Human Perception and Performance*, 1980, *6*, p. 518. Copyright (1980) by the American Psychological Association. Reprinted by permission of publisher and author.]

    Subsequently, Shankweiler (1966) used this same test with temporal lobe patients. He found that right temporal lobectomy significantly reduced performance, especially on the left ear. At the same time, he noted a clear dissociation between performance on the melodies test and on a dichotic digits test similar to that used by Kimura (1961b): Subjects who were better on one ear for the melodies task tended to be better on the opposite ear for the digits task.

    Gordon (1970) used both a melodies test similar to Kimura's (1964) and a chords test, in which 2-sec dichotic chords were followed by four binaural alternatives. He found a significant left-ear advantage only on the chords test. It should be noted, however, that his subjects did not exhibit a particularly large right-ear effect on a digits (three-pair) test.

    The melodies task is not an easy one to understand. It takes time to present the multiple-choice alternatives—some 18–20 sec with Kimura's (1964) task—and memory factors could have a major effect (cf. Yeni-Komshian & Gordon, 1974). A detailed analysis of performance as a function of position in the multiple-choice list would be desirable, but it has not been provided. In addition, the task is very difficult, especially for unskilled musicians: Shankweiler's (1966) patients were performing only slightly above chance level. Kimura's task also permits the subject to deploy attention in a number of different ways. Finally, there is evidence for left- as well as right-hemispheric involvement in some aspects of music (Benton, 1977; Damasio & Damasio, 1977; Gates & Bradshaw, 1977a, 1977b; Wertheim, 1977). In a sodium amytal study, Gordon and Bogen (1974) found that unilateral suppression of the right hemisphere blocked melodic expression with little disturbance of speech, suggesting a right-hemispheric involvement in musical expression. However, amusias are often related to language deficits (Benton, 1977), and receptive dysfunctions can be found following left-hemispheric damage (Wertheim, 1977).

Other investigators have investigated the relative contribution of different aspects of music to the left-ear effect (see Gates & Bradshaw, 1977b, for a thorough review). For example, Spellacy (1970) used dichotic presentations of solo violin melodies, four-note patterns varying in frequency, patterns consisting of tone pulses of different durations, and single organ notes differing in timbre. He tested 32 subjects who had previously been found to show a right-ear advantage on a dichotic word-pair test. In Spellacy's task, subjects heard a dichotic pair, followed after a 5- or 12-sec interval by a single test item. The task was to indicate whether the test item was or was not one of the dichotic stimuli. A significant left-ear superiority was found for the musical material at the 5-sec delay, but not at the 12-sec delay. No other laterality effects were significant, although there were trends for a left-ear effect at the short delay with frequency patterns and for a right-ear effect at the long delay with temporal patterns. The latter trend is of particular note, since Halperin, Nachshon, and Carmon (1973) subsequently reported that ear superiority shifted from left to right as the number of frequency or duration transitions increased. They suggest a left-hemispheric involvement in the perception of complex temporal patterns. Spreen, Spellacy, and Reid (1970) also employed music and frequency patterns, using a 1-sec delay. They found a clear left-ear superiority for both types of material and some tendency for the magnitude of the ear effect to be reduced at higher intensities. Using a reaction time procedure, Kallman and Corballis (1975) found a left-ear advantage for music in unpracticed subjects that dissipated with experience. However, Sidtis and Bryden (1978) reported just the opposite effect with sequences of piano notes.

While musical stimuli generally exhibit a left-ear advantage, temporal sequencing and rhythm are more likely to show a right-ear effect (Halperin *et al.*, 1973; Robinson & Solomon, 1974). A study by Divenyi and Efron (1979) may shed some light on this. They have attempted to segregate the components of dichotic processing. Using pairs of well-defined stimuli, they presented them in the AB order to one ear and the

BA order to the other ear, asking the subjects whether they heard stimuli more like AB or BA. When the stimulus pair was made up of pure tones, all their subjects showed a large ear effect, five to the left and one to the right. A right-ear effect was seen for the /ga/–/ka/ pairing. Divenyi and Efron suggest two components to the ear effect: an idiosyncratic advantage that may be to the left or right for processing spectral information, and a right-ear advantage for the temporal characteristic of voice onset time that provides the voicing distinction between /ga/ and /ka/. If we assume that the spectral component is most often a left-ear effect, then much of the music literature begins to fall into place. When spectral characteristics are critical, as with Gordon's (1970) chords, a left-ear advantage is seen; when temporal characteristics are more important, as with Robinson and Solomon's rhythms, a right-ear effect is observed.

Finally, there is some evidence that musical experience affects performance on these tasks. One of the most frequently cited studies is that of Bever and Chiarello, (1974), who found a left-ear effect in nonmusicians and a right-ear effect in musicians. This study, although often referenced with the dichotic literature, was a monaural identification task, and somewhat different factors may be relevant. Gaede, Parsons, and Bertera (1978) have suggested that it is musical *aptitude,* rather than musical *experience,* that is relevant in determining this shift to the right ear. More recently, Gordon (1980) has reported a left-ear superiority for the perception of dichotic chords in musicians of all levels of competence, although the professional musicians did show more extreme absolute asymmetries than did nonprofessionals.

The left-ear superiority for melodic patterns can be observed with human voices as well as with instrumental material (Bartholomeus, 1974; King & Kimura, 1972). The Bartholomeus study is particularly interesting. She had eight different singers sing sequences of letters to different melodies. As in the multiple-choice procedure of Kimura (1964), each dichotic pair was followed by four alternatives. Two of these alternatives involved the same singers, two the same letter sequences, and two the same melodies, carefully counterbalanced so that the precise combinations that had been heard dichotically did not recur in the test stimuli. This procedure permitted Bartholomeus to test the same subjects on the same material three times, with instructions to identify the melodies, the singers, or the specific letter sequences. She found a left-ear superiority for melody recognition, a right-ear superiority for letter sequences, and no ear difference for voice of singer.

Left-ear advantages have been reported for auditory material other than music. King and Kimura (1972) found a left-ear superiority for such vocal nonspeech sounds as laughing, crying, and sighing. Curry (1967) reported a left-ear effect for dichotically presented environmental sounds (e.g., car starting, toilet flushing, tooth brushing). Curry also reported that this left-ear advantage was reduced in left-handers, as would be expected if it were related to cerebral organization. One problem is that the environmental sounds task is a very difficult one to work with. If the subjects are familiarized with the sounds at the start, or if the sounds are easy to identify, performance is very high. If the subjects are not familiarized with the sounds, they may fail to identify them on the first trials and then always identify them on subsequent presentations. It would seem best to prepare an environmental sounds tape with a large number of different sounds that are used only once at each ear.

Finally, left-ear effects have been reported for the perception of sonar signals (Chaney & Webster, 1966) and Morse code signals (Papcun, Krashen, Terbeek, Remington, & Harshman, 1974). Like the Bever and Chiarello (1974) study, Papcun *et al.* (1974) reported that the left-ear advantage in unskilled subjects shifted to a right-ear advantage in trained Morse operators.

In summary, the results of nonverbal dichotic experiments point toward a right-hemispheric involvement in the perception of environmental sounds, melodies, and chords, but a left-hemispheric involvement in rhythm and in the perception of complex tonal sequences.

Some Concluding Remarks

Despite the concerns we have expressed about procedural details, the dichotic listening procedure has provided us with some of the most robust effects available in contemporary neuropsychological research. Kimura's (1961a) initial finding of a right-ear advantage for verbal material has been replicated dozens of times, and there is little doubt that this right-ear effect is related to cerebral speech lateralization. The left-ear effect obtained for music and environmental sounds are somewhat more ephemeral, but the procedural problems are rather different, and it is not easy to achieve an appropriate level of difficulty.

Even Kimura's (1967) simple model of an occlusion mechanism has remained viable over the years. Although there are many reports of monaural right-ear effects for verbal material, there is little compelling evidence to indicate that the monaural effects are the result of the same processes that produce the dichotic effects. At the very least, the dichotic procedure introduces some factor that makes it much easier to observe ear asymmetries. Thus, for example, there is almost total suppression of ipsilateral input in patients following section of the corpus callosum, yet such individuals have no difficulty with verbal items presented monaurally to the left ear (Milner *et al.*, 1968). This occlusion cannot be complete, however, for hemispherectomized subjects do identify items from the ipsilateral ear (Netley, 1972), and individuals with callosal agenesis do recognize items from both ears (Bryden & Zurif, 1970; Lassonde, Lortie, & Ptito, 1979). Thus, there must be some information arriving along the ipsilateral auditory pathways that people can learn to use with sufficient practice.

Kimura (1961b) showed a direct relationship between the direction of the dichotic ear advantage and speech lateralization as assessed by the sodium amytal test. Other studies involving unilateral cerebral damage indicate that performance on both verbal (Oscar-Berman *et al.*, 1975) and melodies (Shankweiler, 1966) tasks are related to cerebral organization. The evidence for a relation between performance on some of the other dichotic tasks and cerebral organization is rather more inferential. One approach has been to compare groups of right- and left-handers, under the argument that left-hemispheric speech representation will be less common in the left-handers. Using this approach, Piazza (1980) demonstrated that dextrals showed right-ear effects for CV syllables and left-ear effects for melodies and environmental sounds, whereas sinistrals were much weaker in their lateralization. Although the specific patterns of lateralization depended on both sex and familial sinistrality, Piazza's data do suggest that right-hemisphere mechanisms are involved in the processing of both environmental sounds and melodies. Similarly, Nachshon (1978) found a left-ear effect for discrimination of the pitch and loudness of speech sounds in dextrals, but not in sinistrals.

The conclusion is that many of the auditory asymmetries discussed in the preceding pages are in fact related to cerebral organization. The difficulty arises in turning this statement around. Just because a particular task shows a right-ear effect does not mean that it is related to cerebral lateralization. Careful control needs to be exerted over possible extraneous variables (cf. Bryden, 1978), or some verification that we are really dealing with cerebral lateralization needs to be done, such as demonstrating that left- and right-handers behave differently.

The stronger position, that an *individual* showing a particular lateralization effect is necessarily employing the contralateral hemisphere to execute the task is even more dangerous. Variability on all measures of auditory asymmetry is great, and many extraneous factors can dictate the performance of an individual. Without understanding attention, memory, and other such factors that can influence performance, and without controlling for such effects, it is unjustified to assume that dichotic lateralization effects are necessarily the reflection of lateralized cerebral mechanisms in a specific individual.

Do we have a strategy-pure dichotic procedure? It is not entirely clear what the criteria for such a technique should be, but there are certainly procedures that are far less affected by attentional biases and strategies than others. The free recall of dichotic lists is a particularly weak approach, with a vast number of factors that are known to influence performance. The dichotic fusion procedure (Repp, 1977) offers one approach to verbal presentation that appears to be unaffected by the deployment of attention, although one would like to see stronger evidence that the laterality effects obtained with this procedure are related to cerebral lateralization. The attentional monitoring procedure, whereby the subject is instructed to monitor one ear at a time and report only the items from that ear (Bryden *et al.*, 1980; Piazza, 1980), also controls for many of the extraneous factors, although there are initial practice effects in learning how to attend to one ear. Despite this problem, it seems to provide a fruitful approach and should be employed more frequently.

If one had to provide a general description of auditory laterality effects, one would say that right-ear effects are obtained with speech material and on tasks that require fine temporal discrimination, whereas left-ear effects are obtained for music, environmental sounds, and tasks that require the integration of information across time and the audible spectrum. Perhaps Semmes's (1968) distinction between focal and diffuse systems comes closest to capturing this distinction: A right-ear effect occurs when the task requires attention to fine temporal detail, whereas a left-ear effect occurs when detail is less important than a holistic integration.

Such a general statement may be an oversimplification, since several assumptions are implicit in any attempt to provide such a summary. First, it assumes that there is a single left-hemisphere laterality effect and a single right-hemisphere laterality effect. Furthermore, it assumes a notion of complementary specialization: If verbal processes are lateralized to the left hemisphere, then nonverbal mechanisms are necessarily lateralized to the right hemisphere. The evidence for these assumptions is relatively sparse.

At a very broad level, there is some evidence for complementarity. Right-handers *as a group* do tend to show left-ear effects for music and environmental sounds, whereas left-handers, with less clearly defined speech lateralization, are more unpredictable. When the same subjects are tested on both verbal and nonverbal material, laterality effects tend to be negatively correlated (Piazza, 1980). However, such correlations are often insignificant, and it is hard to tell whether this is due to low test reliability or to a true lack of correlation. Certainly, many individual subjects will show the same lateralization for both verbal and nonverbal material. It remains questionable whether or not hemispheric specialization is anything more than statistically complementary (see Chapter 10).

We also tend to assume that left-ear effects have a common origin and that right-ear effects have a common origin. Kimura's (1961b) work employed lists of spoken digits, but now it is more common to use CV nonsense syllables with specific phonemic contrasts. It is assumed that the right-ear effect obtained with the two types of material is a manifestation of some common underlying mechanism. Yet this need not be the case. Ojemann and Mateer (1979), for instance, have reported that phoneme identification is disturbed by mild electrical stimulation of regions surrounding Broca's area, in superior temporal, inferior frontal, and parietal peri-Sylvian cortex. Errors of reading, naming, and syntactic organization were elicited from other sites in frontal, temporal, and parietal cortex further removed from the final motor pathway for speech. These results indicate that phonemic and syntactic components of language are dependent on different regions of the dominant hemisphere, and they raise the possibility that lateralization effects might be different for tasks involving phonological, syntactic, and semantic distinctions.

A similar point can be made with respect to the right hemisphere. Piazza's (1980) data show clear left-ear effects for both environmental sounds and melodies, but there are some differences between the two tasks, especially in the effect of familial sinistrality in females. While this may simply be measurement error, it is also possible that melodies and environmental sounds depend on somewhat different right-hemispheric mechanisms.

Thus, while the dichotic listening procedure produces some very robust effects, there remain many issues deserving of further investigation.

4

Visual Laterality Effects

Although the dichotic listening procedure was the first approach to laterality in the normal brain to be related to cerebral asymmetry, vision has almost certainly been the most popular modality for laterality research. As with dichotic listening, the basic studies reveal a right-visual-field superiority for words and letters, and a left-visual-field superiority for a variety of tasks that do not involve language processes. Chapter 2 provided a general review of visual procedures, together with some cautions about their interpretation. This chapter examines the findings from visual laterality studies in more detail. The initial section deals with those experiments that have used verbal material. Subsequently, a variety of nonverbal tasks are examined, and finally those experiments that have used both types of material are considered.

Verbal Laterality and Handedness

One way to supply some credibility to the contention that visual laterality measures are in fact related to cerebral lateralization in normal subjects is to compare the performance of left- and right-handers. As indicated earlier, left-handers as a group are much less likely to have left-hemispheric speech representation than are right-handers. Thus, a visual laterality effect that results from lateralized cerebral processes should show a reduced or reversed effect in a large sample of left-handers. In some ways, it is surprising how rarely this approach has been used, although left-handers do tend to be in short supply. One might also note that such studies require fairly large samples of left-handers, given that many left-handers have left-hemispheric speech representation and that there will be some error of measurement (Segalowitz & Bryden, forthcoming).

With single-letter material and unilateral presentation, Bryden (1965) found evidence that left-handers did not show the right-visual-field superiority observed in right-handers. Similar results were found by Bryden (1973), and Zurif and Bryden (1969) found differences between familial and nonfamilial left-handers. In these three studies, all conducted at the University of Waterloo, 72% of the right-handed subjects were more accurate in the right visual field, but only 46% of the left-handers were. Haun (1978) also found that left-handers showed a left-visual-field superiority in a vocal reaction time study using single letters.

In a further experiment involving single-letter stimuli, Cohen (1972) found that left-handers exhibited no visual-field effect on a name matching task, whereas right-handers were faster when the letters appeared in the right visual field. However, only six subjects of each handedness type were used.

Words have provided somewhat less compelling data. With horizontal displays, Orbach (1967) found that right- and left-handed Israelis differed in laterality effects for Hebrew words, but both groups showed a right-visual-field superiority for English words. Bradshaw and Taylor (1979) found faster vocal naming latencies in the right visual field, which were reduced among sinistrals. No difference was observed between familial and nonfamilial left-handers. With a vertical display, Levy and Reid (1978) found a reversed visual-field effect in left-handers as compared to right-handers for CVC syllables. Levy and Reid also found that sinistrals who wrote with an inverted writing posture resembled the right-handers, whereas those who wrote with a normal or upright posture were quite the reverse. Bradshaw and Taylor (1979) found that writing position showed a trend in the opposite direction in their study. Further, the difference between left- and right-handers is not always evident (Goodglass & Barton, 1963).

Rather fewer studies have assessed the influence of handedness in the bilateral presentation procedure, but they have generally shown that right-handers show a right-visual-field superiority, whereas left-handers yield mixed results (Higgenbottom, 1973; McKeever & VanDeventer, 1977b; Piazza, 1980; Schmuller & Goodman, 1979). In some studies, it is the familial left-handers who show the weak or reversed laterality effects (Piazza, 1980; Schmuller & Goodman, 1979), whereas in others it is the nonfamilial left-handers (Higgenbottom, 1973; McKeever, 1979; McKeever & VanDeventer, 1977a, 1977b; VanDeventer, & Suberi, 1973). McKeever et al. (1973) also found a reduced effect in right-handers with a familial history of sinistrality. Zurif and Bryden (1969), with a bilateral serial presentation technique, found that familial sinistrals showed a reversed laterality effect.

Left-handers therefore show reduced or reversed laterality effects with both unilateral and bilateral procedures. Since left-handers are rather less likely to have clear left-hemispheric speech representation, this suggests that at least some component of both procedures is related to cerebral speech lateralization. Yet there have been no attempts to determine which procedures most clearly differentiate handedness groups. Admittedly, there is no compelling way of predicting which sinistrals are right-hemispheric for speech (see Levy & Reid, 1978, and Chapter 10), and it may be premature to expect a handedness study to provide any final answers. Nevertheless, it does seem that the visual procedure least influenced by extraneous variables should yield the largest difference between handedness groups.

Verbal Stimulus or Verbal Task?

It is easy to slip into statements, such as "right-visual-field effects are obtained with verbal material," that seem to imply that visual patterns forming alphabetic characters have some privileged access to the left hemisphere or that a verbal processing of alphabetic characters is automatic. Such phenomena as the Stroop effect (Stroop, 1935) do suggest that it is very difficult to avoid some verbal processing of words. Nevertheless, a number of studies do make it possible to distinguish between laterality effects due to the nature of the stimulus and those due to the nature of the task the subject is required to perform.

Kimura (1967), for instance, found a left-visual-field superiority for the enumeration of the number of elements in a display, whether the items consisted of dots or of letters. The simple presence of letter material was not sufficient to induce a right-visual-field effect. In a single-letter identification task, Bryden and Allard (1976) found that letters in certain nonstandard typefaces yielded a reliable left-visual-field effect, whereas more regular typefaces gave the usual right-visual-field superiority. Different operations, and ones that are less dependent upon left-hemispheric language mechanisms, seem to be involved in the identification of the uncommon typefaces.

Perhaps the most common procedure for showing the influence of the task on direction of lateralization is the name matching task (Posner

& Keele, 1967). Posner and Keele asked subjects to make same–different judgments on pairs of letters. They found that response times were consistently faster when the letters were in the same case (e.g., *AA, bb*) than when they were in different cases (e.g., *Aa, bB*). In the first situation, the "same" response could be made on the basis of the physical characteristics of the stimuli, whereas in the latter situation, the stimuli had to be identified and the response made on the basis of the names of the characters. Several investigators have employed this procedure with lateralized stimuli (e.g., Cohen, 1972; R. Davis & Schmit, 1973; Geffen *et al.*, 1972; Kirsner, 1979; Segalowitz & Stewart, 1979; Wilkins & Stewart, 1974). In general, a right-visual-field superiority is observed with name matching, but not with physical matching. Kirsner (1979), however, did find right-visual-field effects for both physical and name matching. Unlike most of the other studies, Kirsner presented his stimuli serially, with the first item appearing in central vision and the second lateralized to one side. Such a procedure may encourage a naming of the initial item and thus generate a right-visual-field effect.

Gibson, Dimond, and Gazzaniga (1972) found a left-visual-field effect for matching successively presented words. In effect, this task is rather like the physical match component of the Posner and Keele (1967) task, although the specific procedure is different. While physical matches for letters have not always yielded a left-visual-field effect (Geffen *et al.*, 1972; Moscovitch, 1979; Segalowitz & Stewart, 1979), the word matching task may be sufficiently more complex to involve right-hemisphere mechanisms.

A rather different approach was used by Klatzky and Atkinson (1971). They had subjects memorize a set of letters. Following this, a number of letters or pictures were shown in the two visual fields. Subjects were asked to indicate whether or not the letters were part of the memory set, or whether the picture was of an object beginning with one of the letters in the memory set. A right-visual-field effect was obtained for the pictures, but a left-field effect for the letters. Klatzky and Atkinson argue that the picture task involved accessing language mechanisms, whereas the letter task could be carried out as a physical matching task.

Right-visual-field effects do not appear simply because verbal stimuli have been used. Rather, the existence of right-visual-field effects depend on the nature of the task being performed by the subject. When the task involves language processing, a right-field effect is observed; when it does not, or when nonlanguage processes become relatively more important, no right-field effect is seen.

Nonverbal Effects

If one can find a right-visual-field (left-hemisphere) superiority for the recognition or identification of words and other alphabetic material, it would seem logical that one could also show a right-hemisphere or left-visual-field superiority for those types of nonlanguage tasks that depend on the integrity of the right hemisphere. It was not long after the first reports of verbal effects appeared that studies of nonverbal tasks began to be published in the literature, and by now dozens of different types of nonverbal tasks have been employed. The left-visual-field effects obtained with such material are not nearly so robust as those found with words, and there are numerous failures to replicate. However, some general patterns do emerge.

One of the first nonverbal tasks to be studied was that of enumeration. Kimura (1966) presented arrays of dots unilaterally and had subjects estimate the number of dots that had appeared. A left-visual-field superiority was found. Further studies used letter material or random shapes (see Figure 4.1), but again the task was to enumerate the number of items, and again a left-field effect was found. McGlone and Davidson (1973) used the same procedure and found that 70% of their right-handed subjects showed a left-visual-field effect. However, a left-field superiority was also observed in 64% of their sinistrals—an insignificant difference. In addition, Bryden (cited by M. J. White, 1972) attempted two replications of the original Kimura (1966) study without success. More recently, Young and Bion (1979) have found a left-visual-field effect in children between the ages of 5 and 11, and Charness and Shea (1981) have replicated the effect in young adults. Furthermore, Warrington and James (1967) have reported that right parietal, but not right temporal, patients are impaired on number estimation. The right-hemispheric superiority for enumeration seems to be a rather fragile phenomenon, but it may be worthy of further investigation.

Kimura's (1966) report of a left-visual-field superiority for enumeration was followed by an immense number of studies reporting left-field effects for a variety of "nonverbal" tasks. Basically, these may be divided into three general areas. Some studies deal with basic sensory processes, such as brightness and color discrimination, others with tasks that may be broadly classified as spatial in nature, and still others with complex visual patterns. Let us examine each of these in turn.

Moscovitch's (1979) information processing model of perceptual laterality suggests that perceptual laterality effects do not emerge until relatively late stages of processing. Such a view would not lead one to

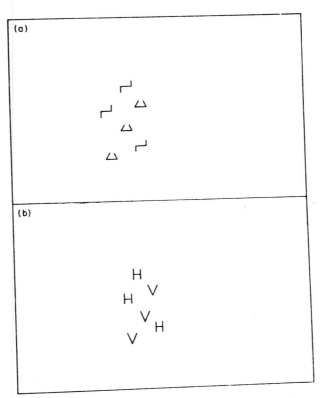

Figure 4.1. Kimura's display for item enumeration. Randomly arranged shapes (a) or letters (b) were presented unilaterally. (From Kimura, D. Dual functional asymmetry of the brain in visual perception. *Neuropsychologia*, 1966, *4*, 275–285. Reprinted with permission of Pergamon Press Ltd.)

expect laterality effects to be observed with simple sensory discriminations or matching tasks. We have already seen that the literature on physical matching of letters is somewhat ambiguous (Cohen, 1972; Kirsner, 1979). Other investigators have concerned themselves with color tasks. A left-visual-field superiority has been reported for color discrimination by Davidoff (1976) and by Hannay (1979), for color detection by Pirot, Pulton, and Sutker (1977), and for the accuracy and latency of matching by selecting the proper colored key to press by Pennal (1977). In contrast, Malone and Hannay (1978) and Dimond and Beaumont (1972) found no visual-field effects on color tasks. Malone and Hannay, in fact, found a right-visual-field superiority when it was possible to assign a name to the colored stimuli. Finally, Meyer (1976) presented evidence that the McCullough color-contingent aftereffect is bigger in the left visual field. The general trend is for studies of color discrimination and matching to show a left-visual-field superiority when color names cannot readily be assigned. This conclusion would be supported by a number of studies that have indicated that defects of both color matching and color sorting are associated with lesions of the right hemisphere (DeRenzi & Spinnler, 1967; Scotti & Spinnler, 1970). Meadows (1974b), however, has argued that bilateral lesions in the region of the occipitotemporal junction are critical for defects of color perception. A similar left-visual-field effect has been reported for brightness matching by Kaushall (1975).

Visuospatial disorders have long been associated with damage to the right hemisphere (Benton, 1969; McFie, Piercy, & Zangwill, 1950), and it is not at all surprising that the search for left-visual-field effects in the normal should concentrate on tasks that have some spatial component. As with the literature on color discrimination, however, there are inconsistencies and failures to replicate throughout the literature.

For example, Kimura (1969) had subjects localize dots presented singly in one visual field or the other. Subjects saw a briefly exposed dot and then were to indicate where it had appeared on a response card containing a set of numbered locations (see Figure 4.2 for a similar response card). She found a left-visual-field superiority, more pronounced in her male subjects than in her females. Quite different results were obtained by Pohl, Butters, and Goodglass (1972): They found a right-visual-field superiority when there was no frame of reference, and no field effect when a frame surrounded the area in which the dots could appear. Bryden (1976a) carried out a number of experiments employing a simultaneous detection and localization task. He included a number of trials on which no dot appeared at all, to provide a measure of the detectability of the dots. Again, no consistent visual-field effects were obtained for either detection or localization. However, Allard and Bryden (1979) did find a left-visual-field superiority with the same procedure, as did Levy and Reid (1978) with a task similar to Kimura's (1969). McKeever and Huling (1970) found that subjects were better at reproducing dot designs, and thus presumably better at localizing the dots, when they appeared in the left visual field. In general, the results of dot localization studies have been inconsistent and equivocal. Kimura (1969) suggests that her female subjects failed to show the left-visual-field effect because they attempted to code the location of the dots verbally. It may well be that the procedure is one in which some subjects find it difficult to avoid verbal strategies.

74	26	10	t t	53	48	69	14	35	97	nn	02	81	49
88	39	47	62	00	16	f f	90	57	31	24	19	65	x x
z z	05	99	28	41	79	34	52	83	66	43	20	73	08
82	13	37	64	92	55	86	r r	60	91	58	11	94	45
95	22	04	72	15	30	77	93	42	03	18	57	56	70
h h	61	38	61	89	27	01	dd	17	75	84	32	98	bb
76	29	44	06	23	50	cc	71	33	46	21	59	07	85
40	12	s s	78	63	87	25	09	68	36	80	kk	54	96

Figure 4.2. Bryden's response matrix for dot localization. A single dot was presented briefly, the response matrix appeared, and the subject had to indicate the number of the square in which the dot had appeared. Dots actually appeared only in the 24 shaded squares. (From Bryden, 1973.)

Another task that involves at least primitive visuospatial abilities is that of perceiving stereoscopic depth. Durnford and Kimura (1971; Kimura & Durnford, 1974) found that subjects were better at aligning the rods in a depth box when the rods were exposed briefly in the left visual field than when they appeared in the right visual field. Furthermore, there was also a left-visual-field superiority for detecting depth in Julesz random-dot stereograms, where binocular disparity is the only available cue for depth. These findings are in agreement with studies by Carmon and Bechtoldt (1969) and Benton and Hécaen (1970) indicating that right-hemispheric damage has a specific effect on the binocular perception of depth. However, Julesz and his colleagues have not been able to replicate Kimura and Durnford's findings (Breitmeyer, Julesz, & Kropfl, 1975; Julesz, Breitmeyer, & Kropfl, 1976). Julesz' studies are very careful ones, and they do report an anisotropy in the vertical direction: Depth is more readily detected in the upper visual field with uncrossed disparity and in the lower visual field with crossed disparity. Julesz *et al.* suggest that the Kimura and Durnford results are dependent on the form component of the task and would reverse if the form seen in depth was a letter. To complicate the matter further, Pitblado (1979) found a left-visual-field effect with small dots and a right-field effect with large ones.

Yet another simple visuospatial task that has been extensively investigated involves the determination of line slant. For example, Kimura and Durnford (1974) presented a single line in one visual field for 40 msec. Subjects were then given a response sheet with 11 lines at different angles to choose from (see Figure 4.3). Accuracy on this task was significantly better in the left visual field. In a further experiment, subjects were asked to detect the presence of a line, using an ascending method of limits procedure. No visual-field effects were obtained for detecting a 45° line in 1 of 14 different positions, but a highly significant left-visual-field superiority was found when 3 different slopes were used at each of 4 different positions in each visual field. In contrast, M. J. White (1971)

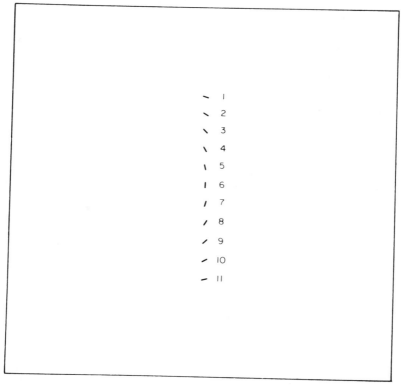

Figure 4.3. Response choices for visual line orientation experiment. A single line appeared unilaterally, and the subject was to select the appropriate orientation from the 11 choices given. [From Kimura, D., & Durnford, M. Normal studies on the function of the right hemisphere in vision. In S. J. Dimond and J. G. Beaumont (Eds.), *Hemisphere function in the brain.* London: Elek Science, 1974. Reprinted with permission.]

found a right-visual-field superiority for determining line slant. This discrepancy may be resolved by a study by Umilta, Rizzolatti, Marzi, Zamboni, Franzini, Carmada, and Berlucchi (1974). They found a right-visual-field effect for line orientation when the orientations were easy to label (e.g., vertical, horizontal, diagonal left, diagonal right) and a left-field effect when the lines were at odd angles and hard to label.

Benton, Hannay, and Varney (1975) found that lesions of the right hemisphere, except for the right prefrontal area, produced deficits on a task very similar to that employed by Kimura and Durnford (1974). As long as the line slant task employs angles that are not easily coded verbally, it seems to provide a fairly robust left-field superiority. It would be interesting to know how left-handers perform on this task, and how it relates to other measures of visual laterality.

Factor analytic studies of cognitive ability have indicated that one of the most clearly spatial factors involves mental rotation—the ability to rotate the visual image of an object from one position to another. Shepard and Metzler (1971) have provided some interesting insights into the processes involved in mental rotation, and by now their figures have become well known. Vandenberg and Kuse (1978) have constructed a paper-and-pencil version of the Shepard–Metzler figures (see Figure 4.4) and have found that it correlates well with other measures of spatial ability. Although there do not seem to be any laterality studies involving the Shepard–Metzler figures, a number of studies suggest a left-visual-field or right-hemisphere superiority for tasks involving some form of mental rotation. For instance, R. Hayashi and Hatta (1978) found a left-visual-field superiority for the rotation of Japanese Kanji ideographs, at least when the subject did not know the orientation in advance. Berlucchi, Brizzolara, Marzi, Rizzolatti, and Umilta (1979) found that speed, though not accuracy, for reading a clockface was better in the left visual field. Finally, Ratcliff (1979) found that patients with right posterior lesions did better than those with left posterior lesions in identifying upright stick figures of a person, but worse on rotated figures. However, as with other nonverbal effects, there are exceptions to the general trend. For example, Hatta (1978b) found a right-visual-field superiority for identifying watch figures when the watch time was wrong and the subject had to readjust the time mentally. It is possible that this task is accomplished by verbally adding or subtracting the correction factor, rather than through mental rotation.

In general, there seems to be fairly good evidence for a right-hemispheric or left-visual-field superiority on a variety of tasks involving visuospatial abilities. The most difficult problem lies in knowing what will be treated as a visuospatial task by the subject. If verbal mediation

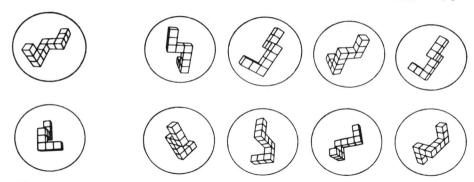

Figure 4.4. Sample items from the Mental Rotations Test to illustrate the requirements of a mental rotation task. In the examples given, the first and fourth choices match the leftmost figure on the top row, and the second and third choices match the leftmost figure on the bottom row. (From Vandenberg, S. G., & Kuse, A. R. Mental rotations: A group test of three-dimensional spatial visualization. *Perceptual and Motor Skills,* 1978, *47,* 559–604. Reprinted with permission.)

can aid in the performance of the task, it may destroy any left-visual-field superiority (e.g., Umilta *et al.,* 1974). Of all the tasks employed, line orientation tasks seem to provide the most consistent results. The most disappointing facet of the existing literature is that there have been no attempts to validate the relation between left-visual-field visuospatial effects and right-hemispheric functioning through the comparison of different handedness groups. The clinical literature suggests that good visuospatial performance is dependent on the integrity of the right hemisphere, although the extent of right-hemispheric dominance for spatial abilities is not so great as the left-hemispheric dominance for language (Hécaen *et al.,* 1981).

The third type of nonverbal visual studies involves the presentation of complex forms. Very often photographs or caricatures of faces are employed, but the complex random polygons scaled by Vanderplas and Garvin (1959) have also been used, as have line drawings of objects.

A variety of different procedures have been used to study face recognition in the lateral visual fields. Geffen *et al.* (1971), for instance, had subjects remember a single face. Then they presented one of five alternatives laterally in one visual field or the other. When subjects used a manual response to indicate whether or not the lateralized face was the same as the one they had memorized, a left-visual-field superiority was obtained. When a vocal response was used, on the other hand, no visual-field effect was observed. Hilliard (1973), on the other hand, presented a single face briefly to one side of a fixation point, followed by a central comparison face. Subjects were to indicate whether or not the comparison face was the same as the briefly exposed test face. Hilliard (1973) also observed a left-visual-field superiority on this task. A slightly different procedure has been used by a number of Italian investigators (e.g., Rizzolatti & Buchtel, 1977). They had subjects learn four faces and respond positively to two of them while withholding response to the other two in a "go–no go" reaction time task. Facial stimuli were presented laterally, but separate blocks of trials were run for each visual field, so that the subject knew where the stimulus would appear on any given trial. Eye movements were monitored, and trials on which the subject was not fixating properly were discarded. This blocking of visual fields is a relatively uncommon procedure and would of course be wholly inappropriate without adequate eye movement control. It is, however, rather like a dichotic monitoring task: Unlike the usual unilateral presentation procedure, in which subjects must decide for themselves how to divide attention between the two visual fields, this approach permits the subject to devote maximum attention to each field in turn. Interestingly, the Rizolatti and Buchtel study found a left-visual-field superiority for men, but not for women.

The stimuli used in face recognition studies have also varied considerably (see Figure 4.5). Hilliard (1973), for instance, used black-and-white photographs, while Geffen et al. (1971) employed facial likenesses constructed from a set used to aid in police identification, Ley and Bryden (1979a) used cartoon faces, and Patterson and Bradshaw (1975) used very stylized line drawings of faces. Despite the differences in the type of material used, a left-visual-field superiority seems to be the rule (Geffen et al., 1971; Hilliard, 1973; Ley & Bryden, 1979a; Moscovitch, Scullion, & Christie, 1976; Rizzolatti & Buchtel, 1977; St. John, 1981; Zoccolotti & Oltman, 1978).

Some of the exceptions to the left-visual-field superiority arise because of the involvement of language systems in the task. Thus, Marzi and Berlucchi (1977) found a right-visual-field superiority for the recognition of famous (nameable) faces, and the left-visual-field effect disappeared when Geffen et al. (1971) used a vocal response. Other right-field effects are not so easily explained. Patterson and Bradshaw (1975), for instance, found a left-visual-field effect when the test and memory figures differed on many features, but a right-field superiority when they were different in only a single feature.

In their review, Sergent and Bindra (1981) observed that right-visual-field superiorities are most consistently obtained when the conditions are such as to require "analytic" judgments. They concluded that left-hemisphere advantages need not involve the language function, but represent a genuine visuospatial contribution of the left hemisphere.

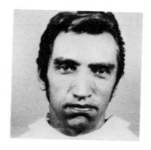

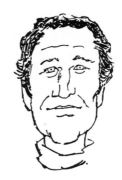

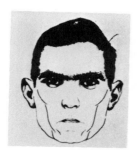

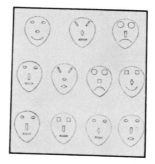

Figure 4.5. Different types of facial stimuli used in face recognition experiments. Upper left: photograph. Upper right: cartoon drawing (Ley & Bryden, 1979a). Lower left: Ident-a-kit (R) face [From Geffen, G., Bradshaw, J. L., & Wallace, G. Interhemispheric effects on reaction time to verbal and nonverbal visual stimuli. *Journal of Experimental Psychology*, 1971, *87*, 415–422. Copyright (1978) by the American Psychological Association. Reprinted by permission of publisher and author.] Lower right: schematic faces. [From Patterson, K., & Bradshaw, J. L. Differential hemispheric mediation of nonverbal visual stimuli. *Journal of Experimental Psychology: Human Perception and Performance*, 1975, *1*, 246–252. Copyright (1975) by the American Psychological Association. Reprinted by permission of publisher and author.]

Ley and Bryden (1979a) have found some evidence to indicate a dissociation between the ability to identify specific faces and the ability to identify the expressions shown. They employed a matching task like that used by Hilliard (1973). In one condition, subjects were asked to indicate whether the central stimulus represented the same character as the laterally presented one; in a second condition, they were asked whether the two faces expressed the same emotion. A left-visual-field superiority was obtained for both tasks, but the effects were statistically independent. Ley and Bryden (1979a) have interpreted this finding as a manifestation of a right-hemispheric superiority in the recognition of emotion (see Chapter 8), but it may simply be another way of assessing complex pattern recognition. The statistical independence could be accounted for by the fact that the tasks involve somewhat different discriminations. Interestingly, Berent (1977) used a very similar task with patients undergoing unilateral electroconvulsive therapy (ECT). In one condition, Berent had subjects study a picture and then indicate which one of three people showing different expressions was the original person. This task was highly vulnerable to right-sided ECT. In a second condition, subjects were asked to pick the picture "most similar" to the study picture, when all three comparison stimuli were photographs of different people and the correct choice was the person showing the same expression as the person in the study picture. Performance on this task was severely impaired by left-sided ECT. Berent's instructions did not emphasize the expression matching required on this task, in contrast to Ley and Bryden's (1979a) instructions, and this difference may have forced Berent's subjects into using a more verbal approach to the task.

The general finding of a right-hemispheric superiority for face recognition is not surprising. Considerable clinical data point to the posterior right parietal or right occipitotemporal region as being critical to agnosia for faces (prosopagnosia) (Benton & VanAllen, 1968; Hécaen & Angelergues, 1962; Meadows, 1974a; Yin, 1970).

The most common alternative to faces as a complex visual form is the set of complex polygons developed and scaled by Vanderplas and Garvin (1959) (see Figure 4.6). These figures range in complexity from 4 to 20 sides and have been scaled for association value. Presumably, forms with low association value would be difficult to encode verbally and thus would make an ideal "nonverbal" stimulus. Dee and Fontenot (1973) found a left-visual-field superiority for complex 12-sided low-association forms, but only after a delay interval of 5–20 sec between the presentation of the lateral stimulus and a set of response alternatives.

Hellige (1978; Hellige & Cox, 1976; Hellige, Cox, & Litvac, 1979) has also made extensive use of the Vanderplas and Garvin figures. Rather consistently, he found left-visual-field effects for 12-sided figures, but either no laterality effect (Hellige, 1978) or a reduced one (Hellige & Cox, 1976) for 16-sided figures. Hellige suggests that these effects are due to subtle differences in stimulus codability. Two possibilities come to

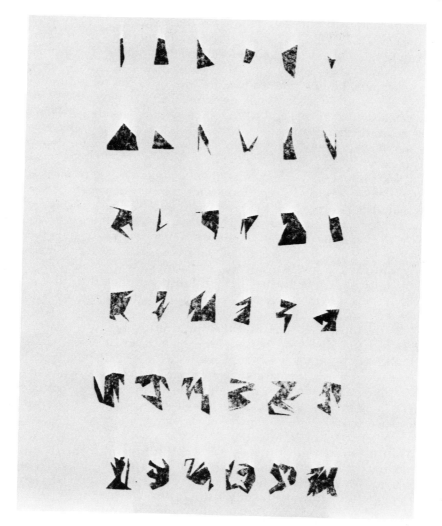

Figure 4.6. Examples of complex polygons used in shape recognition experiments. (From Vanderplas & Garvin, 1959.)

mind. First of all, the Vanderplas and Garvin figures are not bilaterally symmetric, and subjects may obtain a better view of that part of the stimulus nearest the fixation point. The relative information on the left side of the figure may be greater for the 16-sided figures than for the 12-sided figures. Second, the assumption that the number of sides is directly related to stimulus complexity is derived from an early study of Attneave (1957). Under tachistoscopic exposure, the same relation between number of sides and complexity may not hold. Subjects are looking at a figure that subtends less than half a degree (a figure of about 16 mm examined at a normal reading distance of 36 cm) for a duration on the order of 10–20 msec. While discriminability between the figures is reasonably good (Hellige, 1978, reports accuracy levels between 50% and 80%), this is no guarantee that subjects could actually perceive the details of the figure, and quite different factors might determine complexity.

At least under some conditions, then, complex polygons yield a left-visual-field superiority. There thus seems to be a wide variety of nonverbal materials that produce left-visual-field effects. These effects are not as robust as those obtained with verbal material, and there are frequent failures to replicate. Some of the inconsistency may result from the fact that the right hemisphere is not so clearly specialized for visuospatial processing as the left hemisphere is for language (Benton, 1979). Another problem may be the use of verbal response indicators that would involve the left hemisphere and reduce the magnitude of any left-field effect (Geffen et al., 1971).

It is perhaps surprising that there are relatively few studies of the effect of handedness on performance on nonverbal visual tasks. Although there is fairly good clinical evidence for believing that such tasks as face recognition, mental rotation, recognition of line orientation, dot localization, and even color discrimination should show left-visual-field effects, few investigators have attempted to provide any evidence that their specific task actually taps cerebral lateralization rather than some extraneous scanning or attentional process.

With a face recognition task, Piazza (1980) found a left-visual-field effect in dextrals, but a small right-visual-field effect in sinistrals. Right-handers with no familial history of left-handedness showed a strong left-field effect, while nonfamilial left-handers showed the largest right-field effect of any group. The overall handedness difference is at least consistent with the argument that face recognition effects are related to cerebral lateralization. Bryden (1973), on the other hand, found no difference between handedness groups for either dot localization or complex form recognition. In contrast, Levy and Reid (1978) report that right-handers show a left-field effect, and left-handers show the reverse. In addition, Levy and Reid report a major effect of handwriting posture, with inverted left-handers showing a small left-field superiority and left-handers who write with the hand upright giving a large right-field effect. Other than the dot location task, where there has been some prob-

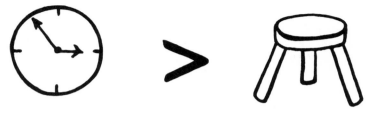

Figure 4.7. The bilateral stimulus presentation technique used by Schmuller and Good-man. The arrowhead at fixation indicates which item is to be reported. (From Schmuller, J., & Goodman, R. Bilateral tachistoscopic perception, handedness, and laterality. II. Nonverbal stimuli. *Brain and Language*, 1980, *11*, 12–18. Reprinted with permission.)

lem with replication (Bryden, 1973, 1976a), and the face recognition task, most investigators have been content to use right-handed subjects and have not dealt with the question of handedness effects.

One exception to this is a study by Schmuller and Goodman (1980). They presented outline drawings of common objects bilaterally, with an arrowhead at the fixation point to indicate order of report (see Figure 4.7). Right-handers and nonfamilial left-handers were more accurate in the left visual field, although the effect was statistically significant only for the right-handers without a familial history of left-handedness. The failure of the other groups to reach significance may be due to the small sample (eight per group). In contrast, the familial left-handers showed a significant right-visual-field superiority.

Dissociation of Verbal and Nonverbal Effects

A second way of providing some converging evidence that the procedures being employed are actually related to cerebral lateralization is to show a dissociation of verbal and nonverbal effects. A number of studies have reported opposite laterality effects for verbal and nonverbal tasks in the same subjects (e.g., Fontenot, 1973, for letters and complex polygons; Klatzky & Atkinson, 1971, for picture names and letter matching; Robertshaw & Sheldon, 1976, for letters and spatial position; M. Gross, 1972, for words and dot matrices; and Hellige, 1978, for words and complex polygons). In these experiments, the same subjects have been given both a verbal task and a nonverbal task at separate times. Without additional information, such experiments do not fully dissociate verbal and nonverbal effects.

One problem with most of the studies that have employed both verbal and nonverbal material with the same subjects is that they have used only right-handers. Since virtually all right-handers are left-hemispheric for speech, intertask correlations on such samples may involve nothing more than intercorrelating one set of extraneous variables with another. A correlation is a measure of shared variance: By restricting the sample to right-handers, one is ensuring that most of the variance in the laterality measures is due to error of measurement and to strategy variables peculiar to the experimental situation, and very little of it to variability in cerebral asymmetry. Thus, one is correlating error variance and situational-specific strategy effects, and it should not be surprising if high correlations do not emerge. Thus, there is no association between visual-field effects for face recognition and those for nonsense trigrams in Hilliard's (1973) study. To look at task intercorrelations, one should increase the variance in cerebral asymmetry by including left-handers or by studying left-handers only and simultaneously controlling the subjects' freedom to develop their own strategies.

One study that accomplishes this has been reported by Piazza (1980). She tested subjects on four different tests: face and word recognition, using a bilateral presentation procedure in which the fixation item cued the subject as to which visual field to report, and dichotic speech and environmental sounds, using a monitoring procedure. In the study, eight subjects were tested in each of eight groups: the various combinations of handedness, sex, and familial history of sinistrality. Laterality coefficients (Halwes, 1969) for each group computed from her data are shown in Table 4.1. Based on the group coefficients, rank-order correlations between verbal and nonverbal tests show a clear negative correlation (−.71 for words and faces, −.69 for speech and sounds, and −.76 for the combination). Thus, her choice of tasks seems to tap complementary aspects of specialization and provide fairly strong evidence that her tasks successfully assess the differing functions of the two hemispheres. Of course, the figures shown in Table 4.1 are based on cell means and may cover up a lot of noise. Piazza (1980) reports that verbal–nonverbal correlations are negative, but usually nonsignificant; however, she apparently used the difference score in her correlations, and this may not be the most appropriate measure of laterality (see Chapter 2).

There are a number of other interesting points in Table 4.1. Fairly clear handedness effects emerge for all tasks, though the specific interaction of handedness and side reported by Piazza (1980) varies and is nonsignificant in her analysis of the word data. If we may be permitted a flight of statistical fancy, the difference between the combined verbal

Table 4.1
Laterality Coefficients (e) for Different Handedness Groups

Group	Words	Speech	Sum verbal	Faces	Sounds	Sum nonverbal	Verbal–nonverbal difference
Males right-handed							
FS−[a]	.237	.143	.380	−.246	−.191	−.437	.817
FS+[b]	.255	.133	.388	−.029	−.010	−.039	.427
Males left-handed							
FS−	.217	.095	.312	.078	.035	.113	.199
FS+	.204	.022	.226	−.071	.085	.014	.212
Females right-handed							
FS−	.274	.141	.415	−.285	−.214	−.499	.914
FS+	.176	.039	.215	.039	−.053	−.014	.229
Females left-handed							
FS−	.109	.061	.170	.101	.114	.215	−.045
FS+	.078	.014	.092	.058	.052	.110	−.018
All right handed	.236	.114	.350	−.130	−.117	−.247	.597
All left handed	.152	.048	.200	.042	.071	.113	.087

Note. Data from Piazza (1980); laterality coefficients (e values) calculated according to Halwes (1969).
[a]No familial history of sinistrality.
[b]Familial history of sinistrality.

laterality measures and the combined nonverbal scores should be related to the pattern of cerebral organization. An individual (or group) with left-hemispheric speech and right-hemispheric nonverbal processes should show a large positive difference between the laterality measures for verbal and nonverbal tasks; those individuals with reversed patterns of lateral specialization should show a large negative difference. From Table 4.1, we can see that the strong lateralization of right-handers is considerably attenuated in those with a familial history of sinistrality. Given the high incidence of left-hemispheric speech representation in dextrals, this is a bit surprising, but relatively little work has been done on dextrals with a familial history of left-handedness. Left-handers are not the mirror image of right-handers, but tend to be rather ambiguous with respect to cerebral organization, all groups showing similar laterality for verbal and nonverbal tasks. It is here that individual, rather than group, data would be very important.

A further problem in trying to dissociate verbal and nonverbal effects is that the negative correlation at the individual level presumes a notion of complementary specialization. While it is true that most right-handers are left-hemispheric for speech and right-hemispheric for visuospatial function, there is no necessary linkage between the two. In left-handers, visuospatial functions remain dependent on the right hemisphere although speech is much more likely to be right-hemispheric (Hécaen *et al.* 1981; Hécaen & Sauguet, 1971). It may therefore turn out that language and visuospatial functions are independent of one another. Such an argument would lead us back to the investigation of right-handers, in whom complementarity is at least statistically the norm, or to comparing the performance of groups exhibiting different patterns of cerebral organization (cf. McGlone & Davidson, 1973).

Other compelling data employing the dissociation of verbal and nonverbal tasks have been provided by Levy and Reid (1978). They used two visual tasks: the unilateral presentation of a vertically oriented CVC nonsense syllable, and the localization of a unilaterally presented dot. In both procedures, a fixation digit was used, and the stimuli were white on black, rather than the more conventional black on white. They report a reciprocal relation between the two tasks, with right-visual-field superiority on one task being associated with left-field superiority on the other.

A major problem with trying to dissociate verbal and nonverbal effects simply by comparing performance under two separate conditions is that many other factors may enter into the laterality effect. For instance, quite different scanning strategies might be used for words and for faces. Kinsbourne (1970, 1973, 1975a) has argued that the simple fact that one expects to perform a verbal task can serve to activate the left hemisphere and make it more receptive to incoming stimuli. Similarly, expecting a nonverbal stimulus can activate the right hemisphere and improve left-visual-field scores. By this argument, some of the laterality effect observed in most studies is the result of selectively priming one hemisphere.

One way around the problem of task set is to intermingle both verbal and nonverbal material in the same experiment, so that the subject does not know on any one trial what type of material is to appear. This way, the subject cannot develop a specific set for the type of material and cannot selectively activate one hemisphere for one type of material and the other hemisphere for a different type of material. One procedure that would accomplish this end is the Posner physical and name matching experiment (Posner & Keele, 1967). We have already seen that this procedure generally produces an interaction of match type with visual field, although the specific laterality effect obtained for physical matches is rather variable. Certainly, the results of such experiments would suggest that name matching involves left-hemispheric processes more than does physical matching.

Hellige (1978) has used a mixed presentation of words and complex polygons. His analysis indicates a significant interaction between field and stimulus type, but the interpretation of this is clouded by the fact that he used two different types of forms (12 and 16 sided). Right-visual-field effects were obtained for both words and 16-sided figures, and a small but insignificant left-field effect for 12-sided figures. It is the 12-sided figures that consistently show a left-field superiority when shown alone. Thus, were one to analyze words and 12-sided figures alone, the interaction between visual field and stimulus type would appear with both pure and mixed lists. Similar results were obtained in a replication experiment, although the left-field effect for 12-sided figures varied as a function of whether or not the subject was precued about the nature of the stimulus. Interestingly, the strong left-field superiority for 12-sided forms in Hellige's (1978) second experiment occurred when the subject did not know which type of stimulus would appear next.

Because extraneous factors such as a slight fixation bias could affect the specific magnitude of the laterality effects in an experiment such as this, the critical point is whether or not an interaction between type of material and visual field exists. Hellige's (1978) data clearly show this for the 12-sided figure and word comparison. Quite different results are found with 16-sided figures, which show strong right-field effects in the mixed lists, but Hellige was unable to find a left-field effect for this type of material when it was presented alone. It simply does not appear to be an appropriate stimulus for extracting right-hemispheric effects. Hellige's data thus seem to provide a clear dissociation between words and 12-sided polygons.

Haun (1978) has also been able to dissociate verbal and nonverbal effects. He had subjects remember a target set of four letters and a simple geometric form, and then presented stimuli laterally in one visual field or the other. Subjects were to indicate whether or not the lateralized stimulus was a member of the memory set. Haun found a clear right-visual-field effect for the letters and a left-visual-field effect for the form.

A rather subtle technique for dissociating left- and right-hemispheric effects involves the use of imagery in word recognition experiments. One of the major ideas in current memory research is that stimuli can be encoded in both a verbal and a visual memory (Paivio, 1969). It is difficult to produce images of abstract words or concepts, but easy to do so for concrete words. Thus, concrete words, which can be dually encoded, are more easily remembered. It is only a small leap to link this research to studies of hemispheric asymmetry and to argue that verbal memory is left-hemispheric and visual memory right-hemispheric. By this argument, concrete and easily imaged words should activate both left- and right-hemispheric processes and thus should yield a smaller laterality effect than abstract material. Such a result has in fact been reported (Ellis & Shepherd, 1974; Hines, 1976, 1977), although Hines (1976) finds it to be true only for familiar words. Further, Schmuller and Goodman (1979) failed to find an imagery effect in their study.

Perhaps the best study in this area is by J. Day (1977). Day carried out three experiments, all of which involved mixed presentation of concrete and abstract nouns, and consistently found a strong right-visual-field effect for abstract material and no laterality effect for concrete material. In one experiment, subjects were shown lateralized words or nonwords in a lexical decision task, where the subject was to indicate whether the stimulus was a word or not. In his second experiment, he presented a category name in central vision, followed by a lateralized noun that either was or was not a member of the category. Some categories (animals, vegetables) were concrete; others (feelings, directions) were abstract. To ensure that the presentation of the category name did not have a priming effect, a third experiment involved simultaneous presentation of category name and subordinate noun. In all three studies, response times were faster in the right visual field for abstract material, whereas concrete material showed little or no laterality effect.

Reaction Time Studies or Error Analysis?

Most of the early studies of visual laterality effects (e.g., Bryden, 1965; Kimura, 1967) investigated the errors made by subjects following brief visual presentation. The increased use of computers and automated timing systems, coupled with the successes of reaction time measurement in cognitive psychology (e.g., Lachman, Lachman, & Butterfield, 1979; Posner & Mitchell, 1967), has resulted in a sharp increase in the number of reaction time studies of laterality effects (cf. Moscovitch, 1979). Are there reasons for preferring one type of study over the other?

In general, reaction time studies are characterized by the use of relatively long exposure durations (100–200 msec), to keep error rates low, and by the use of simple two-choice response alternatives (same–different or yes–no). These permit the use of relatively complex visual stimuli but require that the stimulus set be selected carefully so that the responses are appropriate. In contrast, accuracy studies are more likely to use very short exposure durations, in order to ensure a reasonable number of errors, and to require identification responses, such as naming a letter or word. It is true, however, that two-alternative response instructions can easily be employed in studies using error analyses (cf. Ley & Bryden, 1979a).

Rather similar effects have been reported in reaction time studies and in accuracy studies: The evidence indicates that the two procedures assess similar processes. There is little evidence to indicate that manipulations of exposure duration do much more than alter overall level of accuracy, although there have been no systematic studies with complex material. With very brief exposure durations, the stimulus will be more degraded, and high-frequency spatial information will be lost relative to low-frequency information (Breitmeyer & Ganz, 1976). As a result, one might expect to find that judgments were based more on overall stimulus configuration rather than internal detail when very brief exposures are used (cf. Sergent & Bindra, 1981).

One of the primary justifications for the use of reaction time is that the dependent measure is a continuous variable, permitting somewhat more powerful statistical analyses. However, as seen in Chapter 2, there are relatively strong techniques for analyzing error data, and most treatments of reaction time discard information about individual trials. Thus, some of the power of reaction time measurement may be more imaginary than real. In order to be sure that the task is sufficiently difficult to tax the resources of the subject, some errors must be made, and this leads to a number of problems. Not only must one be concerned about the latencies of wrong responses, but there remains a problem of potential speed and accuracy trade-offs. That is, subjects who emphasize speed may show little reaction time difference between conditions, but a considerable error difference, whereas subjects who emphasize accuracy may show the reverse pattern. Furthermore, many of the experimental paradigms that employ a detailed analysis of reaction time measures have been developed to study the limitations of human resources (e.g., the distinction between physical matching and name matching), and the conceptualizations may not be appropriate at tachistoscopic exposure durations, where the task is data limited as well as resource limited (Norman & Bobrow, 1975).

A second justification for reaction time measurement is that a simple finger movement makes a fine two-alternative nonverbal response, and one might as well measure response time if the equipment is available. While it is certainly true that finger movement is a good nonverbal response, the decision to use response times as the dependent measure may well be an example of letting the technology control the design of the experiment. Although there are often good reasons for preferring to measure response time, there is no good reason to believe that it is a better or more accurate dependent measure than accuracy. In the long run, one must understand the experimental procedure no matter what dependent measure is chosen.

Finally, one should remember a number of things that response time measures do *not* provide. The fact that each hemisphere receives input from the opposite visual field and sends output to the opposite hand (see Figure 4.8) has led many people to argue that the difference between reaction times when stimulus and responding hand are on the

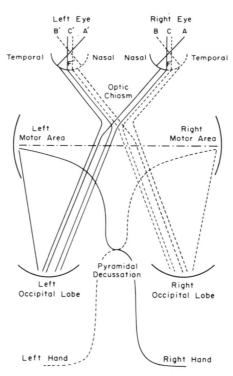

DIAGRAM   OF   CONDUCTION   PATHS

Figure 4.8. Diagrammatic representation of the visuomotor pathways. [From Bashore, T. R. Vocal and manual reaction time estimates of interhemispheric transmission time. *Psychological Bulletin*, 1981, *89*, p. 354. Copyright (1981) by the American Psychological Association. Reprinted by permission of publisher and author.]

same side and when they are contralateral should be a measure of interhemispheric transmission time. Although Swanson, Ledlow, and Kinsbourne (1978) have concluded that behavioral methods are too variable to provide any accurate measure of interhemispheric transmission time, Bashore (1981) has indicated that simple manual reaction time measures to light flashes yield a consistent estimate of interhemispheric transmission time on the order of 3 msec. In more complex situations, however, processing demands, attentional factors, and the like become very important, and estimates of transmission time are too variable to be meaningful (Swanson *et al.*, 1978). Thus, the fact that a response to a left-visual-field verbal stimulus may take 50 msec longer than the same response to a right-visual-field stimulus cannot be interpreted as indicating that callosal transmission takes 50 msec. Rather, one must remember that the left hemisphere is potentially processing a more degraded version of the left-field stimulus than of the right-field stimulus and that this will affect response time. Furthermore, we cannot tell whether the slower left-visual-field reaction time is a result of the right hemisphere doing the task more slowly than the left, or of the left hemisphere doing the task more slowly on left-visual-field input than on the right-field input.

Some General Comments on Visual Laterality Studies

It would be nice if this review of visual laterality studies led to some simple general overview, or to a clear prescription as to how to do laterality studies, but it does not. There are many different procedures that have generated at least relatively consistent visual-field asymmetries. In general, these favor the right visual field for language-oriented tasks and the left visual field for visuospatial tasks. There is considerable presumptive evidence to indicate that functional cerebral lateralization is important in producing these laterality effects. At the same time, it is clear that other factors affect the specific magnitude of the laterality effects observed in any specific experiment. There is no clearly "right way to do it" that can be specified at the present time. One of the reasons for this is that, in many ways, the appropriate experiments have not yet been done. As a result, it is going beyond the evidence to claim that the magnitude of a visual-field asymmetry is a measure of the degree of lateralization of a particular function.

There are a few general procedural points that one can make. As yet, there is no clear evidence that manipulations of exposure duration have any systematic effect, despite some reports to the contrary (e.g., Bryden, 1965; Sergent & Bindra, 1981). At least in the range up to 100 or 150 msec, changes in exposure duration seem primarily to affect overall accuracy; any loss of laterality is likely due to ceiling or floor effects. Similarly, the specific retinal loci, so long as they are foveal or para-foveal, do not appear to be critical. At least within 5° or so of fixation, robust laterality effects can be found (Bryden, 1969; Haun, 1978). Again, the manipulation may serve more to adjust accuracy to an appropriate level than to alter the primary effect.

Obviously, lack of adequate fixation control can do nothing but add noise to the situation. What specific procedure should be used to ensure adequate fixation is another question. Given the proper equipment, one could monitor fixation by some technique of eye movement recording or by directly observing the subject's eyes. The arguments in favor of the use of a central fixation digit do not seem very strong, since processing the central digit may have different effects on the subsequent report of the two visual fields. On the other hand, the use of a small directional arrow to indicate partial report of one field seems to hold promise (Piazza, 1980; Schmuller & Goodman, 1979). Other things failing, uni-lateral presentation certainly provides somewhat better fixation control than bilateral presentation.

Hines (1975) has argued that bilateral presentation is more analogous to the dichotic listening situation used in auditory studies. He feels that bilateral presentation inhibits callosal transfer between the two hemi-spheres and thus gives an independent assessment of the abilities of the two hemispheres. In contrast, unilateral presentation, according to Hines, is more appropriate for measuring the information lost during interhemispheric transfer. His argument is based largely on the fact that, when mixed pairs of words and nonverbal items such as shapes or faces were presented bilaterally, accuracy on any one type of material was more or less independent of the type of material it was paired with. In subsequent studies (e.g., 1976), however, Hines has found very similar effects with unilateral and bilateral presentation. It is also generally true that the pattern of laterality effects obtained with the two procedures is the same. The one advantage of the unilateral procedure is that it does not involve one in the complexities of controlling (and interpreting) order of report, although Piazza's (1980) bilateral procedure also solves this problem. Otherwise, we can see no compelling reasons for favoring one procedure over the other.

In terms of fixation control, one should also note the advantage of trying to dissociate laterality effects through the use of a mixed list presentation of different types of material. If the subject does not know which type of material will be exposed on any given trial, an interaction between stimulus type and visual field cannot arise because fixation is biased differently in the two situations.

Finally, with verbal material, a vertical display rather than a horizontal one seems to be called for, on the grounds that left-to-right scanning patterns may interact with field of presentation (Bryden, 1967b; Heron, 1957). It becomes important, however, to learn more about the factors that are involved in the recognition of vertically displayed words.

Given these points, what can we say about visual laterality effects in general? First, there is little doubt that verbal laterality effects are dependent at least in part on the specialized language functions of the left hemisphere. The problem with any specific procedure lies in knowing how much of the effect is the result of this functional asymmetry and how much is due to extraneous factors. Nonverbal laterality effects are somewhat more elusive. There is at least reasonable evidence, from a variety of different sources, that tasks that broadly tap visuospatial abilities show a right-hemispheric superiority. Some procedures that have been used to tap this domain, such as stereoscopic depth, yield inconsistent and unreliable results. Others, such as mental rotation, have not yet been studied in sufficient detail. At the present time, the most complete evidence that one is actually dealing with a functional cerebral asymmetry comes from the face recognition studies, and there are some reasons to believe that this might be at least partially independent of other visuospatial abilities (Meadows, 1974a). Line tilt and mental rotation seem to be promising visuospatial procedures, but more work needs to be done with them. Finally, the color discrimination data are tantalizing, but there is little in the way of even indirect evidence to indicate that this is really related to a functional asymmetry.

If one is going to continue to work with the normal brain, it seems that more conclusive evidence that these procedures really tap functional cerebral asymmetries is needed. For this reason, it would be important to discover what variables lead some left-handers to be right-hemispheric for speech (cf. Levy & Reid, 1978). If this could be done, one could compare presumptive left- and right-hemispheric speech subjects on a variety of tasks and see which best discriminated the groups. Even now, we might use the same approach on left- and right-handers, on the presumption that the left-handed group will have a lower percentage of left-hemispheric speech representation.

5

Tactual Laterality Effects

For a variety of reasons, somatosensory laterality experiments have not been as popular as auditory and visual ones. Most experimental psychology laboratories are equipped to carry out fairly sophisticated auditory and visual experiments but are less likely to have the equipment for good somatosensory research. Discrimination between simple stimuli is fairly rudimentary, yet when one permits active palpation of stimuli, control over time parameters and the manner of palpation is lost. Nevertheless, there have been a number of studies investigating laterality effects in somesthesis.

Anatomically, the ascending sensory fibers from the skin and joints cross the midline and project to the postcentral gyrus of the opposite hemisphere. There is also sensory representation in the precentral gyrus, the traditional motor cortex (Rasmussen & Penfield, 1947). In addition, there is a second sensory area, along the superior border of the Sylvian fissure in the parietal cortex, in which both ipsilateral and contralateral sides of the body are represented in each hemisphere (Penfield & Rasmussen, 1950). There is also evidence for bilateral representation of the lower part of the face area in the postcentral region (see Corkin, 1978, for review) (see Figures 5.1 and 5.2). Thus, despite the general assumption that the somatosensory system is a completely crossed one, there is reason to believe that some information is projected via ipsilateral pathways (Albe-Fessard, 1967; Kohn & Dennis, 1974b; Semmes, 1969).

The crossed representation of the somatosensory system would lead one to expect right-side advantages for verbal tasks, because of the greater involvement of the left hemisphere, and left-side advantages for nonverbal tasks. Such laterality effects might be tempered in the face region or through the action of ipsilateral input systems.

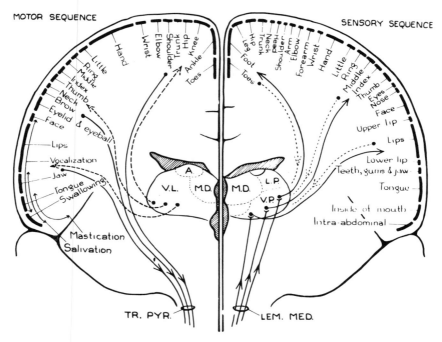

MOTOR SEQUENCE

SENSORY SEQUENCE

Figure 5.1. Cortical representation in the sensorimotor region. [From Penfield, W., & Rasmussen, T. *The cerebral cortex of man.* New York: Macmillan. Copyright (1950) by Macmillan Publishing Co., Inc., renewed 1978 by Theodore Rasmussen.]

Many of the initial studies of somatosensory asymmetry involved measures of pressure sensitivity with von Frey hairs. As one example, S. Weinstein and Sersen (1961) reported that right-handers were more likely to show lower thresholds on the left palm, forearm, and sole than on the right. For the palm, left-handers with a familial history of left-handedness showed the reverse effect, whereas nonfamilial left-handers behaved like right-handers. This pattern was not repeated for the forearm and sole. The sharp distinction between familial and nonfamilial left-handers, however, suggested that these effects were due to some central asymmetry. The general trend toward greater pressure sensitivity on the left recurs in other studies (e.g., S. Weinstein, 1962, 1963). Still other studies, however, fail to show any lateral differences in pressure sensitivity (Carmon, Bilstrom, & Benton, 1969; Fennell, Satz, & Wise, 1967; S. Weinstein, 1968). If there are differences between left and right sides in pressure sensitivity, they are small and inconsistent.

Measurements of two-point threshold have met with a similar fate. The Weinstein (1963) data suggest a lower two-point threshold on the right breast, but later measurements (Weinstein, 1968) indicate that this does not hold across different body parts. There is a slight trend for better two-point limens on the left side of the tongue (McCall & Cunningham, 1971; McNutt, 1975), but the effect is far from statistically significant. In a review of these data, Corkin (1978) concludes that there is no evidence for any lateralization effect in basic somatosensory measures. Since these are very simple tasks not involving any complex cortical processing, such a lack of laterality effects is not surprising. To find somatosensory effects related to cerebral asymmetries, one must look to more complex verbal and nonverbal tasks.

Some somatosensory researchers have followed the path indicated by

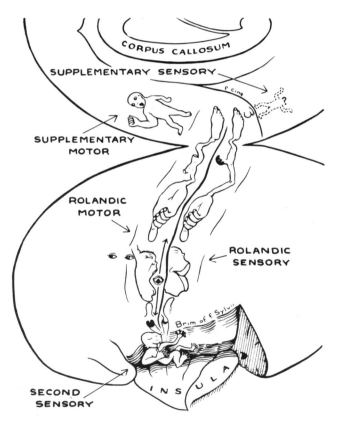

Figure 5.2. Somatic representation in the left hemisphere of the human brain. [From Penfield, W., & Jasper, H. H. *Epilepsy and the functional anatomy of the human brain.* Boston: Little, Brown and Company. Copyright (1954). Reprinted with permission.]

the early visual research (e.g., Kimura, 1966) and have compared the performance of the two hands tested singly. Superficially, this is analogous to the unilateral visual presentation technique, although in somatosensory experiments, the subject typically knows which hand is to be tested on any given trial. Such a procedure permits the subject to devote as much attention to one hand as to the other, which may not be true of the visual situation. Other investigators have been impressed with the success of the dichotic listening procedure and have tried somatosensory analogues to it. While such an approach increases the difficulty level, it also introduces issues of attentional distribution, order of report, and the like. Before judging the approaches, however, let us see what results have been obtained.

Young and Ellis (1979) found a left-hand superiority for judging the number of random dots in an array. Subjects felt an array of raised dots with their middle finger, working rapidly through a block of 10 trials. When the dots were arranged in a linear array, or raised digits were used, no laterality effect was observed. This left-side superiority for dot patterns is similar to the left-hand superiority reported for reading Braille letters (Hermelin & O'Connor, 1971; Rudel, Denckla, & Hirsch, 1977; Smith, Chu, & Edmonston, 1977).

A left-hand superiority has also been reported for the tactual determination of direction. In a typical experiment, a subject feels one or two metal rods embedded in wood with the fingertips of one hand and then selects from a visual display the rod(s) that have the same orientation (see Figure 5.3). In general, right-handed subjects are more accurate on this task with their left hands (Benton, Levin, & Varney, 1973; Varney & Benton, 1975). Varney and Benton (1975) also found that familial left-handers tended to show a right-hand superiority. Benton, Varney, and Hamsher (1978) showed that the same results could be obtained with a tactual matching task. Most importantly, the task seems to be sensitive to lesions of the right parietal lobe (Carmon & Benton, 1969; Fontenot & Benton, 1971). Right-hemispheric damage produces bilateral impairment on the task, whereas left-hemispheric damage results only in an impairment of the right hand.

Evidence for left-hand superiority in tactual form recognition has been obtained by Dodds (1978) and Hatta (1978a).

All these unimanual laterality effects are left-hand (right-hemisphere) effects. There seems to be no published evidence for a right-hand superiority for any verbally related tactual task, although one cannot do very much by feel alone. Identifying digits by touch (Young & Ellis, 1979) is not a sufficiently difficult task to lead to a right-hand effect, and more complex tasks have not been tried.

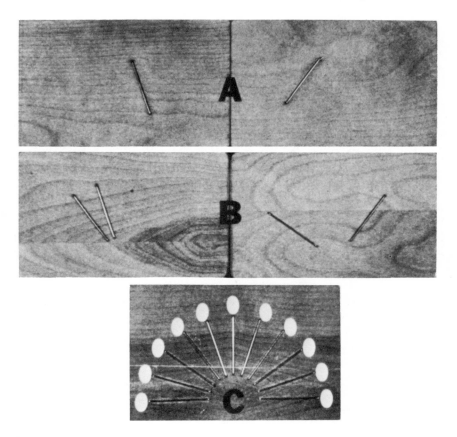

Figure 5.3. Examples of single (top) and double (middle) tactile stimuli presented for detection of tactile orientation. Bottom: the multiple-choice response array. (From Benton, A. L., Varney, N. R., & Hamsher, K. de S. Lateral differences in tactile directional perception. *Neuropsychologia*, 1978, *16*, 109–114. Reprinted with permission of Pergamon Press Ltd.)

Witelson (1974) was perhaps the first to attempt a dichhaptic analogue to the dichotic listening task. She had children palpate two nonsense forms, one with each hand, for 10 sec. Subjects then selected the two forms that had been presented from among six visually presented alternatives. On this task, boys in Grades 1–8 showed a clear left-hand advantage. The same subjects were also tested on a letters task. Here they felt two different letters, one with each hand, for 2 sec, and then a second pair. Following exposure, they recalled the letters they had felt. A right-hand advantage was obtained for this task. In a subsequent study, Witelson (1976b) found that girls did not show the left-hand advantage for haptic form until age 12. Cranney and Ashton (1980) have attempted to replicate Witelson's form data, using both children and adults, without success. In fact, Cranney and Ashton's data indicate a right-hand superiority at most ages and no differences between left- and right-handed subjects.

One of the difficulties with the dichotic listening procedure is that it provides rich opportunities for subjects to employ a variety of different strategies for dealing with the task. Witelson's dichhaptic experiments leave the subject with many of the same opportunities, and strategy effects could easily contaminate the results. For example, in an active palpation task, it is hard to control the specific movements of the two hands: Are subjects actually devoting the same attention to the two hands and making equally effective movements with each hand? In the letters task, one has four letters to report. How does order of report affect the results? Do subjects give the right-hand letters first? With the shapes, is there any bias in the order of selecting the two alternatives?

There have been some attempts to answer these questions. Oscar-Berman *et al.* (1978) tried to deal with the order-of-report issue and with the question of different palpation strategies. They presented two tactual stimuli simultaneously to the palms of the hands, using a passive presentation procedure in which the figure was simply traced on the hand. Subjects were required to identify the two items that had been presented in a specified order, with the left hand being given first on some trials and the right hand first on some. They found a right-hand superiority for letter identification, no difference for digit identification, and a left-hand effect for line orientation. In all cases, the laterality effect was seen on the second hand reported, but not on the first. In dichotic studies, the lack of a first-ear effect is often due to the high accuracy on the first ear recalled (Bryden, 1967a), but this does not appear to be the case in the Oscar-Berman *et al.* (1978) data: Accuracy averaged 78% on the first hand reported and 74% on the second hand. The emergence of a laterality effect on the second hand reported, then, would suggest that haptic laterality effects emerge only after some decay in short-term memory. The Oscar-Berman *et al.* study is also important in showing a dissociation between laterality effects for lines and letters. Unfortunately, they do not carry their analysis to the level of the individual subject, and we do not know whether those people who were better on the left hand for line orientation were the same individuals as those who were better on the right hand for letters.

Another attempt to control some of the relevant factors has been carried out by E. B. Gardner, English, Flannery, Hartnett, McCormick,

and Wilhelmy (1977). They had subjects feel two unfamiliar shapes simultaneously, one with each hand, for 3.75 sec. After a delay of 1.9 sec,
a light indicated which hand was to be reported, and 0.8 sec later, a
further signal indicated whether the response was to be made by pointing with a particular hand or by speaking the number assigned to the
form. In general, the pointing response was faster when the stimulus
was on the left, and the naming response was faster when the stimulus
had been presented to the right hand. Accuracy of the pointing response
was better when the stimulus had been presented to the left hand, but
the same effects were shown in right-handed, left-handed, and ambidextrous subjects. Many of the effects in the E. B. Gardner *et al.* (1977)
study are stimulus–response compatibility effects (e.g., faster response
with the right hand to stimuli presented to the right hand), and these
may have obliterated any hemispheric asymmetries. It is rather discon-
certing to find no differences between handedness groups, since one
would expect that any task clearly related to hemispheric asymmetry
would show handedness effects.

   A somewhat different version of the dichhaptic procedure has been
developed by Gibson and Bryden (1982). They used cutout shapes and
letters made of sandpaper that were moved slowly across the fingertips
(see Figure 5.4). Stimuli were presented in pairs, and subjects were then
cued as to which stimulus to identify first (see Figure 5.5). In the Gibson

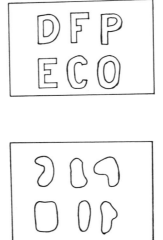

Figure 5.4. Sandpaper shapes used by Gibson and Bryden (1982) for dichhaptic
recognition.

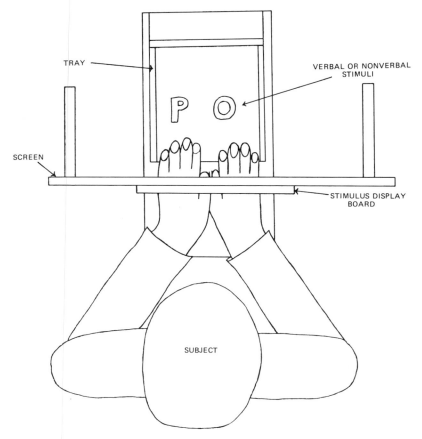

Figure 5.5. Display situation for dichhaptic stimulation used by Gibson and Bryden (1982).

and Bryden (1982) study, 10-year-old children were found to show a right-hand advantage for identifying letters and a left-hand advantage for identifying nonsense shapes. While this procedure has not yet been applied to adult subjects, it holds considerable promise as a technique for investigating tactual laterality effects.

Perhaps the most elegant of the dichhaptic studies has been carried out by Nachshon and Carmon (1975). They tested subjects both unimanually and bimanually on tasks that they describe as "sequential" and "spatial." In their sequential task, the index, middle, and ring fingers were stimulated in random order by tapered metal rods, the three stimuli arriving at .5-sec intervals. Subjects then had to press microswitches next to the rods in the same sequence as they had been stimulated. In the spatial task, one finger was stimulated once, one finger twice, and the third finger not at all. Again, the subject had to indicate the pattern of stimulation by pressing the appropriate microswitches. For bimanual presentation, only the thumb and middle finger of each hand were used. In the sequential task, all four fingers were stimulated in random order, while in the spatial task, one finger was stimulated twice and the other finger of the same hand not at all, and the two fingers of the other hand were stimulated once each. Separate groups of 20 right-handed subjects were tested on the four tasks.

With unimanual presentation, no significant asymmetry was observed, although there was a trend toward fewer errors on the right hand in the spatial task, and significantly more subjects were better on the right hand than on the left. With bimanual presentation, subjects made more errors on the left hand on the sequential task and more errors on the right hand on the spatial task. As was found with dichotic listening, the right-hand advantage found for the bimanual sequential task would tend to implicate the left hemisphere in sequential analysis.

The Nachshon and Carmon (1975) data indicate a dissociation between spatial and sequential tasks, and one that is observed only under conditions of competition. In fact, the data obtained with unimanual presentation are in the opposite direction to what one would expect: a right-hand advantage in the spatial task, and a slight trend toward a left-hand effect on the sequential task. It is unfortunate that Nachshon and Carmon did not use the same subjects for all tasks, since this would make the evidence for a dissociation even more compelling. Further, one would like to have evidence from a sample of left-handed subjects. Nevertheless, Nachshon and Carmon have provided some fairly compelling evidence for an asymmetry of spatial and sequential processes.

The general pattern that emerges from the somatosensory studies is commensurate with that seen in audition and vision. A left-side, right-hemispheric advantage is found for spatial tasks that cannot easily be verbally mediated, such as discriminating line orientation, whereas a right-handed, left-hemispheric superiority is found for verbal mediation (letters) or fine temporal discriminations (as Nachshon and Carmon's sequential task). In particular, the line orientation task seems to be critically dependent on the integrity of the right parietal lobe (Fontenot & Benton, 1971).

It is difficult to know what to conclude from the dichhaptic research. The failure to replicate Witelson's (1974) results by Cranney and Ashton (1980) and E. B. Gardner *et al.*'s (1977) failure to find any difference between handedness groups suggest that there are many problems associated with dichhaptic form recognition that have yet to be solved. At the same time, Oscar-Berman *et al.* (1978), Nachshon and Carmon (1975), and Gibson and Bryden (1982) have found evidence for a dissociation of left- and right-hemispheric effects in studies in which strategy effects have been reasonably well controlled. One would like to know more about how left-handers perform on these tasks and whether the dissociation holds at the individual level as well as the group level. Certainly, somatosensory laterality research has not yet advanced to the point at which one can reliably assess the lateralization of any function through behavioral measures (cf. Witelson, 1976a).

Some General Considerations regarding Perceptual Laterality

The preceding three chapters have reviewed the evidence for perceptual asymmetries in hearing, vision, and touch. Despite the many procedural difficulties, it can be seen that there is good reason to believe that at least some of these perceptual laterality effects reflect the lateral specialization of the human brain. Repeatedly, it has been found that language-related tasks lead to asymmetries favoring the right-side, whereas a variety of nonlanguage tasks lead to asymmetries favoring the left. This chapter will attempt to integrate this material to see if there are any general principles that can be extracted.

Stimulus versus Task Factors

It is very easy to slip into the habit of saying that certain laterality effects are obtained with certain types of material. Doing so carries the implication that there is some special characteristic of the stimulus that leads to the laterality effect. At the same time, one should recognize that stimuli are typically processed in characteristic ways, and it may be the nature of the processing that is applied to the incoming sensory information that leads to the laterality effect. A variety of studies, both auditory and visual, have indicated that laterality effects are determined by the manner in which the stimulus is processed, rather than by the configuration of the stimulus per se. Thus, a pair of letters can yield a right-visual-field superiority when the task is to decide whether or not they have the same name, but a left-field effect or none at all when the task requires a physical match (Cohen, 1972; Geffen et al., 1972; Segalowitz & Stewart, 1979). In dichotic listening, Spellacy and Blumstein (1970) have shown that vowel sounds can produce a right-ear effect when presented in the context of other speech signals, but a left-ear effect when the context involves nonspeech stimuli. Klatzky and Atkinson (1971) have also demonstrated the importance of task factors.

The fact that observed laterality is determined by the demands of the task open up a further problem. In many cases, the same task may be treated differently by different individuals. Thus, for example, Kimura (1969) has argued that the failure of her female subjects to show a significant left-field superiority on dot localization is due to the fact that women approach the task as a verbal problem rather than a spatial one. Segalowitz and Stewart (1979) have used a similar argument to account for sex differences in their study of physical and name matching. It has been suggested that many of the sex differences reported in the literature are due to such strategy effects (Bryden, 1979a). Although there may very well be meaningful individual differences in the ways in which a particular task can be approached, there are few studies that provide any direct assessment of the procedures subjects actually do use. One exception is a study by Seamon and Gazzaniga (1973). Subjects were asked to indicate whether or not a unilateral probe was a member of a prespecified memory set. Subjects given instructions to use a relational imagery strategy to remember the memory set showed a left-field advantage, whereas those led to use verbal rehearsal showed a right-field advantage. To be able to deal with the issue of individual strategies, it is obviously important to have as complete an understanding as possible of the processes involved in the task under investigation.

Attentional Bias as an Explanation of Perceptual Laterality

Throughout the 1970s, Kinsbourne has been developing an integrative theory of functional asymmetry (Kinsbourne, 1970, 1973, 1975a, 1975b; Kinsbourne & Hicks, 1978). Some of the current aspects of Kinsbourne's theorizing are discussed in the chapters on motor lateralization and on lateral eye movements, but his work has also had a major impact on studies of perceptual laterality.

In an initial study, Kinsbourne (1970) investigated the ability of subjects to detect a small gap in a tachistoscopically exposed square. When subjects were required to retain a list of familiar monosyllabic words in memory while performing the gap detection task, accuracy was significantly better in the right visual field. Without concurrent verbal activity, performance was better, though not significantly so, on the left.

Kinsbourne (1970) proposed that verbal activity would activate not only the speech centers of the left hemisphere but a large portion of that hemisphere. As a result, language activity would lead to a tendency to turn the head and eyes to the right, an attentional bias to the right side of space, and a general priming of the left hemisphere that would make it more receptive to incoming stimuli. Even the expectancy for verbal input would serve to activate the left hemisphere. Conversely, a set for nonverbal material would serve to activate the right hemisphere, bias attention to the left, and make the system more receptive to input from the left side.

In terms of the perceptual laterality literature, there are two major predictions from Kinsbourne's position. One is that concurrent activity designed to activate one hemisphere rather than another should lead to predictable shifts in the observed perceptual asymmetries. Thus, verbal activity should prime the left hemisphere and lead to better performance in the right visual field or on the right ear. Such an effect was observed in the gap detection study (Kinsbourne, 1970). Concurrent visuospatial activity, in contrast, should lead to activation of the right hemisphere and superior performance in the left visual field or left ear. Second, because set or expectancy leads to a priming of the appropriate hemisphere, many of the perceptual laterality tasks are self-enhancing. That is, one obtains a right-visual-field superiority for words, not only because right-side input has more direct access to the language centers of the left hemisphere, but also because the set for carrying out processing on verbal material serves to activate the left hemisphere and make it more receptive. By this argument, perceptual laterality effects should be reduced if one eliminates the possibility of priming the system for a particular type of material. Thus, for instance, if both words and sounds are intermingled in a dichotic experiment, the difference in lateral asymmetry between the two types of material should be reduced.

Many experimenters have found at least partial support for Kinsbourne's ideas. For example, Honda (1978) found a left-visual-field effect for determining line orientation: This was eliminated by remembering speech while performing the task, and enhanced by remembering tones. Kershner *et al.* (1977) presented digits bilaterally with different items as fixation control material. When letters were used, a right-field advantage emerged, but a left-field superiority was found when forms were used. Hellige (1978) found a shift toward the right visual field in the recognition of complex polygons when they were intermingled with words or when a concurrent verbal memory load was imposed.

When it has been subject to careful scrutiny, however, Kinsbourne's model has not been quite so successful. Mixed lists do produce concurrent left- and right-hemispheric laterality effects, both visually (Haun, 1978) and dichotically (Goodglass & Calderon, 1977; Kallman, 1978). In fact, Ley and Bryden (1982) have found that it is possible to obtain left- and right-hemispheric effects simultaneously when judgments of content and emotional tone are made on each trial of a dichotic listening task. Likewise, the effects of concurrent activity have not always followed Kinsbourne's predictions (Allard & Bryden, 1979; Boles, 1979; E. B. Gardner & Branski, 1976; Hellige et al., 1979). One problem is that a concurrent activity also serves to occupy some of the limited overall capacity of the system and has effects because of this capacity limitation (cf. Hellige et al., 1979).

The notion that set or expectancy leads to a general priming of one hemisphere at the expense of the other does not seem to be supported by the existing evidence. There is no evidence, for example, that a set for faces would simultaneously enhance the right hemisphere's processing capacity for, say, environmental sounds or line orientation. At the same time, expectancy effects do occur, in the sense that a readiness for verbal material can prime the subject to use a mode of analysis that is appropriate for verbal material. The fact that many laterality effects can be obtained with mixed lists, or are otherwise dissociable (e.g., J. Day, 1977, 1979), would indicate that expectancy effects do not involve a general priming of one hemisphere.

Concurrent activity manipulations are a somewhat different problem. Any concurrent activity takes capacity and therefore reduces the capacity for dealing with the lateralized task. Hellige et al. (1979) found, for example, that a verbal memory load shifted performance on a verbal task to the right hemisphere, the opposite effect from that predicted by a selective priming model. Allard and Bryden (1979) found no evidence for an improvement in detection thresholds with concurrent activity, and Hellige et al. (1979) observed no change in the laterality effect found for judging whether or not two forms were the same with a concurrent memory load. Such experiments indicate that concurrent activity cannot act to make one hemisphere more receptive to incoming stimuli than the other; rather, any effect must be at a later stage of processing (cf. Kinsbourne, 1975a). Just what the effect is, however, seems to depend, not on a general priming mechanism, but on the specific interactions between the lateralization task and the concurrent activity. Kinsbourne's model has not yet reached the point at which adequate predictions can be made about new experimental situations.

Lateralization as a Late Stage of Processing

It has become increasingly common to apply information processing notions to the study of lateralization. Perhaps the most explicit proponent of such a view is Morris Moscovitch (Moscovitch, 1979; Moscovitch *et al.*, 1976). In effect, he argues that early processes (at the sensory, iconic, or echoic level) are not lateralized and that lateralization occurs only at the later or deeper stages of processing. In a face recognition study, for instance, Moscovitch *et al.* (1976) found no laterality effect when the target and comparison faces were presented close together in time, so that the subject could respond on the basis of physical features and did not have to process the target face to any great extent. When, however, a time lag was introduced between the two stimuli, so that the subject had to analyze the target face to some depth, a laterality effect was found. Some support for Moscovitch's notions is provided by a study by Marzi, DiStefano, Tassinari, and Crea (1979), who found no laterality effect in iconic memory, using a partial-report procedure (Sperling, 1960; but see Cohen, 1976). Figure 6.1 shows the essential aspects of the Moscovitch model.

It is not entirely clear whether or not Moscovitch's model is any more than a restatement of the obvious. If language processes are lateralized, for instance, one clearly has to make the task a language task before any lateralization effect is going to emerge. Similarly, if face recognition is lateralized, one must do a face recognition task, and not a stimulus matching task, before any laterality effect will be seen.

Further, it is also not entirely clear that there are no laterality effects at early stages of processing. Certainly the color tasks that show a left-field superiority involve matching at an early sensory level (Pennal, 1977; Pirot *et al.*, 1977), and left-field effects have often been reported for the early stages of letter and word processing (Cohen, 1972; A. R. Gibson *et al.*, 1972; Hellige & Webster, 1979).

The Moscovitch model does seem to lead to the prediction that laterality effects will increase if the final response is delayed and the subject has time to process the information to a later stage or a deeper level. Evidence on this point is equivocal, with some investigators reporting an increment in the laterality effect with delay and others not. Thus, Oscar-Berman *et al.* (1978) find that laterality effects are most evident on the second hand reported in a dichhaptic situation, whereas Bryden (1967a) concludes that such effects are more likely due to ceiling effects on the first ear or hand reported. Some (Dee & Fontenot, 1973) have obtained increments in laterality following a delay; others (Spellacy,

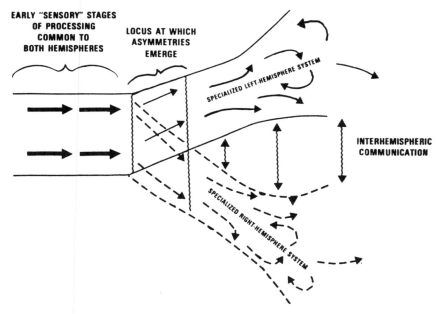

Figure 6.1. Moscovitch's model of information flow in the two cerebral hemispheres. [From Moscovitch, M., & Klein, D. Material-specific perceptual interference for visual words and faces: Implications for models of capacity limitations, attention and laterality. *Journal of Experimental Psychology: Human Perception and Performance,* 1980, *6,* 590–604. Copyright (1980) by the American Psychological Association. Reprinted by permission of publisher and author.]

1970) have found a decrement. There does not appear to be a general principle applicable to all laterality studies. Rather, any delay effect seems to be specific to the particular procedure employed.

However, Moscovitch is correct in the sense that it is necessary to have a detailed task analysis of the procedures that have been used to generate laterality effects. The information processing model makes use of current developments in cognitive and perceptual psychology, and as such represents an up-to-date approach to the issues.

What Is Lateralized?

Table 6.1 provides a summary of the major perceptual laterality effects that have been discussed in the preceding chapters. There are numerous failures to replicate in the literature, and this problem particularly plagues the nonverbal or right-hemispheric effects. Yet in many cases, there is clinical support for the contention that a particular function should show a right-hemispheric superiority. For this reason, a number of right-hemispheric effects are marked in Table 6.1 as questionable. These represent areas of research in which some careful experiments have failed to reproduce the original result.

Is there a general principle underlying the general pattern of effects exhibited in Table 6.1? Psychologists and neurologists have been attempting to describe the differing functions of the two hemispheres in a simple way for many years. Table 6.2 indicates some of the distinctions that have been proposed. Few investigators have been content with so simple a differentiation as verbal–nonverbal. In fact, many tasks that are not obviously verbal lead to a left-hemispheric advantage, such as Carmon and Nachshon's (1973) sequential finger localization task, the dichotic discrimination of tonal sequences (Halperin *et al.*, 1973), and musical sequences in trained subjects (Bever & Chiarello, 1974). At the same time, some superficially verbal tasks produce right-hemispheric effects, such as letter recognition when the items are in novel typefaces (Bryden & Allard, 1976) or embedded in noise (Hellige & Webster, 1979).

It has become popular to describe the left hemisphere as being analytic and sequential in its operations, whereas the right hemisphere is

Table 6.1
Summary of Major Perceptual Laterality Effects

	Left hemisphere superior	Right hemisphere superior
Auditory	Words	Environmental sounds
	Speech sounds, especially stop consonants	Music (melodies)
		Emotional expression in speech
	Rapid temporal changes	
Tactual	Letters	Finger localization
	Sequential finger localization	Random shapes
		Braille
		Line orientation
Visual	Words	Color (?)
	Letters	Line orientation
	Name matches	Dot localization (?)
		Stereopsis (?)
		Mental rotation (?)
		Complex polygons (12-sided)
		Face recognition

(?) indicates that there are good reasons for accepting the asymmetry, but also difficulties in replication.

Table 6.2
Dichotomies Associated with Cerebral Lateralization

Author(s)	Major hemisphere	Minor hemisphere
Jackson (1864)	Expression	Perception
Jackson (1874)	Auditoarticulary	Retinoocular
Jackson (1878–1879)	Propositioning	Visual imagery
Weisenberg and McBride (1935)	Linguistic	Visual or kinesthetic
Anderson (1951)	Executive	Storage
Humphrey and Zangwill (1951)	Symbolic or propositional	Visual or imaginative
McFie and Piercy (1952)	Relations	Correlates
Milner (1958)	Verbal	Perceptual or nonverbal
Semmes, Weinstein, Ghent, and Teuber (1960)	Discrete	Diffuse
Zangwill (1960)	Symbolic	Visuospatial
Hécaen, Ajuriaguerra, and Angelergues (1963)	Linguistic	Preverbal
Bogen and Gazzaniga (1965)	Verbal	Visuospatial
Levy-Agresti and Sperry (1968)	Logical or analytic	Synthetic perceptual
Bogen (1969b)	Propositional	Appositional

Note. After Bogen (1969b) and Corballis and Beale (1976).

seen to be holistic, integrative, and nonsequential. The work of Carmon and his colleagues (Carmon & Nachshon, 1973; Halperin *et al.,* 1973) provides evidence for the importance of the left hemisphere in the perception of sequential relations. (See also Kimura, 1976, for an assessment of left-hemispheric functioning in motor sequencing.) There are also sequential operations involved in the perception of written words or spoken speech. But what is it that makes the perception of a single letter any more sequential or analytic than the perception of a complex polygon? Can the perception of line orientation really be called integrative or holistic?

A variety of studies give some general validity to the analytic–holistic distinction. For example, Cohen (1973) asked subjects to judge whether a set of items were all the same or whether they contained one odd item. With letter material, increasing the number of items in the set resulted in increased reaction times in the right visual field, but not in the left. In contrast, set size had no effect on response time in either visual field when the items were unnameable shapes. Cohen concluded that letter material is processed serially by the left hemisphere, but in parallel by the right hemisphere, whereas shapes are processed in parallel by both hemispheres. Bradshaw, Gates, and Patterson (1976) varied the specific task requirements and he number of items that differed in the set, and concluded that an analytic–holistic dichotomy is more fundamental than a serial–parallel one (see also Bradshaw & Nettleton, 1981).

Martin (1979) presented stimuli in which a set of small letters were arranged in the shape of a large letter. She found that responses to the elements were faster in the right visual field, whereas responses to the global configuration did not favor either field, and argued that analytic processing was more easily carried out by the left hemisphere. Her failure to find a left-field effect for the global or holistic task may have been due to the lack of power of the task to detect such a difference.

The difficulty in evaluating the various dichotomies proposed to describe hemispheric asymmetries is that none of them seem to fit all the data. This "dichotomania" may be more a reflection of experimentalists' desire to see things in contrast than a reflection of the true state of affairs. There are now so many different laterality effects that it is difficult to keep them all in mind. Analytic–holistic and verbal–nonverbal distinctions may have their greatest value as mnemonic devices that enable one to remember what effects have been found with what tasks. At the same time, they may be one of the great menaces to laterality research, since such dichotomies often carry excess meaning and unintended associations. What starts out as a metaphorical description winds up being taken seriously and leads us to believe that there is documentary scientific evidence that the right hemisphere is creative or artistic, or that Western civilization has been dedicated to the development of the left hemisphere.

In fact, there is remarkably little reason to believe that a single dichotomy will ever adequately describe all the differences between the two hemispheres. There is little reason to believe that each hemisphere acts in a unitary fashion and that one can ultimately discern that a particular hemisphere is analytic, or linguistic, or integrative, or what have you. We have perhaps become too impressed with the dramatic effects produced by section of the cerebral commissures and forgotten that there are local differences within the hemispheres, as well as between them.

In other words, there may not be a single overriding principle that can explain or describe all laterality effects. What we may have, rather, is a diversity of different laterality effects, interrelated but not perfectly correlated with one another. We know that the areas of the right hemisphere primarily involved in prosopagnosia, for instance, are not those involved in music perception. Why should we expect the left-ear effect for music to have the same basis as the left-visual-field effect for faces? We know that different parts of the left hemisphere are involved in phonetic analysis and semantic analysis (Ojeman & Mateer, 1979). Why should the dichotic laterality effect for stop consonants have the same basis as the visual effect for word recognition? Should we ever document a relation between perceptual and anatomical asymmetries, do we expect the posterior parietal region to show an asymmetry just because the temporal planum does?

This is not to take a defeatist attitude about laterality research on the normal subject. Rather, it is an argument that we have been looking at things in an overly idealistic way and that we have been overwhelmed by the left–right differences while forgetting about regional differences within each hemisphere. What we need to do is isolate the laterality differences we think are important and study them in detail, rather than attempting to find new ones. Further, most researchers involved with laterality effects in normals have become overcommitted to the study of the "modal" individual: the right-handed subject with left-hemispheric speech representation. To study the interrelations between laterality variables, we need a group of subjects who are maximally different. By this argument, we should study the performance of groups of left-handers, rather than groups of right-handers, and we should study their performance on several laterality tasks at the same time, attempting to dissociate different factors.

7

Asymmetry of
Motor Performance

One of the newest topics of interest to researchers concerned with brain asymmetries is the area of asymmetry of control for motor performance. The motor performance research done to date is quite unlike the research into perceptual asymmetries described earlier. Research into functional asymmetries in the sensory systems has been guided by the hope that the discovery of the type of information best analyzed by the left and right hemispheres will eventually lead to a rule that will capture the essence of the left–right dichotomy. The work on motor asymmetries that will be discussed in this chapter consists of research generated by three different sets of investigators, all attempting to answer very different questions through studying motor performance. Attempting to synthesize the findings of these three sets of investigators is no simple task. As well, studies of perceptual asymmetries have shown excellent correspondence between performance deficits seen in brain-damaged subjects and performance asymmetries seen in normal subjects with special experimental techniques. This is not the case for motor asymmetries: There is a marked lack of correspondence between performance problems in brain-damaged subjects and studies involving normal subjects.

Early Studies

Early anatomical work showed that there exists bilateral representation of all but the most distal musculature (Brinkman & Kuypers, 1972). This means that either hemisphere has the potential to control all of the body except the fingers of the side ipsilateral to the hemisphere. However, the work of Maria Wyke (1966, 1967, 1968, 1969, 1971a, 1971b) showed that the effects of right and left damage were not symmetrical, as anatomical considerations would suggest. Wyke studied performance on a wide variety of motor tasks, from rapidly tapping a key to precision pegboard tasks, in patients with unilateral brain damage. Wyke found that patients with right-hemispheric damage showed the pattern of performance that anatomical considerations would suggest: poor performance on the left hand controlled by the damaged right hemisphere. Patients with left-hemispheric damage also showed poor performance on the contralateral hand—the right hand in this case. As well, patients with left damage showed poor performance on their left hands—a bilateral performance problem. The pattern that emerged from Wyke's work was clear: Right-hemisphere damage resulted in a performance decrement on the contralateral left hand only, whereas left-hemisphere damage resulted in a performance decrement on both left and right hands.

Wyke's work led directly to the series of studies on motor asymmetries carried out by Kimura. In a direct extension of the Wyke research, Kimura and Archibald (1974) tested patients with right- or left-hemispheric damage on a task involving copying hand postures demonstrated by the experimenter. Note that this task involves a subject moving only his or her hand—no key tapping or tracking or other moving of implements is required. Kimura and Archibald found that both groups of patients were able to produce individual hand postures with no difficulty. However, patients with left-hemispheric damage were unable to produce sequences of the same set of hand postures that they had been able to produce in isolation. Right-hemispheric-damaged patients had no trouble with hand positioning. The production problem of the left-damaged group was seen for both left and right hands—again, a bilateral deficit. That the problem of the left-damaged group was a production problem rather than a memory or recognition problem was confirmed when the left-damaged group was able to recognize the correct sequence of hand postures when produced by someone else.

In another study, Kimura (1977) demonstrated the bilateral problem for generating a series of motor responses of a patient with left-hemisphere damage in yet another way. In this experiment, patients were tested on a manual sequencing task involving three component movements: a button push with the index finger, a vertical bar pull using four fingers, and a horizontal bar push with the thumb. As would be expected, left-damaged patients were much poorer than right-damaged patients at learning the task with either hand. The manual sequencing task allowed Kimura to quantify the type of errors made by both groups of patients in performing the task. A good number of two types of errors was found in the performance of the left-damaged group: perseverative errors (repeating the movement just performed) and amorphous errors (movements not clearly related to any of the tasks at hand). Right-damaged patients made no perseverative or amorphous errors. Both groups made equal numbers of sequencing errors—producing the right response at the wrong time. The problem of the left-damaged group, then, seemed to be related to the production of a series of different limb positions.

As well as comparing right- and left-damaged subjects in this study, Kimura was able to compare aphasic and nonaphasic patients within the left-hemisphere group. Although all left-hemispheric patients were impaired on the manual sequencing task, the aphasic patients were clearly more impaired than were the nonaphasics. This suggested to Kimura that oral movements were just as susceptible to disruption due to damage to a left-hemisphere movement generator as were hand movements. The relationship between oral and brachial performance deficits was confirmed by Mateer and Kimura (1977). They found that nonfluent aphasics were impaired on single oral movements, production of single phonemes, and speed of repeating a single syllable, as compared to left-damaged nonaphasic patients.

Kimura showed, then, that an intact left hemisphere is critical for generating a series of movements involving either oral or brachial musculature. That this left-hemispheric system is responsible for generating commands for both arms is shown by the bilateral deficit seen with damage to the system.

Studies with Normal Subjects

Kimura (e.g., Kimura, 1979; Lomas & Kimura, 1976) has also studied the nature of the left-hemispheric movement generator by using normal, intact subjects. The logic of studying motor asymmetry in normal subjects is not as straightforward as the logic of studying the perceptual asymmetries. For both audition and vision, the verbal stimulus that gains most direct access to left-hemisphere language analyzers will be reported fastest or with greatest accuracy. Translating into motor performance, this logic would argue that the limb having the most direct access to a left-hemispheric movement generator would perform fastest or with greatest accuracy. In other words, the right hand would perform best or fastest in motor tasks, an observation that needs little experimental confirmation. The study of motor asymmetries, then, is confounded by the fact that the hands do not start off performing at all equally. Experimenters in motor asymmetries have, by and large, tended to avoid the question of handedness as much as possible and to develop ways of manipulating brain activity experimentally while observing the effects of the ongoing activity on motor performance.

More specifically, experimental neuropsychologists interested in motor asymmetries have frequently used an interference or dual-task paradigm to investigate motor asymmetries in normal subjects. In these studies, a subject is given a task, such as reciting nursery rhymes or humming, that can be performed at the same time as he or she is engaged in performing a motor task. Presumably the interfering task keeps a part of the brain busy so that it cannot contribute to performance of the motor task. If the interfering task and the motor task require the same brain structure, "something's gotta give," resulting in poorer performance on one of the tasks. The interference paradigm then might be thought to create a "temporary lesion" in a perfectly normal subject. But the interference paradigm must be handled with great care in order to make appropriate inferences about behavior.

The interference paradigm is really a special instance of the dual-task experiment that has a long and noble tradition in experimental psychology. The dual-task experiment has been used to study a great variety of issues, including selective attention, fluctuations in attention demands of a variety of information processing tasks, the psychological refractory period, and automaticity. Control considerations in the dual-task or interference paradigm require four dependent measures: speed and/or accuracy of both the primary and secondary tasks performed alone and speed and/or accuracy of both tasks when they are performed together. All four (or eight, if it is reasonable to measure both speed and accuracy) measures of performance are crucial in order to know for certain how adequately a subject is maintaining performance in the face of interference. Since the interference paradigm is used by experimenters studying motor asymmetries, performance on the interfering task is often evaluated very superficially. Frequently, no single-task performance measure of the interference task has been taken, leading experimenters to assume that subjects are performing the interference task to the best of their ability in the dual-task situation. In fact, a subject could be dividing processing resources between motor and interfering tasks so as to preserve performance on the motor task, which would result in an underestimate of the amount of interference being produced. In other words, in order to know that the temporary lesion is producing an effect, an experimenter must create an interference task that is measurable in both single- and dual-task situations.

In addition, the inferences to be made from experiments using the interference paradigm depend on what you think you are interfering with. The notion of a temporary lesion implies that the interference task is occupying a particular brain structure and is creating structural interference. There is at least one other way of thinking about performance decrements caused by doing two things at once. Drops in performance may be the result of exceeding the overall capacity of the information processing system: The interference task may be creating capacity interference. In summary, the interference paradigm is complex, requiring careful control observations, a judicious selection of experimental tasks, and some theoretical notion as to the nature of the interference, whether it is structural or capacity interference.

Applying the interference task to the study of motor asymmetries should result in a straightforward finding. If an interference task causes structural interference, bilateral performance decrements should be seen on the motor task.

The data generated from interference task studies have been complex and confusing, to say the least. Kinsbourne and Cook (1971) had subjects balance a dowel on their right or left index finger for 250 sec or until the dowel fell. In a single-task control condition, subjects balanced best with their right hands. When speaking a sentence while dowel balancing, performance on the right hand decreased, whereas left-hand performance actually improved. A verbal interfering task, then, resulted in a drop in performance for only the right hand.

Lomas and Kimura (1976) attempted to replicate and extend the Kinsbourne and Cook finding. They required their subjects to balance a dowel on their left or right index fingers under three conditions: a single-task control in which the subject simply balanced the dowel, one interference condition in which a subject balanced while reciting nursery rhymes, and a second interference condition in which a subject balanced while humming a tune. Speaking is a left-hemispheric speciality, and humming is presumably a right-hemispheric task. If motor sequencing is a function of a left-hemisphere system, speaking should cause a decrement in performance, whereas humming should cause no effect. The findings of Lomas and Kimura were quite different from those of Kinsbourne and Cook (1971). Female subjects showed no effects of interference across conditions. Male subjects showed poor performance on the right hand while speaking, thus replicating Kinsbourne and Cook, but the male subjects also showed poor performance on *both* hands while humming. Results from the dowel balancing replication, then, were not the picture of clarity that one would have hoped for. Arguing that the dowel balancing task was not the most appropriate means for probing the nature of a motor generator, Lomas and Kimura changed the motor task to finger sequencing. Subjects were instructed to depress four keys sequentially in the required order (index, middle, ring, and little finger) as many times as possible in a 15-sec trial. Again, finger sequencing was performed alone, while repeating nursery rhymes, or while humming. For finger sequencing, humming produced no change in performance, whereas speaking depressed right-hand performance in right-handed subjects. For left-handed subjects, performance on both hands dropped for both humming and speaking. Again the data present a confusing pattern.

In a final attempt to extract order, Lomas and Kimura performed a third experiment. The motor tasks used in this experiment consisted of single finger tapping (hitting a telegraph key as many times as possible) and sequential arm tapping (hitting sequentially the four keys used for finger sequencing using a whole arm movement rather than a finger movement). Inteference tasks consisted of speaking and humming. Single finger tapping speed was slower for both hands when performed with speaking. Arm sequencing speed was slower for the right arm in the speaking condition. A summary of the rather complex pattern of results from the Lomas and Kimura (1976) study is presented in Table 7.1.

As this table shows, for every motor task tested, speaking produced a performance decrement for the right hand. Indeed, the right-hand decrement seems to be the most consistent feature of the data. Lomas and Kimura, then, working with normal subjects, have shown a consistent unilateral effect of a verbal interfering task rather than the bilateral effect seen with damage to the left hemisphere.

Table 7.1
Interference Task Effects Shown by Lomas and Kimura (1976)

	Interference task	
Motor task	Speaking	Humming
Dowel balancing	R hand (males)	R and L hand (males)
Finger sequencing	R hand (R handers)	No effect
	R and L hand (L handers)	R and L hand
Arm tapping	R hand	No effect
Single finger tapping	R and L hand	No effect

More recently, Lomas (1980) has returned to this problem. He compared the effects of speaking on both sequential arm tapping and sequential finger tapping with and without visual guidance. When the apparatus was concealed from the subject's view, speaking produced a unilateral decrement on the right hand. With visual guidance, however, the results were much less consistent, with speaking during finger tapping having a unilateral effect on the left hand in one experiment and on the right hand in a replication study. In general, though, the effects of speaking are confined to the right hand.

A theoretical notion that would, at first blush, seem to account for unilateral interference effects is the "functional space" concept of Kinsbourne and Hicks (1978), the second group of investigators studying motor asymmetries. According to the notion of functional space, two different tasks will interfere if they both require the same brain structure. Conversely, two similar tasks requiring the same structure should cause no interference. To the degree that the two tasks being attempted require similar functional units, then, interference will be seen. Note that the proposed overlap is in terms of *functional* units, rather than neuroanatomical units. This means that there is no a priori method of determining what tasks will interfere. "Functional space" is described after the fact: If two tasks interfere, there must be overlap in some neural structure. Functional space would seem to have little predictive theoretical power. This does not mean that proponents of the functional space notion have nothing to say. These investigators have produced an interesting series of studies examining the nature of interference effects on motor performance dating from the Kinsbourne and Cook (1971) dowel balancing study described earlier. In general, studies on functional space support the idea that the interference effects of speaking on motor performance are unilateral rather than bilateral. One problem with many of the interference task experiments generated from the functional space position is the lack of a single-task control observation for the interfering task. As described earlier, without some indication of how hard a subject is working at the interference task in the dual-task situation, any inferences about the nature of interference are difficult. Ideally, a subject would be performing at the *single-task level* for the interfering task in the dual-task situation. Given freedom to allocate his or her resources at will, one subject may decide to switch between interfering and motor tasks, while another subject may choose to lock onto the interference task. Certainly then, single-task control observations for both interfering and motor tasks are essential in these studies. A case could be made for interference tasks that are more readily quantifiable, more amenable to measurement, than humming or repeating nursery rhymes.

Another theoretical problem with the functional space position is the idea that all interference is the result of structural interference. As outlined earlier in this chapter, an interference task could be causing performance decrements due to capacity interference. It would seem critical to attempt to disentangle capacity and structural interference effects in interference effects experiments.

Despite the objections to the notion of functional space raised in the preceding paragraphs, the fact remains that these experimenters have, over a variety of experiments, shown that speaking influences motor performance on the right hand only, the same sort of unimanual effect observed by Lomas and Kimura (1976). Why the discrepancy between the effects of unilateral brain damage and the effects of a temporary lesion as created by an interference task?

A series of studies by Rodney (1980) seem to provide a partial answer to the different effects of real or temporary lesions on motor performance. As has been argued, the interference paradigm can be difficult to control. While not solving all the control problems, the Rodney experiments are more satisfying than most.

Rodney started by replicating the finger sequencing task done by Lomas and Kimura (1976). Recall that this task required that a subject depress four telegraph keys sequentially from index to little finger as many times as possible in 15 sec. Interfering tasks consisted of humming and repeating nursery rhymes. Using the same dependent measure as had Lomas and Kimura—the number of "good" sequences produced in each 15-sec trial—Rodney found exactly what the previous study had found. Performance on the right hand dropped only when the verbal interference task was being performed; again, a unilateral interference effect was shown. Rodney then considered interference effects on a number of other dependent measures for the finger sequencing task. Counting the total number of keys pressed in a 15-sec trial, Rodney showed that subjects were able to make more key presses in control and humming conditions than while speaking. The number of errors in sequencing showed that the right hand was more accurate in the control and speaking conditions than in the humming condition. In other words, both speaking and humming produced interference effects; speaking slowed subjects down, whereas humming caused them to make mistakes.

Rodney felt that some of the problems subjects were having in the interference task trials were due to subjects not having learned the motor sequence before being asked to execute the sequence while doing the interference task. Because the sequencing task had not been practiced prior to introduction of the secondary tasks, the subjects' left-hand performance was so bad in control trials that it had little chance to decrease performance in interference trials.

In a second study, Rodney (1980) gave subjects 1 day of practice on the motor task. On the practice day, subjects performed 20 trials with each hand on the finger sequencing task. On a second day, subjects performed the actual experiment: finger sequencing alone, while humming, and while speaking. Results of the practiced subjects showed no differences between hands or conditions for the number of good responses produced. Nor were there any differences in the number of errors a subject made in the three experimental conditions. Once a subject was practiced on the motor task, interfering tasks exerted no influence over the accuracy of response. The rate of responding, however, continued to show effects of interference. Speaking produced a significant reduction in the number of key presses a subject made with either hand. As well, in the speaking interference condition, there was a significant increase in the time between the termination of one sequence and the initiation of the next, regardless of performing hand. Rate of response measures showed a slowing of performance with speaking that was bilateral in nature. Rodney's findings with finger sequencing argue that subjects should be practiced on the motor task before interfering tasks are introduced. With practice, left-hand performance reaches some degree of proficiency and is thus able to reflect any influence of right-hemisphere loading.

Rodney's (1980) data, then, seem to reflect interference from speaking that is bilateral in nature and more closely in line with what would be expected from the studies of patients with unilateral brain damage. There is another possible explanation for Rodney's data—the old problem of capacity interference. Rather than similar brain structures mediating performance on both speaking and motor sequencing, speaking could simply be a more difficult interfering task than humming. By this argument, humming does not disrupt performance because humming and motor sequencing are not difficult enough to exceed a subject's available capacity.

Evidence for capacity interference in motor performance has been provided by Summers and Sharp (1979), who investigated the effects of a verbal, a spatial, and a verbal–spatial interfering task on a bimanual motor task, a unimanual motor task, and single finger tapping. The result of interest to the present discussion is the similar performance decrement found for the interfering tasks. Despite the fact that verbal and spatial tasks require the resources of opposite hemispheres, Summers and Sharp found essentially equivalent interference effects for verbal and spatial tasks on motor sequencing. The authors contend that their data strongly suggest generalized capacity interference rather than structural interference.

In a third study, Rodney (1980) attempted to disentangle capacity and structural interference effects. The motor sequencing task used for this experiment consisted of a manual sequencing task similar to the manual sequencing board used by Kimura (1977). Rodney's task components consisted of six elements: a plug that had to be pulled out of one socket and inserted into a second socket, a knob that had to be turned through 290°, a round knob on a metal rod that had to be pushed in or pulled out, a round knob on a metal slide that had to be moved through 180° on a semi circular track, a breaker switch that had to be thrown, and a round knob that had to be moved in a diagonal track (see Figure 7.1). Subjects moved the components in the appropriate fashion as quickly as possible with right and left hands for a 40-trial practice session. On a second day, subjects performed the manual sequencing task alone and with a variety of interfering tasks.

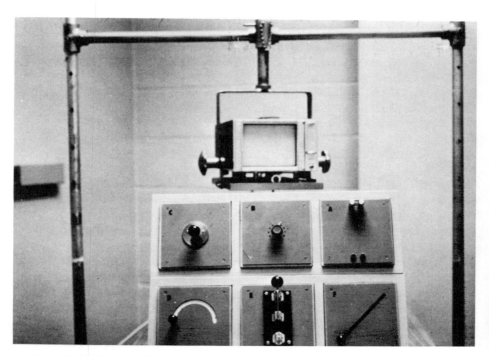

Figure 7.1. The manual sequencing task employed by Rodney (1980). The subject was to operate in sequence the six switches, knobs, and levers shown at the bottom of the photograph.

Table 7.2
Interference Tasks Employed by Rodney (1980)

Structural interference	Capacity interference		
	Easy task	versus	Difficult task
Vocal interference	Repeating a single word		Repeating six words
versus			
Motor interference	Single finger tapping		Four finger sequencing

In order to investigate structural interference, Rodney had subjects perform the manual sequencing task while speaking or while performing a second motor task. If structural interference exists, a second motor interfering task should provide more interference than a vocal interfering task.

Capacity interference is more difficult to manipulate. It would be a simple matter to manipulate capacity interference if there existed some metric for assessing task difficulty: Clearly, a more difficult secondary task should demand more capacity than a simple secondary task. Lacking a clear metric for difficulty, Rodney chose two motor and two vocal tasks that seemed intuitively to represent hard and easy tasks. The actual interfering tasks chosen and the design of the study are illustrated in Table 7.2.

Subjects performed the manual sequencing task while performing each of the interfering tasks. Were structural factors predominant in interference, subjects should show less interference for vocal than for motor interference tasks, regardless of the level of difficulty of the task. Were capacity factors predominant, subjects should show less interference for easy than for difficult interference tasks, regardless of the mode, motor or verbal, of the interfering task.

Rodney (1980) found significant interference effects for both structural and capacity conditions. Both structural and capacity interference were reflected by a slowing in response for both hands. Clearly, then, both structural and capacity interference are factors in motor sequencing task, and both sorts of interference show bilateral effects for subjects practiced in the primary motor task. Rodney's experiments provide two guidelines for experimenters utilizing the interference paradigm to study motor asymmetries:

1. Practice subjects on the primary motor task.
2. Include a capacity interference control condition, to ensure that structural interference is occurring over and above capacity demands of simply doing two things at once.

The two guidelines emerging from Rodney's (1980) research, as well as the myriad of other factors that must be controlled for cogent use of the interference paradigm as outlined earlier, would lead to the conclusion that the interference paradigm is a mite unwieldy in its application to the study of motor asymmetries.

As well as cleaning up procedural issues, Rodney's (1980) work provides some hints about the functional nature of the lateralized system. The system does not seem to be important in one-shot movements—Kimura's brain-damaged patients could produce a single hand posture. The lateralized system is brought to bear when a series of movements must be produced; but what aspect of producing a series of movements does the functional system control? At least two aspects of a series of movements would seem to be contenders. Movements in a sequence might be considered as a structured series of smaller motor elements or features. The left hemisphere might be crucial for selecting and stringing the motor features together: The left hemisphere could be seen as a master motor programmer. Alternatively, producing a series of movements also requires on-line monitoring at some level of the current position of the limb. In performing a skill such as Kimura's or Rodney's manual sequencing tasks, subjects in all probability never produce exactly the same movements twice. Some system must monitor the current state of the hand and arm in order to initiate the next movement required by the task. The left-hemispheric system, then, might be responsible for this on-line feedback monitoring.

In her third study, Rodney (1980) found that interference effects were greater when a subject was between elements in a task than when a subject was actually engaged in performing the requisite movement. Greater between-element interference would suggest that the left-hemispheric system is most susceptible when programming or evaluating feedback, but it allows no conclusion about which factor is influenced most. Few other data exist to allow a decision about programming versus feedback monitoring; however, Kimura (1979) feels programming is the role of the lateralized system.

Sussman and his colleagues (Sussman, 1971, 1979; Sussman & MacNeilage, 1975; Sussman & Westbury, 1978) have carried out a series of studies that would suggest that feedback evaluation is an important element of the left hemisphere. This work represents the last of the three approaches to the study of lateralized motor performance to be considered here. The experimental task used by Sussman is vastly different from the interference tasks employed by other investigators of motor asymmetries. In Sussman's work, a target tone that a subject is to track is presented to one ear. This target tone may vary in either frequency or amplitude. A cursor tone—the tone that a subject tracks with—is presented to the other ear. The subject's task is to match variations in the target tone by changing the tone under his or her control. Subject's accuracy is evaluated by calculating the difference between target and cursor tones.

When the cursor was controlled by a transducer that changed lateral tongue movements into cursor changes, subjects were more accurate in tracking when the cursor was presented to the right ear and the target was presented to the left ear, over the condition in which the cursor was presented to the left ear and the target to the right ear. This pattern of results could be due to a right-ear, left-hemisphere superiority for cursor control or to a left-ear, right-hemisphere superiority for target tone analysis. In order to discover which explanation was most appropriate, a second experimental condition was run. In this condition, a subject controlled the cursor tone with his or her right hand. All else in the experiment remained the same: A subject heard cursor right and target left as well as cursor left and target right. Were the same pattern of data found for hand tracking as for tongue tracking, the controlling factor to the lateralized superiority would be the ear of target analysis, because the nature of the target analysis did not change across experimental conditions. Were a different pattern of results found in the hand tracking condition, the important factor in producing the experimental effect would be the motor system controlling the cursor. When subjects tracked with the right hand, there were no significant differences in tracking performance as a function of which ear received the cursor tone. More recent studies have shown a small but significant advantage for manual tracking when the cursor was presented to the right ear (Sussman & Westbury, 1978).

Sussman (1979) trained subjects to perform the tracking task without an auditory cursor. Substituting white noise for the cursor signal, he found superior tracking when the target signal was presented to the right ear.

Sussman and MacNeilage (1975) argue that "right ear effects for tasks involving speech articulators were due to the presence in the left hemisphere of a special speech related auditory–sensorimotor integration mechanism [p. 138]." They argue that pursuit auditory tracking and speech production are similar in two ways. First, an auditory signal under a subject's control must be compared to an acoustic standard. Second, both speech production and auditory tracking "require a generalized ability to control the motor system in terms of the acoustic consequences, presumably with concurrent use of somatic sensory information . . . this ability can be regarded as the possession of an auditory–motor algorithm which makes possible the voluntary control over sound generation necessary to achieve the standard [p. 146]."

Sussman, then, would attribute left-hemispheric prepotency in motor production to a left superiority in matching ongoing performance to a standard that can be either internal (phonemes of speech) or external (a target tone). The key construct in the Sussman position is the matching of ongoing motor activity to a standard—that is, in evaluating feedback in terms of goals. This position would seem to describe the performance of Kimura's left-damaged patients as well. The patients might well be able to generate the individual motor elements required but unable to monitor exactly where in the production they are. With normal subjects, the interference paradigm might reduce a subject's ability to attend to the results of feedback comparison, resulting in a drop in performance.

The nature of the left hemisphere's involvement in motor performance as motor programmer or as feedback evaluator remains to be determined.

8

Lateralization of Emotional Processes

In the preceding chapters, the concern has been almost exclusively with the lateralization of cognitive processes. In recent years, attention has turned to the lateralization of affective processes, and many investigators have suggested that there are differences between the two hemispheres in their involvement in the perception and production of emotional behavior. Among proponents of this view, there are two opposing camps. According to one interpretation of the data, the right hemisphere is more involved than the left in all aspects of emotional behavior (e.g., Ley & Bryden, 1981). The alternative view is that the right hemisphere plays a special role in mediating negative emotions, while the left hemisphere is implicated in positive emotions (e.g., D. H. Tucker, 1981). Let us consider the evidence for these two viewpoints.

Dichotic Listening Studies

A number of dichotic listening studies have been carried out that suggest an asymmetry in the recognition of emotional stimuli. For instance, Haggard and Parkinson (1971) asked subjects to identify both the emotional value and the verbal content of sentences that were dichotically presented in competition with a continuous speech babble of many voices speaking at once. Their stimuli consisted of six sentences read in four emotional tones: angry, bored, happy, and distressed. They found a small left-ear advantage in identifying the emotional tone of the sentence, but not in identifying its content. In a similar experiment, Carmon and Nachshon (1973) presented nonverbal stimuli dichotically: the cries, shrieks, and laughter of a child, of an adult female, and of an adult male. They then showed their subjects nine cartoons depicting the three characters in each of the emotional states and asked their subjects to indicate which sounds they had heard. Again, a small but significant left-ear advantage was observed.

Bryden, Ley, and Sugarman (1982) dichotically presented musical passages differing in affective value. They required their subjects to monitor one ear and judge the affective quality of the sound they heard at that ear. Subjects were more accurate in categorizing the music as positive, negative, or neutral when it was heard at the left ear. Furthermore, positive stimuli were judged as more positive when they were heard at the left ear, and negative stimuli were judged as more negative when heard at the left ear. Both positive and negative stimuli, then, were judged as more highly emotional when heard at the left ear.

One of the most compelling experiments was conducted by Ley and Bryden (1982). They employed a number of short sentences spoken in happy, sad, angry, and neutral voices. These sentences were dichotically paired with neutral sentences of similar semantic content. Subjects were instructed to attend to one ear and to report both the emotional tone of the target sentence and to indicate its content by checking off items on a multiple-choice recognition sheet. Virtually every subject showed a left-ear advantage for identifying the emotional tone of the voice and, at the same time, a right-ear advantage for identifying the content.

Beaton (1979) has also investigated emotional asymmetry using a dichotic listening procedure. He presented passages of music or poetry to one ear while playing white noise to the other. Subjects judged each of the passages for pleasantness, soothingness, and cheerfulness. In general, passages were judged as more pleasant when they arrived at the left ear, regardless of whether the overall tone of the passage was positive or negative. Rather similar results were obtained with the cheerful–depressing scale, though the differences were not statistically significant. Music, but not poetry, was judged more soothing when it arrived at the left ear. Beaton (1979) suggests that the right hemisphere adopts a more pleasant outlook, although the Bryden *et al.* (1982) data do not substantiate this view. However, Beaton tested different subjects with left-ear presentation and with right-ear presentation, so that no statement about the effect within individuals is possible.

In a study involving monaural rather than dichotic presentation, Safer and Leventhal (1977) presented prose passages with positive, negative, or neutral content. These passages were read in three tones of voice: positive, negative, or neutral. They found that subjects listening on the left ear rated the passages in terms of the tone of voice employed, whereas those listening on the right ear used the content cues to evaluate the passage.

We have earlier commented on the possibility of attentional biases in dichotic listening experiments. The possibility of such biases exists in many of the studies discussed in the preceding paragraphs, although Bryden *et al.* (1982) and Ley and Bryden (1982) avoided this particular problem by using a monitoring procedure. The Ley and Bryden (1982) study is particularly valuable, in that content and emotion judgments were shown to have opposite effects in the same subjects. Thus, the majority of the dichotic listening studies point to a specialized right-hemisphere involvement in the perception of emotional stimuli.

Lateral Tachistoscopic Presentation

Most studies employing lateral tachistoscopic presentation have used pictures or drawings of faces expressing different emotions. Since many studies have shown that face recognition is generally better in the left visual field (e.g., Hilliard, 1973; Patterson & Bradshaw, 1975; Rizzolatti, Umilta, & Berlucchi, 1971), some of the emotional judgment effects may be due to a general right-hemispheric superiority in processing faces.

Suberi and McKeever (1977) asked subjects to study and memorize either emotional or nonemotional faces and then to judge whether a unilaterally presented face was a target face or not. They found faster reaction times to emotional stimuli presented in the left visual field. In addition, the left-visual-field superiority was greater for subjects memorizing emotional as opposed to nonemotional faces.

Buchtel, Campari, DeRisio, and Rota (1978) required subjects to make discriminative reactions to differing facial expressions. Their subjects were told to respond as quickly as possible to happy faces or to sad faces. Unknown to the subjects, faces showing neutral expressions were also included in the stimulus set. The stimuli were presented laterally, but in blocked trials, so that subjects could anticipate the location of the stimulus on any given trial. Response times were faster to both happy and sad faces when the stimuli appeared in the left visual field. Curiously, false positives to neutral stimuli were faster in the right visual field. While the general findings would seem to indicate a right-hemispheric superiority for the processing of emotional expression, the use of blocked trials makes the claim of unilateral presentation rather suspect.

Strauss and Moscovitch (1981) have also carried out reaction time experiments using facial stimuli. They employed photographs of six individuals showing three different facial expressions: happy, sad, and surprised. On each trial, the subject saw two lateralized photographs, one above the other, and was to judge whether or not the faces showed the same expression. As did Buchtel *et al.* (1978), Strauss and Moscovitch (1981) used a "go–no go" procedure, in which half the subjects responded only when there was a match and half only when the expressions differed. Strauss and Moscovitch found faster response times in the left visual field when the expressions were the same, but little difference between the two fields when different expressions were portrayed. They also ran a similar experiment in which subjects were to judge whether or not the same character, rather than the same expression, was portrayed in the two photographs. Although the detailed pattern differed somewhat, faster response times were again found in the left visual field when the same expression was shown in the two photographs. Note that similar effects were produced by the same stimuli in the two experiments, although the response requirements to stimulus pairs containing different faces showing the same expression were quite different in the two studies.

In a third study, Strauss and Moscovitch (1981) had subjects memorize a set of target faces all exhibiting a single expression. Pairs of lateralized stimuli were again presented, and the subject was required to determine whether or not either of the two faces exhibited the target affect. As before, some subjects responded only to positive instances and others only to negative instances. In general, women showed a left-visual-field advantage in this study, whereas men did not. In sum, then, Strauss and Moscovitch's (1981) study is rather inconclusive: A left-visual-field superiority for emotional expression appeared in a number of situations, but it was not stable across all conditions, varied with sex, and was not clearly dissociable from a left-visual-field effect for face recognition.

A clear dissociation between the categorization of emotional expression and categorization of objects was shown by Landis, Assal, and Perret (1979). They presented an outline drawing of a face or a familiar object in central vision and, at the same time, a lateralized photograph of a face or object. Subjects were to decide whether or not the drawing and photograph represented the same meaning. When the stimuli represented objects, decision times were faster in the right visual field; when they represented different emotional expressions, response times were faster in the left visual field.

Ley and Bryden (1979a) presented cartoon drawings of five adult male characters, each showing five emotional expressions ranging from very positive through mildly positive, neutral, and mildly negative to very negative. Subjects were shown a single face laterally presented and then a second face in central vision. They were required to judge whether or not the two faces showed the same expression, and whether or not they represented the same character. Significant left-visual-field superiorities were found for both judgments of expression and for recognition of the character. A subsequent covariance analysis indicated that a significant left-visual-field superiority for the emotion judgments remained when the effects of the face recognition had been partialled out. This finding would give at least provisional support for the notion that the left-visual-field effect for emotional expression was independent of that for simple face recognition. In addition, Ley and Bryden (1979a) found that the magnitude of the left-visual-field effect for the emotion judgments varied with the degree of emotion expressed: Left-field effects were largest for the extreme positive and negative stimuli.

Safer (1981) has reported an experiment very similar to that of Ley and Bryden (1979a). Subjects were required to make same–different judgments about the emotions expressed in two facial photographs. Some subjects were told to label the initial stimulus with a verbal description, others to try to feel the emotion expressed. As in the Ley and Bryden experiment (1979a), subjects showed a left-visual-field superiority. However, this effect was significant only for males. Furthermore, subjects given empathy instructions showed a larger left-field effect than did those given the verbal labeling instructions. Safer suggests that women are more able to benefit from the verbal codes for emotion.

Further evidence for a sex difference in the lateralization of affective processes comes from a study by Graves, Landis, and Goodglass (1981). They presented four-letter words, varying in frequency, imageability, and emotionality, along with nonwords, in a lexical decision task. As would be expected from the verbal nature of the task, a general right-visual-field superiority was observed. However, this right-field superiority was reduced for the emotional words in men, but not in women. In men, emotionality was the major predictor of response times in the left visual field, and frequency was the major predictor in the right visual field. For the women, in contrast, imageability was the best predictor of left-field latencies, and both frequency and emotionality were relevant in the right field. While the data from the women are difficult to interpret (see Chapter 14), the data on males would suggest that even words can access right-hemispheric systems specific to emotionality.

A rather different approach was employed in a series of studies by Ley (1980b; Ley & Bryden, 1979b, forthcoming). In these studies, subjects were initially tested on a lateralized perceptual task. They were then asked to memorize a list of words, with different groups of subjects being given lists of varying emotional tone and imagery value. Subjects were told that they would have to recall these lists, but, prior to recall, they were retested on the lateralized task. The data of interest are the changes in performance on the lateralized task from the initial testing to the retest when the word list was being held in memory. Ley carried out two experiments using this general procedure: In one (Ley & Bryden, 1979b), a face recognition task was used as the lateralization task; in the other (Ley, 1980b), dichotic stop consonant CV syllables were used. The major findings in the two experiments were the same: Both imagery and affect influenced the relative lateralization of the test material. Subjects who were given either emotionally positive word lists (e.g., kiss, party, friend) or emotionally negative word lists (e.g., noose, corpse, snake) to remember showed a shift to the left side (right hemisphere) in performance. Thus, with the face recognition tasks, the left-visual-field superiority was enhanced by affectively positive or negative word lists, while the same word lists reduced the dichotic right-ear advantage (see Figure 8.1). A similar enhancement of right-hemispheric performance was produced by high-imagery lists (e.g., ink, limb, pencil), as opposed to low-imagery ones (e.g., shy, bland, evident). Statistically, the imagery and

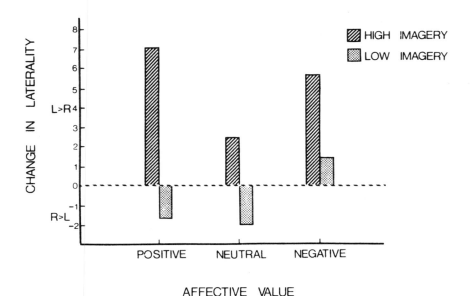

Figure 8.1. Shift in laterality on a face recognition task following the study of word lists varying in imagery and emotional content. (From Ley & Bryden, forthcoming.)

affect effects were independent, indicating that both factors had a distinct contribution to the change in performance. These results are rather different from those obtained in other studies of lateralization and emotion. Rather than showing a right-hemispheric superiority for recognizing emotion, they indicate that processes involved in remembering a list of emotionally charged words serves to activate the right hemisphere and improve relative performance for stimuli directed to that hemisphere. This priming effect suggests a generalized activation effect of the sort postulated by Kinsbourne (1970, 1975a). In this case, however, verbal material has not selectively primed the left hemisphere, as Kinsbourne has proposed, but the right hemisphere. Such findings, taken with those of Graves *et al.* (1981), would suggest that words high in imagery or emotionality have some right-hemisphere components to their representations.

In general, then, the visual-field studies are in agreement with the dichotic studies in showing a general right-hemispheric superiority for emotion judgments. The fact that similar results can be obtained with diverse procedures, and the dissociation of verbal and emotional effects shown by Ley (1980b), provide some fairly convincing evidence that the right hemisphere plays a special role in the perception of emotional stimuli. It is not so clear that this is the result of some precognitive recognition of affect, as suggested by Zajonc (1980). While some studies have shown an enhanced right-hemispheric effect for emotional, but not neutral, stimuli (e.g., Ley & Bryden, 1979a), other studies have found that the use of emotional material enhances the right-hemispheric effect for neutral stimuli as well (e.g., Bryden *et al.,* 1982). Certainly, the results of Ley's priming studies would suggest that thinking about emotional material produces a general activation of right-hemispheric processes.

It is also difficult to separate a right-hemispheric superiority for emotion recognition from the more general right-hemispheric superiority for nonverbal tasks that require holistic integration of information. Ley and Bryden (1979a) and Safer (1981) have attempted such a separation by having subjects match face stimuli with respect to both the emotion shown and the individual represented. The two tasks, however, may require the integration of somewhat different physical information, thereby leading to different confusions and a different pattern of results. In fact, one should not be surprised to find that similar mechanisms underlie asymmetries in both emotion and complex pattern recognition. Judgments of emotion, after all, involve the integration of information from a wide variety of different sources and therefore may provide an ideal example of the holistic or integrative perceptual process (Gazzaniga & LeDoux, 1978; Zajonc, 1980).

Lateralization of Emotional Expression

Although the dichotic and tachistoscopic studies have been concerned with the lateralization of emotion perception, there also exists evidence that the expression of emotion is asymmetric. Campbell (1978) and Sackheim, Gur, and Saucy (1978) had subjects pose for full frontal photographs. They then cut these photographs down the middle, reversed the halves, and produced left-side and right-side composites of the original faces (see Figure 8.2). Subjects judged that the left-half composite was more emotional than the right-half composite. Similarly, Borod and Caron (1980) videotaped posed facial expressions and found that judges rated the left side as more expressive. Moscovitch and Olds (1982) have also found that more expressive movements are made with the left side of the face, both in the laboratory and in a field setting.

The Moscovitch and Olds (1982) study is particularly illuminating since the asymmetry of expression was found only in right-handers and not in left-handers. Such a result provides support for the argument that the effect is related to cerebral asymmetry. Further, the tendency to gesture with the right hand while speaking (Kimura, 1973a, 1973b) was observed only when speech was not also accompanied by facial expressions, suggesting that the act of making a facial expression led to an activation of the right hemisphere.

Clinical Observations on Lateralization of Emotion

If the right hemisphere is more sensitive to emotional stimuli, representation of emotions should also be more fully developed in the right hemisphere than in the left. Instances of extreme emotional upset should lead to symptoms that would reveal this greater involvement of the right hemisphere. One example of intense emotional upset exists in the conversion type of hysterical neurosis, when symptoms of some physical illness, such as limb paralysis, appear in the absence of an underlying organic pathology. The physical symptoms serve a defensive or symbolic function, enabling the individual to avoid or to express fantasy in stressful experiences. Conversion hysteria may result in sensory, motor, or visceral symptoms, as with hysterical blindness, paralysis, or nausea.

If the right hemisphere is more involved in emotion, one might expect to find a preponderance of left-sided hysterical symptoms. Four studies have supported this view. Galin, Diamond, and Braff (1977) and

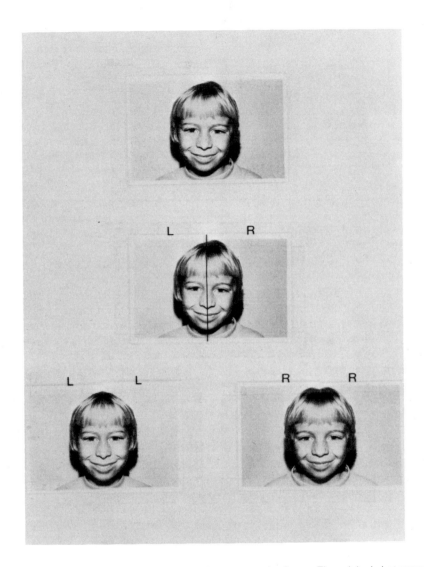

Figure 8.2. The construction of left and right composite faces. The original photograph is mirror imaged, and the two left halves paired to make the left composite, the two right halves paired to make the right composite.

Stern (1977) have reported that left-sided symptoms are twice as prevalent as right-sided ones among hospitalized hysterical psychiatric patients. Similar findings have been found in retrospective archival examinations of case studies by Ley (1980a) and by Axelrod, Noonan, and Atanacio (1980).

Hysterical conversion symptoms would seem to have an exclusively psychological etiology or basis, despite the reality of overt physical disability. Anosognosia is a somewhat different disorder that, like hysteria, seems to have a strong psychological component and specific sidedness differences in its manifestations, but unlike hysteria has a definite neurological basis. Anosognosia is a condition in which a patient with a severe neurological deficit, such as a hemiplegia or a hemianopia, is unaware of, is indifferent to, or simply denies the disability. An interesting aspect to this disorder is that sidedness differences and corresponding emotional reactions are apparent. Critchley (1953), for instance, concludes that anosognosics frequently display a disability of the nondominant (right) hemisphere and that anosognosia for hemiplegia is found with left but not right paralysis. Similarly, Flor-Henry (1976) asserts that it is an old neurological observation that euphoric indifference is a feature of cerebral tumors of the nondominant hemisphere. According to Hécaen's (1962) statistics, anosognosia is seven times more frequent with right-hemispheric damage than with left-hemispheric disturbance.

E. A. Weinstein and Kahn (1955) also conclude that anosognosia is much more prevalent following right-hemispheric damage than following damage to the left hemisphere. They suggest that the denial is an emotional reaction to the deficit, to the patient's social attitudes toward illness, or to symbolic aspects of the disability. At the same time, they are careful to point out the danger of attributing the emotional effects to the intact right hemisphere. For instance, the greater incidence of denial after right-hemispheric lesions may be due to aphasic symptoms masking the anosognosia following left-hemispheric injury.

For our purposes, however, the important point is that a characteristic emotional reaction seems to occur following injury to the right hemisphere. The parallel with hysterical conversion neuroses is obvious.

Effects of Unilateral Brain Lesions

In the 1930s, clinicians were reporting observations on the emotional behavior of patients affected by unilateral lesions. The usual description of the response to left-hemispheric damage was described as a catastrophic reaction (Alford, 1933; Goldstein, 1939). In contrast, right-hemispheric responses were considered to be ones of indifference. Gainotti (1969) compared the incidence of these two types of responses in 150 cases of unilateral brain damage. Catastrophic reactions were reported for 62% of the left-hemisphere cases, but for only 10% of the right-hemisphere cases. Conversely, the incidence of indifference reactions was 38% with right-hemispheric damage and only 11% with left-hemispheric damage. Catastrophic reactions included such emotional behaviors as crying, swearing, anxiety reactions, and suggestive behavior. Indifferent reactions included explicit indifference, joking, minimization, and anosognosia. In a subsequent study of 160 lateralized cerebrovascular lesions, 80 to the left and 80 to the right, Gainotti (1972) again found a strong association between catastrophic reactions and dominant lesions, as well as between indifferent reactions and nondominant lesions.

Hécaen (1962) also found a greater incidence of catastrophic reactions in left-hemisphere lesions (25.7%) than in right-hemisphere lesions (12.9%). Indifference to failure was found in only 16.5% of left-hemisphere cases and in 33% of right-hemisphere cases.

However, Ross and Mesulam (1979) have reported on two patients who lost the ability to modulate the affective components of speech following right-hemispheric damage. Their report would indicate that the right hemisphere exerts an effect on all types of affective speech, whether positive or negative. It therefore stands in agreement with the general pattern observed in dichotic and tachistoscopic studies of normal subjects. Furthermore, DeKosky, Heilman, Bowers, and Valenstein (1980) have reported that right-hemispheric patients are poorer than those with left-hemispheric damage at discriminating emotional faces or naming emotional scenes.

In general, though, clinical observations of patients with unilateral brain lesions suggest that there may be a particular emotional reaction that is characteristic of injury to each hemisphere. Other evidence also points to this asymmetry of affective response.

Terzian (1964) demonstrated that intracarotid injection of sodium amytal produces different behavior in patients when injected on the dominant as opposed to the nondominant side. The procedure is typically used prior to surgery to assess hemispheric dominance for language. Terzian observed that severe emotional reactions often accompanied the dissipation of the anesthetic and that specific emotional responses typified lateralization of the injections. Injections of the dominant hemisphere were distinguished by the appearance of characteristic emotional reactions of the depressive–catastrophic type. Injections of the nondominant side evidenced emotional reactions of the opposite type, euphoric–maniacal.

Terzian's findings have been corroborated by Rossi and Rosadini (1967) and by Alema, Rosadini, and Rossi (1961). Alema *et al.* (1961) indicate that the lateralized affective response was seen most clearly in patients without brain damage. However, Milner (1974) has failed to observe any lateralization of emotional response to sodium amytal.

Further support for the possible asymmetry of affective responses comes from research on the efficacy of electroconvulsive shock treatment (ECT). If there are hemispheric differences in emotionality, one might expect that therapeutic outcomes would differ as a function of which hemisphere received the shock. Reviews by Galin (1974) and Robertson and Inglis (1977) suggest that unilateral nondominant ECT is therapeutically more effective than bilateral ECT and also minimizes the memory disturbances and confusion that follow conventional bilateral ECT.

Deglin (1973) also offers some interesting evidence as to the effects of unilateral ECT on emotion recognition. He reports that nondominant ECT disrupted the ability to recognize the emotional tone of vocal expressions. At the same time, right-hemisphere ECT led to positive, happy responses from the patient, whereas left-hemisphere ECT produced distressed and fearful responses.

One Hemisphere or Both?

One major difference exists between the clinical studies on emotion and the majority of the normal studies. In the clinical studies, characteristic emotional responses follow the invasion of either hemisphere. Patients show catastrophic responses and depression following either damage to or suppression of the left hemisphere, whereas right-hemisphere disturbance leads to euphoria or indifference reactions. Such findings would suggest that both hemispheres are involved in emotional reactivity, although in different ways. In contrast, the majority of studies with normal subjects indicate that the right hemisphere has a specific role in the appreciation of emotion.

Several interpretations of these data are possible. First of all, it may well be that lateralization is different for the perceptual and expressive components of emotion (Ley & Bryden, 1981). Most of the normal studies involve the recognition of emotional stimuli (e.g., Carmon & Nachshon, 1973) or the influence of affective priming material on the

recognition of other stimuli (e.g., Ley & Bryden, 1979b). By this argument, the right hemisphere has primacy for the recognition and reception of emotional stimuli, while each hemisphere has a characteristic role
in the expression of affect. Tucker (1981) has taken a position similar to
this in suggesting that the right hemisphere is responsible for the initial
elaboration of emotional arousal, whereas the left hemisphere serves to
regulate the responsivity of the right hemisphere. The fact that a left-
sided dominance has been observed in studies of facial expression
(Moscovitch & Olds, 1982) would seem to belie any distinction based on
a difference between expression and reception.

It is also true that the majority of studies showing a right-hemisphere
effect for both positive and negative affect have involved relatively benign manipulations of affect, whereas those showing a dissociation of
the affective reactions of the two hemispheres involve rather stronger
emotional experiences. Again, however, there are exceptions to this
generalization, as in the face recognition study of Reuter-Lorenz and
Davidson (1981).

A third possibility is that the change in emotional expression following left-hemispheric disturbance may be only a by-product of the language effects that occur as a result of the damage. Disturbances of
speech and language may be particularly frustrating to patients and lead
to behaviors that are classified as depressive. By this argument, the left-
hemispheric disturbances are secondary to the language disturbance
and do not represent a true lateralization of emotion.

It is also possible that we are dealing with several different laterality
effects. The tasks employed to detect emotional asymmetry in normals
often involve the recognition of complex stimuli, and they may lead to
right-hemisphere effects, not because the stimuli are emotional, but because they involve complex pattern recognition. Such an explanation
does not seem to hold for the priming studies, such as those of Ley and
Bryden (1979b). However, Heilman and Van Den Abell (1979) have suggested that the right hemisphere dominates activation. The presentation
of an affectively loaded priming list may serve to increase general
arousal more in the right hemisphere than in the left and thus lead to the
right-hemisphere improvement noted by Ley and Bryden (1979b). In
addition to pattern recognition and activation components, it remains
possible that there is an underlying specialization of the two hemispheres for different emotional states—the left for positive affect and the
right for negative (Tucker, 1981). The wealth of different results, then,
could be explained by the interplay of these different factors. This, of
course, is highly speculative, and there remain a variety of fruitful questions to ask about the lateralization of emotional processes.

Physiological Measures
of Asymmetry

The extreme difficulty of separating hemispheric and experimental effects with behavioral measures of lateralization of function has led many investigators to search for more direct measures of hemispheric asymmetry. Not surprisingly, such people have turned to various measures of the physiological activity of the brain. In most cases, work along these lines has employed some measure of the electrical activity of the brain, such as the ongoing electroencephalogram (EEG) or the average evoked response (AER) to some stimulus, recorded from scalp electrodes. In the past few years, technical advances have made it possible to record regional cerebral blood flow (rCBF) and to assess local metabolic rates in the brain. These techniques have also found application in the study of hemispheric asymmetry.

For the beginning investigator, the electrophysiological techniques have an almost seductive appeal. There is something intuitively "scientific" and "objective" about the use of electrodes, amplifiers, and recorders, about watching a pen produce a permanent record of some mysterious events going on inside the brain that cannot be achieved in a dichotic listening or tachistoscopic recognition paradigm. Yet electrophysiological studies are just as subject to problems, artifacts, and poor experimental design as are behavioral ones, and problems of interpretation arise with electrophysiological data just as with behavioral data.

In the normal subject, electrophysiological techniques involve recording from the surface of the scalp the electrical activity in the underlying brain tissue. Of necessity, this activity is summated over a large number of neurons and may well incorporate dendritic potentials and nonneural electrical activity as well as axonal potentials. Interpreting changes in such activity is not always an easy task. Most of our dependent measures in electrophysiological studies involve changes in the amplitude of activity, in the spectral composition of the activity, or, in the case of the evoked response, in the latency of the response. Yet we have no particularly strong reasons for believing that bigger or faster responses are necessarily important for behavior (Wall, 1975). A proper understanding of electrophysiological changes will depend on a comprehensive theory of brain activity, and we are presently far from achieving this goal. The interpretation of electrophysiological data is further confused by the fact that the changes we observe may be correlated with a particular stimulus event but have nothing to do with the process in which we are interested (Uttal, 1973).

What then should one expect to find from electrophysiological studies? From the clinical evidence and from the preceding chapters, one should expect to find evidence for more active neural processing in the left hemisphere when the subject is engaged in language-related activities and more active processing in the right hemisphere when the subject is engaged in certain types of nonlinguistic activities.

Asymmetries of electrical activity may arise from such simple things as a difference in skull thickness or a biased placement of a reference electrode. Thus, it is important to look for a *dissociation* of asymmetries, such that activity over one hemisphere is greater under one condition, while the reverse is true under another condition, in the same subjects. To make a case that what we are measuring is related to functional asymmetry, it is important to show some form of dissociation or task dependence. As a further step, one would like to show that the electrophysiological asymmetry has something in common with other asymmetries. The sodium amytal technique provides a way of assessing speech lateralization, and we know that we can expect to find a small number of people who are right-hemispheric for speech. If electrophysiological measures are truly related to functional lateralization, then we should expect to find that the electrophysiological asymmetry reverses in individuals with known right-hemispheric speech.

Because the sodium amytal test is contraindicated for use with normal subjects, this last suggestion may be unrealistic. If we can only be certain of speech lateralization in neurological patients with known cerebral abnormalities, we may not have an appropriate group on which to test the reversal of an electrophysiological asymmetry. An alternative approach is to isolate a group of normal subjects in whom the presumptive incidence of right-hemispheric speech is very high and compare them to a group in whom the presumptive incidence of left-hemispheric speech is very high. As indicated earlier, virtually all right-handers have left-hemispheric speech representation. Left-handers have a much higher incidence of right-hemispheric speech and so represent a possible comparison group, but the incidence is not so high that the contrast is ideal (see Chapter 10). Perhaps a more fruitful approach would be to link electrophysiological measures with some of the behavioral techniques described in Chapters 2–6.

Electroencephalographic Measures

The most striking characteristics of ongoing EEG recorded from the scalp are the high-amplitude rhythmical waves occurring in the 8–13 Hz frequency range, termed *alpha* activity, and the relatively high-frequency (13–30 Hz) low-amplitude activity, called *beta* activity. Normally, alpha is particularly prevalent when the subject is relaxed and has his or her eyes closed, and it is often interpreted as a sign of inhibition of activity in the areas in which it is found (Andersen & Andersson, 1968). Beta activity, in contrast, is usually found in aroused, alert conditions and is taken to indicate an activated cortex.

As this should indicate, the spectral composition of the EEG is often of primary concern in its analysis. Although alpha and beta activity will be of primary concern here, many other types of waves and rhythms have been identified (Lindsley & Wicke, 1974, p. 26). In addition, one is often concerned with the amount of activity shown by the EEG, as measured by the integrated amplitude or *power* of the wave. Power can be measured either across the full frequency spectrum or within one of the typological categories, such as alpha.

It has become commonplace to describe the recording sites employed in terms of the International 10–20 system (Jasper, 1958). This notation system is illustrated in Figure 9.1. The comparable sites in the right hemisphere are assigned even numbers (i.e., C_4 is homologous to C_3). Positions along the midline are assigned the subscript z.

In bioelectrical recording, one is recording the electrical potential difference between a site of interest and some "neutral" or "silent" area. Unfortunately, no truly silent area exists, and the location of the reference electrode thus becomes of critical importance in studies of asymmetry. Reference electrodes placed on or near the skull may pick up brain activity, those placed elsewhere may pick up such artifacts as heart rate or eye movement. The most common reference points employed in asymmetry research are the nose, linked earlobes, or a midline point (C_z).

The earliest studies of EEG asymmetry were concerned with lateral differences in activity while the subjects were at rest (e.g., Cornil &

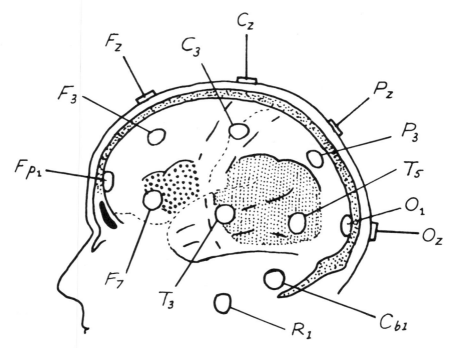

Figure 9.1. Human brain viewed from the left, showing the main landmarks in the International 10–20 system for noting electrode sites. The subscript z denotes a midline position. A subscript 1 marks the left earlobe and C_{b1} the left mastoid. The large-stippled section is Broca's area, the small-stippled area is Wernicke's area. The dotted line underlying C_3 is the central sulcus. [From Marsh, G. R. Asymmetry of electrophysiological phenomena and its relation to behavior in humans. In M. Kinsbourne (Ed.), *Asymmetrical function of the brain.* Cambridge: Cambridge University Press, 1978. Reprinted with permission.]

Gastaut, 1947; Raney, 1939). The results of these studies were ambiguous, with many indicating a greater EEG amplitude over the right hemisphere, but with no clear-cut relation to handedness. Butler and Glass (1976) reviewed this work and concluded that lateral differences in resting measures of total amplitude or alpha amplitude are most likely a product of the recording and analytic techniques, rather than a feature of the resting EEG.

Butler and Glass (1974) and Glass and Butler (1973) recorded alpha activity from occipitoparietocentral areas while subjects were engaged in mental arithmetic and found a suppression of alpha over the left hemisphere. Opening the eyes did not produce a comparable asymmetry of alpha suppression. The right-handed subjects in the study produced marked asymmetries, whereas the left-handers ($N=7$) showed no consistent asymmetry. While this study does not involve a clear dissociation of different activities, nor does it have any behavioral check on the cognitive activity of the subjects, the distinction between the left- and right-handed subgroups does provide some independent verification that the alpha suppression is related to functional cerebral asymmetry.

A more thorough and systematic series of studies was carried out during the 1970s by Galin, Ornstein, and their co-workers. In the initial study (Galin & Ornstein, 1972), EEG recordings were taken from four electrode placements: T_3, T_4, P_3, and P_4, all referenced to C_z. Subjects performed a number of different cognitive tasks, selected to tap the functions of the two hemispheres and to provide a control for movement artifact. The verbal tasks were writing a letter and mentally composing a letter while fixating. The spatial tasks were a block design task in which the subject had to memorize a two-dimensional geometric pattern and then reconstruct it with multicolored blocks, and a modified version of the Minnesota Paper Form Board test, in which the subject was presented with a sectioned figure and asked to choose mentally which of five assembled figures could be constructed from the sections.

EEG recordings were divided into 1-sec epochs, and those in which gross artifacts had occurred were deleted. The average power over the 1–35 Hz band was then determined for each acceptable epoch. From these averaged power values, the ratio of right- to left-hemispheric activity (R/L ratio) was determined for each task and electrode placement (P_4/P_3; T_4/T_3). The results, for nine right-handed subjects without familial history of sinistrality, are shown in Table 9.1. Data for the temporal leads are based on eight subjects.

Although there is a general tendency for the power ratios to be

Table 9.1
Mean R/L Power Ratios for Varying Electrode Placements, Tasks, and Degree of Motor Involvement

Task	Parietal	Temporal
Spatial tasks		
Blocks (motor)	1.15	.83
Form board (mental)	1.15	.90
Verbal tasks		
Written letter (motor)	1.30	1.01
Mental letter	1.21	1.02

Note. From Galin and Ornstein (1972).

greater than 1, indicating more power in the right hemisphere, especially at the parietal leads, the ratio is consistently higher for verbal tasks than for spatial tasks. That is, if greater power can be considered indicative of more synchronous activity and thus of less involvement in the task, the relative involvement of the right hemisphere was greatest in the spatial tasks and that of the left hemisphere greatest in the verbal tasks. No significant effect of motor activity, nor interaction of motor activity with task, was observed.

This initial study provides the dissociation between right- and left-hemispheric tasks that we consider critical for such studies. Furthermore, it actively engages the subjects in observable behavior, so that there is some external check on whether or not they are doing as instructed.

A subsequent experiment employing the same tasks and electrode placements indicated that the greatest differences in EEG asymmetry occurred in the alpha band (8–13 Hz) (Doyle, Ornstein, & Galin, 1974). This study also indicated that somewhat clearer distinctions between verbal and nonverbal tasks were obtained with the temporal placements (T_4/T_3) than with the parietal placements (P_4/P_3).

Doyle *et al.* also investigated a number of additional tasks: serial arithmetic, verbal listening, tonal memory, and manipulating an $x-y$ plotting toy (Etch-a-Sketch®). At the temporal site, the alpha power ratios for both blocks and Etch-a-Sketch® were significantly lower than for any of the verbal tasks. Alpha ratios while composing a mental letter were higher than for any of the nonverbal tasks, and those recorded when writing a letter exceeded all but those for the tonal memory task. In general, asymmetries were more clear-cut for those tasks with a motor component: blocks, Etch-a-Skech®, written letter, and serial arithmetic.

In subsequent research, this group has found even more marked task-dependent asymmetries with central placements (C_4/C_3). In addition, left-handers have been shown to exhibit different patterns of asymmetry than right-handers (Johnstone, Galin, & Herron, 1979).

Galin, Johnstone, and Herron (1978) investigated the effects of task difficulty on the block design task. They employed 14 different block designs of graded complexity and found both higher alpha power and higher R/L ratios with increasing difficulty. In some ways, this seems to be an anomalous result: Writing yields a high R/L ratio, and blocks a low one. This indicates that there is relatively more alpha in the right hemisphere during writing, presumably showing that the left hemisphere is more involved in this task. At the same time, block designs of increasing difficulty yield increasingly greater R/L ratios, though never as high as the writing condition. This would seem to suggest that the right hemisphere becomes *less* involved in a spatial task as the task becomes more difficult. As alternatives, Galin *et al.* (1978) suggest that the more difficult task may proceed at a slower rate or may involve activity in areas that were not recorded.

Interpretation of these data is further confused by the results of analyses of individual subject data. For each individual, Galin *et al.* (1978) ranked the order of difficulty of the block designs, both in terms of subjective estimates of difficulty and in terms of time to complete the design. These rankings were then correlated with EEG alpha power measures from each individual recording site and from the R/L ratios (C_4/C_3, P_4/P_3). Of the 16 subjects, 7 showed some significant correlation between task difficulty and alpha power in the right hemisphere. However, 7 subjects, including 4 of those who showed right hemisphere increases, also showed correlations between task difficulty and alpha power in the left hemisphere, and 5 subjects showed no significant correlations at all. In 4 subjects, the R/L ratio correlated positively with item difficulty, but one showed a significant correlation only at the parietal leads. In fact, examination of the individual correlations (Galin *et al.*, 1978, p. 465) suggests that alpha power increases with task difficulty over both the left and right hemispheres, especially at C_3 and C_4.

The pattern of correlations with item difficulty not only raises many questions about how changes in alpha power in the two hemispheres should be interpreted but also raises serious questions about the use of EEG asymmetry as a measure of functional specialization. If power ratios change within individuals as a function of task difficulty, then differences between individuals on a fixed task may not provide a "pure" measure of cerebral asymmetry but may be contaminated by how difficult the task is for the subject.

This same group of investigators reported a study dealing with a variety of visuospatial tasks (Ornstein, Johnstone, Herron, & Swencionis, 1980). They employed tests of mental rotation, face recognition, picture completion, arc–circle and circle–circle matching, and part–whole assembly, as well as a verbal test involving definitions of words, while recording from both central (C_3/C_4) and parietal (P_3/P_4) regions, referenced to C_z. In general, alpha power was relatively greater in the left hemisphere for spatial tasks than during the verbal tasks, indicating a differential involvement of the two hemispheres. Effects were greatest at the parietal leads. Interestingly, mental rotation showed a pattern rather like the verbal task, suggesting that it may involve left-hemisphere processes. Furthermore, the circle–circle matching task was more right-hemispheric than the arc–circle task. Ornstein *et al.* (1980) suggest that the strategy used is more critical than the task itself and that the mental rotation task is sufficiently complex to encourage an analytic, verbal strategy.

This section has concentrated on the work of Galin and his colleagues, not because it is the only work in the area, but because it is representative of the current state of knowledge and because Galin and his associates have attempted to address some of the questions that have emerged in earlier chapters. More detailed reviews of work on EEG asymmetries have been published by Butler and Glass (1976), Donchin, Kutas, and McCarthy (1977), Donchin, McCarthy, and Kutas (1977), and Marsh (1978). The evidence does indicate that relatively more power is observed in the alpha band in the right hemisphere during verbal activities, such as writing, whereas relatively more power is observed in the left hemisphere during spatial activities, such as solving a block design problem. Furthermore, Johnstone *et al.* (1979) have found that their EEG measures distinguish between individuals of putatively different cerebral organization (i.e., right- and left-handers). Thus, the evidence is relatively strong that EEG measures can be used to provide at least a global assessment of cerebral organization.

At the same time, measures of EEG alpha asymmetry seem to be subject to experimental effects in the same way that behavioral measures are. The fact that EEG asymmetry is affected by task difficulty must be considered. Furthermore, the evidence indicates that EEG asymmetry is more pronounced when there is motor involvement in the task. Despite the valiant attempts to remove any possible motor artifact, the pattern of arm and hand movements involved in solving a block design problem are different from those involved in writing. Perhaps some of the EEG alpha asymmetry arises from the motor components of the tasks employed (Gevins, Zeitlin, Doyle, Schaffer, Yingling, Callaway, & Yeager, 1979).

Although task-dependent differences in alpha asymmetry exist, it remains unclear just how they are produced and how they are to be interpreted. Despite the promise of the approach, EEG measures must be viewed with as much caution as the behavioral ones. It would be rash to assume that differences in EEG measures *must* reflect differences in cerebral organization.

Averaged Evoked Potentials

The EEG is a measure of the ongoing activity in the brain, without specific reference to any particular event taking place in the subject's world. When specific stimulus events occur, they produce consistent changes in the electrical activity of the brain. Normally, these are too small to be seen against the background of ongoing EEG activity. However, if one presents the same stimulus repeatedly at known points in time, records the EEG during the time interval following the stimulus, and averages this over a number of trials, one finds particular electrical changes that are related to the occurrence of the stimulus. Electrical activity that is unrelated to the stimulus tends to act as noise and to be averaged out over a number of trials, leaving *event-related potentials*. This is the method of the *averaged evoked response* (AER). A typical AER, in this case to a flash, is shown in Figure 9.2. Some of the general characteristics of an AER are shown in this figure.

Following the stimulus, there is an initial negative peak, usually occurring between 80 and 120 msec after the onset of the stimulus. Following this, there is a positive peak occurring between 140 and 240 msec and then a late positive peak occurring some 270–400 msec after the onset of the stimulus. These peaks are identified either by numbering them serially (i.e., N1, P2, P3) or by indicating their direction and approximate latency (e.g., N100, P300).

A variety of different measurement techniques have been applied to AERs. It is common to measure the latency and amplitude of the various peaks, or the difference in amplitude between one positive peak and an adjacent negative one. Wall (1975) has viewed this tendency somewhat caustically, arguing that there is little evidence that "faster" or "bigger" is necessarily better. An alternative approach has been to perform a point-by-point comparison of the AERs obtained under two different conditions, with a view to isolating the loci at which the waveforms differ. While there are some advantages to this approach, it encounters the statistical problems associated with multiple comparisons, as well as questions about whether one should expect time parameters to be the same in different individuals. As AER research advances, more sophisticated methods of data analysis are being employed (Chapman, McCrary, Bragdon, & Chapman, 1979; Desmedt, 1977; Donchin, Kutas, & McCarthy, 1977).

Many of the cautions applicable to EEG research are also pertinent to AER studies. Generalized hemispheric asymmetries observed in the AER to some simple stimulus, such as a click or a flash, are not likely to be of major significance in understanding the nature of functional cerebral asymmetry. There are too many simple explanations, such as differential skull thickness, and too little knowledge of what the subject is doing while watching a flash or listening to a click to obtain very much in the way of clear-cut evidence about cerebral asymmetry.

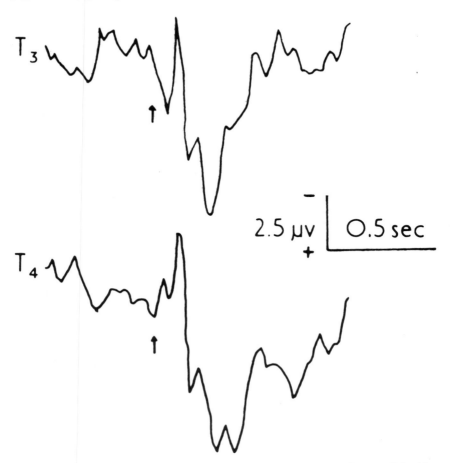

Figure 9.2. Average evoked potentials recorded from the temporal area, elicited by a dim red light at the arrow. [From Marsh, G. R. Asymmetry of electrophysiological phenomena and its relation to behavior in humans. In M. Kinsbourne (Ed.), *Asymmetrical function of the brain.* Cambridge: Cambridge University Press, 1978. Reprinted with permission.]

Most of the early work using AERs that actually employed a task that might be expected to engage one hemisphere or the other involved auditory stimuli. In the auditory domain, stimuli can be presented binaurally, while the subject is engaged in tasks that are either language related or not. Visually, the choice of appropriate tasks has been somewhat more difficult to accomplish.

One of the earliest studies to investigate task dependence in the auditory AER was that of C. C. Wood, Goff, and Day (1971). In one task, they required subjects to discriminate between synthesized versions of the syllables /ba/ and /da/; in a second task, they required a pitch discrimination between two versions of /ba/ with differing fundamental frequencies. Recordings were taken from central (C_4/C_3) and temporal (T_4/T_3) sites, referenced to linked earlobes. The design permitted a comparison of the AERs produced by the common /ba/ syllable under two different conditions—one in which the stimuli were being treated linguistically (the phoneme discrimination), and one in which they were to be treated nonlinguistically (the pitch discrimination). Wood *et al.* found, at both recording sites, a difference between the speech and tonal conditions in the left hemisphere but not in the right. The largest differences occurred between 100 and 200 msec and were generally reflected in the amplitude of the N1–P2 difference. Although this study is highly suggestive and employs a most ingenious task, Friedman, Simson, Ritter, and Rapin (1975) have been very critical of the statistical analysis employed. The use of linked ears as a reference may also have produced biases, since temporal lobe activity may have been picked up at the supposedly neutral site. In a similar vein, Morrell and Salamy (1971) found larger N1 deflections to nonsense words in the left hemisphere, but their work employed no nonlanguage control.

Friedman *et al.* (1975) asked subjects to listen attentively to words or to respond to one specific target while listening to a series of words. They found that the P300 amplitude increased with increased task demands, but there were only isolated and unsystematic lateral asymmetries.

Attempts to record AERs in situations more analogous to the dichotic listening procedure have met with only partial success. Tanguay, Taub, Doubleday, and Clarkson (1977), using consonant–vowel syllables, and Mononen and Seitz (1977), using clicks, found that monaural inputs lead to larger AERs in the hemisphere opposite the ear stimulated. Neither study observed any hemisphere effect. Similarly, Haaland (1974) found that the positive component of the AER was larger over the right hemisphere when listening to speech stimuli. However, no differences were found between dichotic, diotic, and monaural conditions.

Hink, Hillyard, and Benson (1978) had subjects perform a dichotic phoneme discrimination task while attending to one ear. Although they found no systematic hemisphere differences, they found that the N1 component of the AER was enhanced to all stimuli presented to the attended ear, whereas the P3 component was enhanced in the attended ear to those stimuli that were designated as targets.

This research leaves us in a rather ambiguous position. On the one hand, C. C. Wood *et al.* (1971) have isolated task-dependent differences in the left hemisphere. However, these have proven difficult to replicate (Friedman *et al.*, 1975). Studies employing dichotic procedures not only have not found the source of the robust right-ear effect found in behavioral studies but also have indicated that specific components of the auditory AER are attention and task demands (Hink *et al.*, 1978). While certainly effects are taking place, the early auditory AER research leaves us with more problems and questions than answers.

A much more sophisticated statistical approach to dealing with auditory evoked responses has been employed with considerable success by Molfese and his colleagues (e.g., Molfese, 1980; see also Chapman *et al.*, 1979). In this procedure, the asymmetry of electrocortical responses to nonlateralized stimuli is investigated. In a typical experiment, the average evoked response is determined for each subject at each of several recording sites and under each condition. The data matrix of k AERs by n time points is then subjected to a principal components analysis, and a set of orthogonal factors are extracted. These factors are then rotated according to varimax criteria to improve their distinctiveness. The factors resulting from one such analysis are shown in Figure 9.3 (Molfese, 1980). As the next step, factor scores are calculated for each of the original AERs. These factor scores can then be subjected to analysis of variance to determine if any of the effects involving sites, hemispheres, or conditions reach acceptable levels of significance. In the data shown in Figure 9.3, for example, Factor 8 showed a significant conditions by hemisphere interaction, indicating that stimulus-related events were occurring with a latency of about 350 msec in one hemisphere but not in the other.

Using this general approach and a careful selection of stimulus materials, Molfese has been able to show that events correlated with second-formant transition information are found only in the left hemisphere (Molfese, 1978a), even in newborn and preterm infants (Molfese & Molfese, 1979a, 1980). In contrast, events correlated with distinctions in voice onset time are found in the right hemisphere (Molfese, 1978b; Molfese & Hess, 1978; Molfese & Molfese, 1979b). These right-hemispheric events have been found even when nonspeech stimuli are used (Molfese, 1980). Finally, Molfese (1979) has noted that both left and right hemispheres show responses that distinguish between meaningful and nonsense sounds, and has even isolated one component that suggests a subcortical component in semantic processing. This research represents the most impressive use of AER techniques to determine the important asymmetries in the perception of speech and speechlike sounds. Molfese's work would suggest that the left hemisphere is specialized for

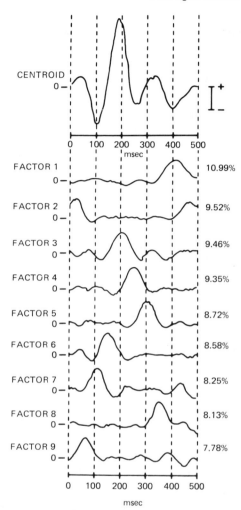

Figure 9.3. The centroid (group averaged AER) for a speech signal, and the nine orthogonal components identified by principal components analysis. (From Molfese, D. L. Hemispheric specialization for temporal information: Implications for the perception of voicing cues during speech perception. *Brain and Language*, 1980, *11*, 285–299. Reprinted with permission.)

detecting the rapid second-formant transitions of speech and indicates that these mechanisms are present even in neonates.

Another promising solution to some of the problems in auditory AER research has been provided by Shucard, Shucard, and Thomas (1977). Rather than asking subjects to deal with auditory stimuli in different ways, these investigators studied the AER to click stimuli while subjects were involved in tasks expected to engage one hemisphere more than the other. AERs to pairs of tone pips were recorded from the temporal region (T_3 and T_4), using a vertex reference (C_z). As a verbal task, subjects listened to prose passages selected for their lack of imagery. They were required to respond to certain target words in each passage. As a nonverbal task, subjects heard musical passages and were required to identify simple melodies when they occurred in the selection. Shucard *et al.* report that left-hemisphere AERs were significantly *greater* in amplitude than right-hemisphere AERs during the verbal condition, whereas the reverse was true during the musical condition. Since C_z produces high-amplitude responses to auditory stimuli, and since the AERs represent voltage differences between C_z and the recording sites, the authors argue that the greater-amplitude AERs actually represent *lower*-amplitude responses at the T_3 recording site for verbal stimuli and at the T_4 site for musical stimuli. This work is encouraging in the identification of a task-dependent hemispheric asymmetry, but the interpretation is far from obvious. It is clear that this approach merits further work.

As with auditory AERs, the initial work on hemispheric asymmetry and visual AERs involved nonlateralized stimuli. In one of the earliest studies, Buchsbaum and Fedio (1969) presented subjects with computer-generated words, random dot patterns, and simple geometric designs while recording from occipital electrodes (O_1, O_2, referenced to ipsilateral earlobe). Stimuli were constructed from light blue dots, presented on a blue black background, and included three-letter words, random dot patterns constructed by rearranging the dots in the letters of the words, and simple but meaningless designs. Subjects simply observed the stimuli as they were presented.

For each recording site, evoked potentials were grouped to produce four AERs, two associated with the verbal stimuli and two with the nonverbal stimuli, on each of 2 days. A discrimination index (zeta) was then calculated: A positive zeta value indicates that the two independent replicates of the AER from the same stimulus resemble each other more than they resemble the dissimilar stimulus. All types of stimuli had better replicates in the right hemisphere than in the left, but AERs from the left hemisphere were more distinct for verbal and nonverbal stimuli than those in the right hemisphere. In addition, verbal stimuli had shorter AER latencies. Like the study of C. C. Wood *et al.* (1971) in the auditory domain, this study provides evidence of a task-dependent asymmetry.

Poon, Thompson, and Marsh (1976) had subjects perform two tasks in response to briefly presented letter pairs. In one condition, subjects simply responded as soon as they saw the letters; in the other, they indicated whether both letters were vowels or consonants or whether there was one of each. AERs were recorded from T_3 and T_4, referenced to linked earlobes. In the vowel–consonant task, larger N1 and P2 amplitudes were found over the left hemisphere, while only the P2 component showed a significant asymmetry during the simple reaction time task. In addition, the vowel–consonant task yielded larger P2 and P3 components overall than did the reaction time task.

Rugg and Beaumont (1978b) have also attempted to show distinctions in the visual AER between verbal and nonverbal stimuli. As a verbal task, subjects were asked to detect targets that included a letter containing the sound "ee"; as a visuospatial task, they were asked to detect targets containing a bilaterally symmetric nonsense pattern. Recordings were taken from a point one-quarter of the way between occipital (O_1, O_2) and posterior temporal (T_5, T_6) loci, referenced to C_z. Rugg and Beaumont found that P1 had a shorter latency in the right hemisphere than in the left for both stimulus types and that the P230–N265 amplitude was greater in both hemispheres during the letter task than during the visuospatial task. While the authors conclude that the right hemisphere was preeminent in early stages of processing, there are no task by hemisphere interactions in this study, and thus it fails to provide a clear replication of the findings of Buchsbaum and Fedio (1969).

Other investigators have attempted to duplicate the lateralized presentation of visual stimuli that yields behavioral asymmetries. Rugg and Beaumont (1978a) had one group of subjects signal letters containing the sound "ee" and another indicate letters containing a right angle. Recording sites were the same as in the previous study. Significant hemisphere by visual field interactions were found for P1 and N1 under both conditions: The hemisphere contralateral to the visual field stimulated produced these components at a shorter latency than did the ipsilateral hemisphere. Such findings are not unexpected in light of the anatomy of the visual system. The two conditions are different in that the N1–P2 amplitude in the left hemisphere differed as a function of field of presentation in the verbal tasks but not in the spatial task, and the P2–N2 amplitude was greater in the left hemisphere in the spatial task but not in the verbal one. Although there is again evidence for task-dependent hemispheric differences, the significance of these findings is not immediately clear.

Somewhat shorter latency hemispheric differences were found by Ledlow, Swanson, and Kinsbourne (1978). They had subjects identify letter pairs that were either physically identical or identical in name only, while recording from occipitoparietal sites (between O_1 and P_3,

O_2 and P_4, referenced to linked mastoids). Interactions of task with hemisphere occurred for P130 and N170 components. In both cases, the left-hemisphere amplitudes were smaller for different-case pairs than for same-case pairs, whereas the reverse was true in the right hemisphere.

While these studies provide evidence for task-dependent hemispheric differences, the significance of the findings is not easy to assess. In different studies, hemispheric asymmetries are manifested in different components of the AER, and there is not even any general agreement on the approximate latency of the significant effects: Some studies find their effects as early as 130 msec after the stimulus onset, others as late as 350 msec.

An alternative approach to the recording of visual AERs is to use a simple stimulus, such as a flash, and engage the subject in different mental activities presumed to activate one hemisphere or the other. Beaumont and Mayes (1977) had subjects either count the letters in nursery rhymes containing either an "ee" sound or a curve while recording flash-evoked potentials from central (C_4/C_3) or parietal (P_4/P_3) sites, referenced to C_z. They found no task by hemisphere interactions, although a number of lateral asymmetries were found, extending as late as 380 msec. Galin and Ellis (1975) found verbal–spatial differences in the early components (N100–P150) of flash-evoked potentials but concluded that their measure of EEG alpha power was more sensitive to task differences than was the AER.

Papanicolaou (1980) used the photic probe technique while subjects performed detection tasks based on semantic, phonetic, or acoustic cues. During recording, subjects monitored a word list and signaled the presence of words containing a particular stop consonant, a particular category of word, or a particular acoustic change, such as an intensity change. The same word lists were used for each of the detection instructions and for a control condition in which no response was required. AERs were recorded from frontal (F_7/F_8), temporal (T_3/T_4), and a point near the supramarginal and angular gyri approximated by the midpoint between T_3 and P_3 or T_4 and P_4, all referenced to linked earlobes. The primary measure in this study was the amplitude shift from P1 (average latency 92 msec) and N1 (average latency 133 msec). As compared to the control condition, P1–N1 amplitude decreased in the left hemisphere and increased in the right hemisphere for both phonetic and semantic tasks, but remained essentially unchanged for the acoustic detection task. These changes seem to be rather more pronounced at the T_3–P_3/T_4–P_4 locus and least at the T_3/T_4 locus. This study is particularly interesting in that it suggests that activation of the left hemisphere (reducing the P1–N1 amplitude) may inhibit input of information to the right hemisphere (enhancing P1–N1 amplitude).

One other series of studies, that of A. E. Davis and Wada (1974a, 1977a, 1977b, 1978), is relevant, if only because of the problems it raises. Davis and Wada have studied AERs to click and flash stimuli through a procedure called coherence analysis. This technique provides a measure of the similarity of AER waveforms at different loci. Davis and Wada have also employed epileptic subjects of known speech lateralization in their studies, so that some evidence can be obtained about which aspects of the AER are in fact related to speech lateralization. In their initial study (1974), they found that occipito–temporal coherence for click responses was greater on the speech-dominant side in the majority of their subjects (8 out of 10 epileptics, 10 out of 12 normals). For flash responses, greater occipitotemporal coherences were found on the side contralateral to speech representation. In a further study (A. E. Davis & Wada, 1977a), the largest coherences were found to occur between homologous sites in the two hemispheres (O_1, O_2; C_5, C_6), but these did not vary as a function of speech lateralization or modality. The basic findings of the earlier study (A. E. Davis & Wada, 1974) were replicated, with the additional observation that flash stimuli produced large interhemispheric coherences between the temporal area on the speech side and the opposite occipital area.

A. E. Davis and Wada (1978) have used their data on patients with known speech lateralization to construct a discriminant function to distinguish between left- and right-hemispheric speech representation. They then obtained click- and flash-evoked AERs from normal left- and right-handed subjects and used the discriminant function to classify the normals with respect to speech lateralization. All 12 left-handers and 10 of 12 right-handers showed presumptive evidence of left-hemispheric speech representation. This would suggest that the relation between handedness and speech lateralization is even weaker than indicated in the aphasia literature (Rasmussen & Milner, 1977; Chapter 10). Of course, it may be quite inappropriate to attempt to build a discriminant function on the basis of data obtained from epileptic brains and apply it to normal subjects. Furthermore, the use of simple flash and click stimuli may not be the best way of engaging the two hemispheres differentially.

In summary, the AER literature is marked by an inconsistency of results and a diversity of approaches and analytic procedures. No very elegant summary can be made at the present time, other than to say task-dependent asymmetries do exist. Certainly, one cannot view the use of AERs as a substitute for behavioral work. The coherence analyses employed by Davis and Wada, however, seem to have particularly great potential, offering the possibility of mapping out the progress of information through the brain.

Regional Cerebral Blood Flow (rCBF)

Local increases in blood flow in the brain indicate increased metabolic activity in the gray matter and thus provide a measure of local neural activity. The intracarotid injection or inhalation of radioactive ^{133}Xe introduces an inert radioactive substance into the blood stream (Risberg, 1980; F. Wood, 1980). Regional blood flow can then be monitored by positioning scintillation counters at the surface of the head, and some estimate can be made of local blood flow, although it does take about 2 min to obtain accurate measures. Carmon, Lavy, Gordon, and Portnoy (1975) had subjects listen to verbal or musical material while the investigators monitored cerebral blood flow. They found that blood flow increased in the right hemisphere while the subject listened to music and in the left hemisphere while the subject listened to verbal material. However, Knopman, Rubens, Klassen, Meyer, and Niccum (1980) found an increase in left-hemispheric flow for both verbal and nonverbal auditory tasks. Their nonverbal task involved listening for changes of intensity and may not have been as appropriate for eliciting right-hemispheric activation as that used by Carmon *et al.* (1975). R. C. Gur and Reivich (1980) also found increased left-hemispheric flow during a verbal task (analogies). Although they found no significant group increase in right-hemispheric flow while subjects were doing a picture completion task, those subjects who showed an increased right-hemispheric flow also performed better on the task.

Local metabolic rates can also be assessed by adding a radioactive marker to glucose, although about 45 min is required to obtain accurate measures. These techniques involve a very low level of radioactivity, and evidence seems to be that they can be used safely. They provide an interesting possibility for assessing metabolic aspects of local brain activity. However, it would be very difficult to have a subject maintain any specified cognitive activity for 45 min, and therefore, the procedure is unlikely to be very useful in localizing specific cognitive events.

Summary

The preceding pages have provided a general overview of various electrophysiological and metabolic techniques that have been employed to assess brain activity and to examine those studies that have investigated hemispheric asymmetry. Measures of gross EEG, visual and auditory AER, and cerebral blood flow have been applied to questions of hemispheric asymmetry. These studies all point in the direction of showing task-dependent hemispheric asymmetries. There is general agreement that activity is in some way greater in the left hemisphere during verbal activities and greater in the right hemisphere during nonverbal activities. Yet surely we knew this many years ago from clinical studies of brain injury.

At the present state of knowledge, the physiological studies have generated almost more confusion than knowledge. While they may provide a more direct assessment of ongoing cerebral activity than do behavioral measures, physiological measures are also subject to task effects that are often left uncontrolled. Before these measures can be truly useful, greater behavioral sophistication is required in the physiological experiments.

One very simple demand that we might have is that the physiological measures tell us whether a particular normal subject has speech represented in the left hemisphere or in the right. Johnstone *et al.* (1979) indicate that EEG alpha power ratios can be used to distinguish between left- and right-handers, with there being a presumption that left-handers are more likely to have right-hemispheric speech. In contrast, A. E. Davis and Wada (1978) find evidence indicating that virtually all normals are left-hemispheric for speech, regardless of handedness. Neither group has yet provided compelling evidence that the electrophysiological techniques provide any better measure of individual differences in cerebral organization than do the behavioral techniques.

We have also posed the question of *what* is lateralized. The physiological research has not taken full advantage of the behavioral work and has done little more than to corroborate the very global distinction between verbal and nonverbal processes. If the behavioral studies raise questions about just what aspects of language function are lateralized to the left hemisphere, or what aspects of spatial function are lateralized to the right, the physiological studies are sufficiently elementary in approach and diverse in their findings as to provide little help in answering the questions.

Likewise, the physiological research is too ambiguous and inconsistent to provide any clear answers about the mechanisms of lateralization. Interhemispheric effects observed at a single pair of homologous recording sites are unlikely to yield much of a clue to mechanism. The coherence analysis procedure employed by A. E. Davis and Wada (1977a) exhibits great promise, but it has not yet been applied to sufficiently complex stimuli to provide any significant theoretical advance.

Questions about the importance of differing patterns of cerebral organization are fundamentally behavioral ones and must be approached behaviorally. Physiological techniques can potentially provide us with a good procedure for classification, although they have not yet done so. To date, there have been few attempts to study the relation between physiological indexes of lateralization and other behaviors (although O'Connor & Shaw, 1978, have reported a relation between EEG alpha coherence and field dependence).

In conclusion, then, the physiological measures remain intrinsically appealing, but they have not yet provided good answers to the primary questions about cerebral lateralization in the normal brain. To do so, one must have more systematic studies and a better integration of physiological techniques and behavioral questions.

10

Handedness and Its Relation to Cerebral Function

In the chapters on perceptual asymmetries, the value of comparing the performance of left- and right-handers has been repeatedly emphasized. Because the incidence of left-hemispheric speech representation is lower in left-handers than in right-handers, this comparison provides one way of determining whether or not the behavioral task is related to cerebral lateralization. To make use of this approach, one must understand something about handedness and its measurement. Further, as will be seen, the relation between handedness and speech lateralization is not a simple one, and even clear-cut differences between left- and right-handers must be viewed with some caution.

Certainly, handedness is the best known and most studied human asymmetry. The vast majority of us are right-handed in the sense that we prefer to use our right hand for unimanual activities and are more proficient with it. We use our right hand for writing, for drawing, for throwing, and for manipulating small objects. There remains, however, a stalwart proportion of us who are left-handed and who use the left hand for those activities that are performed unimanually. The incidence of left-handedness is generally considered to be between 5% and 12%, although the specific figures vary considerably as a function of the source of the sample and the procedure for measuring handedness. Hécaen and Ajuriaguerra (1964) tabulate a number of studies in which the incidence of left-handedness varies from 1% to 30%, with a median at about 7%. In more recent large surveys of handedness, Annett (1973) reports a figure of 11.64% for young adults in the United Kingdom, Bryden (1979c; see Table 10.1) one of 10.39% for comparable subjects in Canada, and Hardyck, Goldman, and Petrinovitch (1975) a value of 9.9% among California schoolchildren. These surveys also indicate a slightly greater incidence of left-handedness in males than in females.

157

Table 10.1

Incidence of Left-Handedness in Respondent and Relatives

	Males		Females	
	N	Percentage left-handed	N	Percentage left-handed
Respondents	2784	11.53	2098	8.86
Fathers	2784	7.36	2098	7.63
Mothers	2784	5.32	2098	4.91
Brothers	1813	13.68	1346	13.00
Sisters	1754	10.72	1303	9.29

Note. Data from Bryden (1979c).

Historically, left-handers have always been with us. In this context, it is customary to quote the Bible (Judges 20:15–16) and the 3% incidence of left-handedness among the armies of the tribe of Benjamin. Coren and Porac (1977) have reported that the incidence of left-handedness as portrayed in works of art has remained constant at about 7–8% since prior to 3000 B.C. The scholarly and humorous review by L. J. Harris (1980) serves as a further reminder that the issue of left-handedness has a long history.

If the incidence of left-handedness has not changed in any systematic way over many centuries, short-term trends may be quite different. In both Annett's (1973) and Bryden's (1979c) surveys, the incidence of left-handedness was much higher in young adults than in their parents (see Table 10.1). The data of Rife (1940) and Chamberlain (1928) show an incidence of left-handedness in the range 4–7%, comparable to the parental data in the Bryden and Annett studies. These data would suggest that the frequency of left-handedness has risen from about 5% to about 11% during the twentieth century, at least in the United Kingdom and North America. Those who were born in the early part of the century often have many tales to tell about being strapped for writing with the left hand or having their left hands tied behind their backs in school. The social pressure to make the child write with the right hand and to conform to the norm may have been far greater in the first half of the century than it is now. A. J. Harris's (1958) handedness questionnaire includes a question about whether the subject has been forced to switch hand usage, indicating that this was not an uncommon case in his experience.

If social pressures against left-handers are in fact being relaxed, the data obtained in family studies of handedness will be changing over time. In the earlier studies, such as those of Chamberlain (1928) and Rife

(1940), many individuals would have been classified as right-handed who would now develop as left-handers. Only now would we approach a state of genetic equilibrium.

In addition to these short-term changes in the incidence of left-handedness, there may also be considerable variation from one culture to another. For example, Hatta and Nakatsuka (1976) report a frequency of 3.1% for left-handers in Japan, and Dawson (1977) gives values of around 10% in primitive hunting and fishing societies, such as those of the Alaskan Eskimo, the Australian Arunta, and the Hong Kong boat people. In contrast, Dawson reports figures of 1–3% among primitive agricultural societies, such as those of the Hong Kong Hakka, the Katanganese, and the Temne of Sierra Leone. Dawson suggests that the agricultural societies are culturally strict and conforming, whereas the hunting and fishing societies are much more permissive, and that this leads the agricultural societies to demand that their children conform to the norm of right-handedness. In agreement with the Japanese study, Teng, Lee, Yang, and Chang (1976) found only 1.5% left-handers among Taiwanese schoolchildren. In California, Oriental schoolchildren show a 6.5% incidence of left-handedness (Hardyck *et al.*, 1975)—greater than in China or Japan, but less than in their Caucasian classmates. Teng *et al.* report a considerable pressure in Taiwan to change hand use from the left to the right. Their data, and those of Dawson, indicate that social pressure can have a profound influence on the measured incidence of left-handedness.

The majority of studies of the incidence of left-handedness have used rather crude measures of handedness, generally asking subjects only which hand is used for writing or which hand is preferred. In other areas, such as aphasiology, where it is thought important to be aware of any possible sign of left-handedness, almost any eccentric use of the hands can be taken as evidence for latent left-handedness (cf. Luria, 1965). Luria, for example, suggests that if the left arm is uppermost when the arms are folded in front of the body, one is potentially left-handed. While this, like many other behaviors, may show an asymmetry, there is little evidence to indicate that it is related to other aspects of hand usage or to cerebral lateralization. Annett (1975) has wisely pointed out that the criterion for calling subjects left-handed is often very broad indeed in neurology.

Many researchers are dissatisfied with the classification of individuals into such simple categories as right- or left-handed and have attempted to develop more systematic and quantitative measures of handedness. Such studies have followed two different paths: the measurement of hand preference, and the measurement of relative hand proficiency. The next sections examine the successes and failures of these two different approaches. One difficulty that plagues both approaches, however, is the absence of any independent external criterion. One cannot claim that one measure of handedness is better than another if the only measure of validity is that the test distinguishes between those who call themselves left-handed and those who do not.

Hand Preference Measures

By far the most common way of assessing handedness is through a hand preference inventory. In such an inventory, a list of unimanual activities is compiled, and the subjects either are asked which hand they prefer to use to carry out the activity or are asked to demonstrate how the activity is performed. The simplest version of such a test is to ask the subjects which hand they prefer to use, and let it go at that. This allows classification of subjects as left- or right-handed, and possibly as ambidextrous. Such a division corresponds to our everyday usage and has satisfied the vast majority of researchers carrying out studies of handedness and its relation to other variables (e.g., Trankell, 1955; Zangwill, 1960).

Other investigators have recognized that there are different degrees of handedness and have constructed inventories to assess this fact. It is not uncommon to encounter a right-hander who will continue to use his or her right hand regardless of how awkward it might be. In contrast, most left-handers are rather flexible in their hand usage and frequently shift to the right hand when it becomes more convenient. In part, this is because we live in a right-handers' world, and many devices are made to be operated by the right-handed. It is difficult, for example, to use a normal pair of scissors left-handed. This certainly contributes to the greater flexibility of the average left-hander, as well as providing an opportunity for shops in large metropolitan areas to cater explicitly to the left-hander. In any event, everyday experience tells us that there are varying degrees of both left- and right-handedness.

Many different hand preference inventories have been constructed, and it is pointless to attempt to survey all of them. Of those in common use at the present time, perhaps the three most popular originate with Annett (1970a), Crovitz and Zener (1962), and Oldfield (1971). As shown in Table 10.2, each of these questionnaires asks slightly different questions. In addition, the instructions for the three tests are somewhat different. Annett (1970a) asks which hand is habitually used for performing the activity—right, left, or either. Thus, the test as a whole can

Table 10.2
Items Used on Representative Hand Preference Questionnaires

Annett (1970a)	Crovitz & Zener (1962)	Oldfield (1971)
Writing	Writing	Writing
Throwing	Throwing	Throwing
Scissors	Scissors	Scissors
Toothbrush	Toothbrush	Toothbrush
	Drawing	Drawing
Match for striking		Match for striking
Upper hand on broom		Upper hand on broom
Tennis racquet	Tennis racquet	
Hammer when nailing	*Nail for hammering	
	Knife when cutting food	Using knife without fork
Guiding thread to needle	*Holding needle when threading	
Unscrewing jar lid	*Holding bottle to uncap	
Upper hand on shovel		
Dealing cards		
	*Holding potato to peel	
	Pitcher to pour	
	Glass when drinking	
	*Dish when wiping	
		Lid to open box
		Spoon

*Activities for which the right-hander normally uses the left hand; scoring is reversed.

yield a score ranging from 12 lefts to 12 rights. Annett herself believes that we grossly underestimate the incidence of mixed-handedness in the population, and classifies individuals as left- or right-handed only if they answer all 12 questions consistently. However, it would be possible to derive a laterality quotient from the responses by subtracting the "left" responses from the "right" responses and dividing by 12. This would yield a score that would range from +1.00 (very right-handed) to −1.00 (very left-handed).

In the Crovitz and Zener (1962) test, subjects are instructed to mark one of six response boxes, labeled "Always use left hand," "Usually use left hand," "Use both equally," "Usually use right hand," "Always use right hand," and "Don't know." The items are scored from 1 to 5, with the strong right-handed response given a score of 1. One should note that on this test five of the items are reversed, in the sense that the strong right-hander will perform the activity with the left hand. These items are, of course, scored in reverse fashion. With 14 items, scores can range from 14 (strongly right-handed) to 70 (strongly left-handed).

"Don't know" responses are fortunately rare, but an appropriate score can be obtained be extrapolating from the items that were answered.

In the Oldfield questionnaire, subjects are provided with two columns, marked "Left" and "Right." They are asked to indicate the preferred hand with a + mark, using + + when the preference is so strong that they would not use the other hand unless forced to and marking a + in each column when they are truly indifferent. The number of +'s in each column is then summed, and a laterality quotient derived by dividing the difference between the two columns by the sum, yielding scores that range from +1.00 (strongly right-handed) to −1.00 (strongly left-handed).

One difficulty with this procedure is that it weighs items differently according to how many + marks have been assigned to it. Bryden (1977) used a 5-point scale for scoring the test, assigning values from 1 for a "right + +" to 5 for a "left + +." This provides scores ranging from 10 (extremely right-handed) to 50 (extremely left-handed).

As Table 10.2 indicates, the three tests involve somewhat different items. Only four items are used on all three tests, and eight more occur on two of the three tests. Clearly, there is some disagreement as to the best items for assessing hand preference.

Of the three, the Oldfield is perhaps the most carefully developed. Oldfield started with a pool of 20 items and reduced this to 10 only after extensive testing. The final items were selected as providing the best discrimination between left- and right-handed subjects. This again illustrates our criterion problem: If we select items because they differentiate between self-professed left- and right-handers, we can never hope to improve on self-classification as a technique. The only thing a carefully worked-out handedness questionnaire will provide us with is a measurement of gradations in hand preference. Perhaps, however, that is the best to which we can aspire.

One of the necessities of a good test is that it be both reliable and valid. A test is reliable if subjects give the same answer at a subsequent testing. While one of the problems with handedness questionnaires is that there is no external criterion for validation, the individual items can have validity in the sense that the responses actually correspond to the behavior of subjects in real situations. The tests shown in Table 10.2 are intended as paper-and-pencil tests, and subjects must be able to visualize how they perform the activities in order to respond to the questions. In some cases, subjects may have difficulty in doing this and give responses that do not correspond to the way they actually behave.

These issues have been addressed by Raczkowski, Kalat, and Nebes (1974). They administered a 23-item questionnaire, including most of the items shown in Table 10.2, to a large sample of undergraduates. A month later, 47 of the original subjects were given individual performance tests on the 23 items, and 27 of these were asked to fill out the original questionnaire a second time. Of the 23 items, the question on dealing cards proved to be the only item on which *all* subjects gave the same answer on both administrations of the questionnaire and also performed the task in the way they had claimed. One of the poorest items was "Which hand is on the top of the handle when you sweep the floor with a straight broom?"—an item that appears on both the Oldfield and Annett questionnaires. Only 78% of the subjects actually performed the task in the way they had claimed on the first administration of the questionnaire, and only 74% gave the same response on the two questionnaires. The Raczkowski *et al.* study also identifies a number of other common items for which the questionnaire–performance agreement was less than 90% (e.g., holding a glass when drinking or a pitcher when pouring, and the two items pertaining to footedness rather than handedness) or for which the test–retest agreement was less than 90% (e.g., holding a match when striking it). The results of this study provide some clear guidelines for selecting questionnaire items.

In a further attempt to refine existing handedness questionnaires, Bryden (1977) administered both the Crovitz and Zener (1962) and Oldfield (1971) questionnaires to a sample of 1107 undergraduate students. Of these subjects, 984 gave answers to all 24 items, and the data from these subjects were subjected to a factor analysis. Three distinct factors were identified. One factor was specific to handedness as described in terms of familiar activities and included such items as writing, drawing, throwing a ball, using a toothbrush, and holding a tennis racquet. A second factor was specific to the Crovitz and Zener questionnaire and included primarily those items that were reverse scored: Apparently many subjects do not pay enough attention to the test to catch these items. While Crovitz and Zener intentionally included such items to ensure that their subjects read the questionnaire, the items seem only to lead to enough confusion to make their value dubious. The third factor included such items from the Oldfield questionnaire as using a broom, striking a match, and holding a box lid. These are all rare activities that subjects have difficulty in visualizing, and they tend to be relatively unreliable (Raczkowski *et al.*, 1974). K. White and Ashton (1976) have also identified two separate factors on the Oldfield questionnaire. If handedness is to be considered a unitary factor, items loading on the secondary factors should also be dropped from standard handedness questionnaires. An association analysis carried out by Annett (1970a) found that the items loading on Bryden's first factor, with the exception of using scissors, clustered together.

Given these considerations of reliability, validity, and loading on a common factor of handedness, there seem to be five items that are clearly pertinent to handedness as we normally understand it. These are writing, drawing, throwing, using scissors, and using a toothbrush. A shortened handedness questionnaire using these items (see Table 10.3), using the Oldfield instructions since they do not encourage extreme responses to the same extent as the Crovitz and Zener instructions, seems to be the best preference measure of handedness that we now have available (Bryden, 1977).

One further problem remains. Existing handedness questionnaires are constructed to weight each of the items equally. Yet individuals do not perform the various activities equally often. Most of us write every day, but some may not throw a ball from one month to the next. Does it mean something different for right-handers to say that they "usually" write right-handed than to say that they "usually" throw right-handed? For some of us, throwing is a rarely exercised skill; for others, throwing left-handed may be a means for developing the ability. Yet our questionnaires make no attempt to weight the items by the relative frequency with which the activities are carried out. In fact, it is the relatively low-frequency activities that show inconsistency of response and low validity. For those who believe that any sign of left-hand usage, however rare, is symptomatic of latent left-handedness or ambilaterality, such items are of importance. On the other hand, if we are attempting to obtain an index of the relative frequency with which the two hands are

---

Table 10.3
A Simplified Hand Preference Questionnaire

Instructions: For each of the activities listed below, indicate with a + which hand you normally use to perform the activity. If you would only use the other hand when forced to, mark a + +. If you would use both hands equally often, place a + in each column.

	Left	Right
Writing a message		
Drawing a picture		
Using a toothbrush		
Throwing a ball		
Using a pair of scissors		

Scoring: Assign 1 for L+ +, 2 for L+, 3 for a + in each column, 4 for R+, and 5 for R+ +. Sum the scores, subtract 15, and divide by 10. This will yield a score ranging from −1.00 (extreme left-handed) through +1.00 (extreme right-handed).

---

used in daily activities, then some weighting of a few reliable items is needed.

At present, neither of these goals have been achieved. There is no hard evidence to indicate that inconsistent items, such as the upper hand on a broom, are diagnostic of anything. On the other hand, even the five items recommended by Bryden (1977) do not represent equally frequent activities. All things considered, however, these five items seem to represent the best available measure for assessing hand preference.

Performance Measures

Virtually any hand preference measure reveals a few individuals who are difficult to classify: They are usually described as showing weak hand preference or as being ambilateral. The existence of such individuals indicates that handedness is not a discrete variable, with people being either right-handed or left-handed, but a continuous one, with all degrees of lateralization being represented in the normal population. Such considerations make it desirable to have a measure of handedness as a continuous variable. Of course, a hand preference inventory such as that suggested in the preceding section does provide a graded measure of handedness, but it does not sample the activities in a representative way. Further, when administered as a questionnaire, it measures what people say they do rather than what they actually do. It is true that one can observe performance on a simple set of five items, such as those shown in Table 10.3, but this is often not done.

These considerations have led many investigators to conclude that some simple measure of the relative skill of the two hands would provide a better assessment of handedness. Such a measure would involve observation of the actual performance of the subject and would provide a continuously graded measure of handedness. Attempts to develop such measures have usually employed measures either of relative hand strength (Woo & Pearson, 1927) or of the relative speed of some fine controlled movement (Annett, 1972, 1976; Peters & Durding, 1978).

Since hand strength can be so clearly modified by practice and depends so much on the daily activities of the subject, and since most of the items on preference questionnaires involve fine motor control, most of the recent studies have involved some task involving fine movement control.

On most of these tasks, the distribution of hand differences is a more or less normal one, with the mean displaced to the right so that on the average the right hand is somewhat superior to the left (Annett, 1976). To some, the very fact that performance measures yield a normal distribution while preference questionnaires produce a J-shaped distribution is an argument for preferring the performance measure. It is not clear, however, that this is anything more than a matter of statistical convenience. With only very minor assumptions, it is easy to see how a performance measure could yield a normal distribution and a preference questionnaire yield a J distribution although both tests measured the same underlying variable. Figure 10.1 shows the distribution of manual asymmetry of a performance task. Now suppose that all subjects who have a performance differential between the two hands greater than some threshold value, k, show a marked preference for the use of the more skilled hand. Intermediate preference scores will be observed in only those subjects whose skill differential is between $+k$ and $-k$. Such a relation between skill and preference would lead to a large number of strongly right-handed subjects, a smaller peak for the left-handers, and a few distributed through the middle range—a J-shaped distribution of preference.

Annett (1967, 1972) has taken a somewhat different approach to reconciling the differences between the distributions of hand preference and hand skill. She has argued that the incidence of ambilaterality, or mixed-handedness, is very much higher than is usually claimed and that the proportion of left-handed, right-handed, and mixed-handed indi-

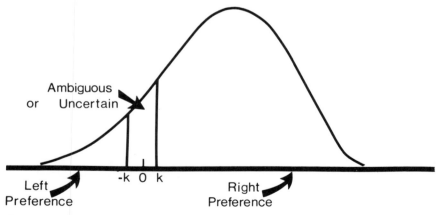

Figure 10.1. An illustration of how a continuous distribution could underlie a J-shaped distribution. If individuals in the range $+k$ to $-k$ are classified as "ambiguous," relatively few cases will fall in this category, and a J distribution of left, ambiguous, and right will result.

viduals actually fits a binomial distribution. This would be expected if one were cutting an underlying normal distribution into three categories. In order to accomplish this, Annett classifies any individual who carries out *any* activity with the nondominant hand as "mixed-handed." Thus, for instance, a right-hander who claimed to use a broom with the left hand on top would be classified as "mixed." Given the problem of reliability associated with some of the items on preference questionnaires (Raczkowski *et al.*, 1974), this would seem to be a rather questionable practice. On the other hand, if the classification of "mixed" subjects is based only on highly reliable items, such as those shown in Table 10.3, Annett's argument is basically the same as that propounded above. It remains to be seen, however, whether the admission of a large number of subjects to the "mixed" category has any predictive validity. This topic will be considered in further detail in the section on the genetics of handedness (see Chapter 11).

Using a peg moving task, Annett (1976) has reported a very close agreement between skill differences and hand preference. Peters and Durding (1978) have found similar agreement using a tapping task. Other researchers have not found such consistency. For example, Todor and Doane (1977) had subjects tap two adjacent targets as rapidly as possible. They manipulated task difficulty by altering the size of the targets and the separation between them. Correlations with hand preference decreased as task difficulty increased. Provins and Cunliffe (1972) report a correlation of .70 between a composite measure of motor performance and a preference questionnaire. While this is clearly significant, it is not impressively high, accounting for only about 50% of the variance. One problem may be that the relation between hand preference and skill may vary as a function of hand preference. Lake and Bryden (1976) found a very high overall correlation between a dot tapping task and a preference measure, but this correlation was zero when the left-handed subjects were considered separately.

One of the most thorough studies of manual proficiency is that of Barnsley and Rabinovitch (1970), who administered a set of 32 different tests to a sample of 50 males and 50 females. Separate factor analyses of the dominant and nondominant hand scores for each sex revealed 10 distinct factors. These can be described as reaction time, speed of arm movement, wrist–finger speed, arm–hand steadiness, arm movement steadiness, aiming, finger tapping, dexterity, stated hand preference, and a motivational factor. More interestingly, Barnsley and Rabinovitch also computed ratio scores for each of the dependent measures. Factor analysis of these scores yielded no meaningful or interpretable factors. In other words, the measures of relative hand proficiency on various tasks did not correlate with one another sufficiently for any meaningful factors to be isolated. By implication, the degree of lateralization of hand proficiency is not unifactorial, and different measures of hand proficiency measure differently lateralized characteristics. At first glance, this would seem to bode ill for any attempt to measure handedness in terms of proficiency. However, Barnsley and Rabinovitch conclude that handedness does appear "to be a single dimension characterized by the superior performance of the preferred hand [1970, p. 360]," largely on the grounds that all their factors except reaction time and speed of arm movement differentiate between preferred and nonpreferred hand performance. They suggest that this dimension is the production of highly practiced and overlearned skills in the preferred hand. Barnsley and Rabinovitch also argue that preference questionnaires are not appropriate for assessing relative proficiency, on the grounds that a distinct factor involving stated hand preference emerged, orthogonal to the hand proficiency factors.

If Barnsley and Rabinovitch's conclusions are correct, then virtually any measure of hand proficiency will do as a performance measure, and one need worry only about the relation between hand proficiency and hand preference. However, a performance measure must show reliability just as much as a preference measure. Provins and Cunliffe (1972) administered a number of motor tests of hand proficiency and found test–retest reliabilities ranging from .15 to .94 for the difference between hands. Only handwriting (the time taken to write out the alphabet six times) and tapping (the number of taps of a telegraph key made in 10 sec) showed significant reliabilities. A dexterity test somewhat similar to Annett's peg moving task showed a reliability of only .38. The fact that some individuals report that they have been forced to learn to write with their right hand would suggest that a handwriting measure would be heavily contaminated by social pressures. Thus, a tapping task would seem to be the best choice for a performance measure of handedness. High reliability for tapping tasks has also been reported by Todor and Doane (1977) and by Peters and Durding (1978).

In conclusion, then, there is at least reasonable evidence for a correlation between hand preference measures and hand proficiency measures. Hand proficiency measures have the advantage of being continuously distributed and of requiring the subject to perform the task rather than simply to state a preference. Of the various measures proposed, those involving speed of tapping seem to have the highest reliability. Whenever possible, it would seem desirable to use a performance measure of handedness, but enough questions remain that a brief preference inventory should almost certainly be administered as well.

Left-Handedness and Hemispheric Specialization

An adequate description of left-handedness becomes of psychological importance only if the incidence of left-handedness is related to other behavioral traits. Over the years, the left-hander has been accused of many things: lower intelligence, poor reading ability, impaired spatial ability (cf. Corballis & Beale, 1976; Hardyck & Petrinovitch, 1977; Hécaen & Ajuriaguerra, 1964; Levy, 1969), a higher incidence of birth stress (Bakan, Dibb, & Reid, 1973), a greater tendency toward alcoholism (Bakan, 1973), and a greater incidence of mental retardation, cerebral palsy, and other pathologies (Satz, 1972). However, a very large-scale study by Hardyck, Petrinovitch, and Goldman (1976) showed no sign of cognitive defect in the left-handed. In their thorough review of left-handedness, Hardyck and Petrinovitch (1977) conclude that the evidence associating left-handedness with behavioral deficit is very weak. At the same time, most contemporary theorists (e.g., Corballis & Beale, 1976; Levy, 1969; Satz, 1972) would argue that any deficit shown by left-handers is a result, not of sinistrality per se, but of the abnormal localization of function in the brains of left-handers.

As indicated earlier, it has long been known that speech functions are primarily localized in the left hemisphere of normal right-handed individuals. More recently, it has become clear that certain aspects of spatial and musical abilities are localized in the right hemisphere of right-handers (Hécaen & Albert, 1978; Milner, 1974). Historically, it was first thought that left-handers would show the mirror-image cerebral organization (Penfield & Roberts, 1959; Roberts, 1968). As cases of aphasia in left-handers following left-hemispheric damage accumulated, it became clear that this was not the case.

Satz (1980) has reviewed the literature on aphasia in left-handers and has concluded that speech is bilaterally represented in many left-handers. His survey indicates that aphasic disturbances are found following unilateral brain damage more often in left-handers than in right-handers, and he concludes that some 40% of left-handers have bilateral speech representation.

Because Satz (1980) included data from a number of studies reporting only on left-handed cases, where the incidence of aphasia was abnormally high, Segalowitz and Bryden (forthcoming) have reevaluated the relation of aphasia and handedness, using only those studies in which both left- and right-handers were investigated. Including only these studies results in a rather lower estimate of the incidence of aphasia in left-handers than indicated by Satz (1980) (see Table 10.4). In right-handers, the ratio of left-hemispheric speech to right-hemispheric speech

Table 10.4
Incidence of Aphasia following Unilateral Brain Injury (%)

	Side of lesion	
	Left hemisphere	Right hemisphere
Right-handers	62.1	3.0
Left-handers	52.8	25.1

Note. Data from Segalowitz and Bryden (forthcoming).

should be the same as the incidence ratio—that is, 62.1:3.0. This ratio is obtained when 94.5% of the right-handers have left-hemispheric speech representation. Furthermore, it indicates that aphasia results from unilateral damage to the dominant hemisphere in only about 65% of the cases. If this same incidence rate holds for left-handers, the 52.8% of left-handers who show aphasia following unilateral left-hemisphere damage represent 65% of all the sinistrals with some left-hemispheric involvement. Similarly, the 25.1% who show aphasia following right-hemispheric damage represent 65% of those with some right-hemispheric involvement, either bilateral or right dominant. These figures lead to estimates of 61.4% left-hemispheric speech, 18.8% right-hemispheric, and 19.8% bilateral representation (see Table 10.5).

The development of sodium amytal techniques for the assessment of speech lateralization (Wada & Rasmussen, 1960) has made it possible to obtain data on the relation between handedness and speech lateralization from large samples of subjects. Studies employing this technique reveal that the majority of left-handers, like right-handers, have speech in the left hemisphere (Milner, Branch, & Rasmussen, 1964; Rossi & Rosadini, 1967), although the data are somewhat discordant from those

Table 10.5
Incidence of Left, Right, and Bilateral Speech Representation Derived from Unilateral Brain Injury Data (%)

	Speech lateralization		
	Left	Bilateral	Right
Right-handers	95.5	—	4.5
Left-handers	61.4	19.8	18.8

Note. Data from Segalowitz and Bryden (forthcoming).

presented by Satz (1980). Table 10.6 shows data that indicate that 96% of right-handers and 70% of left-handers show left-hemispheric speech lateralization. It is again true, however, that the incidence of right-hemispheric speech is much higher in the left-handers than in the right-handers and that bilateral speech representation is a characteristic almost wholly associated with left-handedness.

Yet another approach to estimating the distribution of speech lateralization has been to investigate the incidence of dysphasia following unilateral ECT in patients undergoing treatment for depression, but without signs of organic disorders. Among 30 left-handers, left-hemispheric speech is reported in 70%, right-hemispheric speech in 23%, and bilateral representation in 7%. It is worth noting the general agreement in the figures arising from three very different techniques of assessing lateralization (Segalowitz & Bryden, forthcoming; Rasmussen & Milner, 1977; Warrington & Pratt, 1973).

The patterns shown in Tables 10.4, 10.5, and 10.6 indicate only a weak relation between handedness and speech lateralization. They do indicate that a large sample of left-handers would be expected to contain many more individuals with right-hemispheric or bilateral speech than a comparable group of right-handers and therefore that one should expect to find a difference between left- and right-handers on any behavioral measure related to speech lateralization. If we assume that some of the variance in our behavioral measures is unrelated to cerebral lateralization, it may take sample sizes as large as 50 to show a laterality difference between left- and right-handers (Segalowitz & Bryden, forthcoming) (see Figure 10.2).

It would be much easier to link behavior to cerebral lateralization if we could specify which left-handers have right-hemispheric speech lateralization. Several variables have been suggested as relevant. One possibility is that the left-handers with a familial history of left-handedness are those who show reversed hemispheric specialization. Using dichotic

Table 10.6
Relation of Handedness to Speech Lateralization as Determined by Sodium Amytal (%)

	Left	Bilateral	Right
		Speech representation	
Right-handers	96	—	4
Left- or mixed-handers	70	15	15

Note. Data from Rasmussen and Milner (1977).

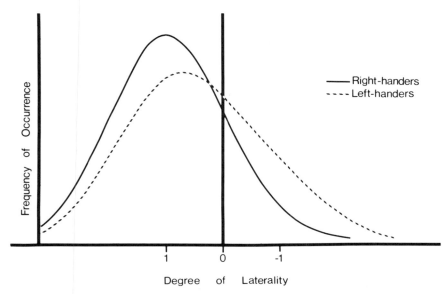

Figure 10.2. Hypothetical distribution of laterality scores for left- and right-handers, assuming the distributions of cerebral lateralization discussed in the text and a standard error of measurement of 1 unit for the laterality measure.

listening and visual hemifield procedures with normal adults, Zurif and Bryden (1969) found evidence to support such a contention. In a clinical population, Hécaen and Sauguet (1971) also found evidence to suggest that it was familial sinistrals who show reversed functional specialization. Other studies (e.g., Bryden, 1973; Lake & Bryden, 1976) have not been so clear-cut.

An alternative is that strong left-handers differ from weak left-handers. Annett's (1967, 1972, 1975) arguments concerning the distribution of handedness would suggest that many self-classified left-handers—those who show weak hand preference—properly belong in her "mixed" category. One might expect that lateralization patterns would be different in strong and weak left-handers. Dee (1971), using a dichotic listening procedure, has reported that weak left-handers show a left-ear advantage, whereas strong left-handers, like right-handers, show a right-ear advantage. Although Hécaen and Sauguet (1971) suggest that weak left-handers are also likely to show familial sinistrality, McKeever and Van-Deventer (1977b) failed to demonstrate any relation between degree of left-handedness and familial sinistrality. Furthermore, A. W. Knox and Boone (1970) and Satz et al., (1967) have reported that it is the strong left-handers who *fail* to show a right-ear advantage in dichotic listening.

A third suggestion comes from Levy (Levy & Nagylaki, 1972; Levy & Reid, 1976, 1978). She suggests that those individuals who write with their hands in an upright position, like most right-handers, have speech and motor movement controlled from the contralateral hemisphere, whereas those who write in an overhand or "hooked" pattern have ipsilateral control. Thus, left-handers who use the hooked pattern are left-hemispheric for speech and should show the same lateral asymmetries as do right-handers. Conversely, those who write in an upright fashion should show right-hemispheric speech. Levy and Reid (1976, 1978) have reported data indicating that writing posture predicts cerebral lateralization in 95% of the cases, using visual hemifield procedures to assess cerebral lateralization. However, other researchers have not been so successful in finding an association between hand posture and cerebral lateralization (Bryden, 1979b; Moscovitch & Smith, 1979). Moscovitch suggests that hand posture may be specifically related to visual control of movement.

Few studies have considered all three of these variables in their attempt to determine how the brains of left-handers are functionally organized. Bryden (1979b) has studied 40 left-handers on tasks involving perceptual asymmetry. He found that familial history was the most successful factor in predicting direction of lateralization, though none were particularly compelling. At present, we can conclude only that left-handers are less likely to demonstrate clear-cut cerebral organization than are right-handers.

It remains possible that left-handers differ from right-handers in performance, not because of differing hemispheric specialization, but because they are left-handed. As one possibility, left-handers may pay more attention to the left side of space, and this could occur regardless of which hemisphere is specialized for speech (although such an effect could also be related to speech organization: cf. Kinsbourne, 1974b). In order to assess such a notion, one would need independent measurement of handedness and speech lateralization, and such data are hard to come by. However, Kimura's (1961a, 1961b) original study of speech lateralization and dichotic listening provides some relevant data. She administered a dichotic free-recall task to clinical patients with speech lateralization previously determined by the sodium amytal test. In her analysis of the data, she found that speech lateralization significantly affected the direction of the ear advantage, whereas handedness did not. However, Bryden (1978) has reexamined these data, calculating group laterality coefficients for each of the hand–speech combinations. His results are shown in Table 10.7. While it is clear from this table that the direction of ear advantage is primarily determined by the speech-

Table 10.7
Laterality Coefficients for Groups Differing in Handedness and
Speech Lateralization

Handedness	Speech lateralization		
	Left	Right	Average
Left	.106 (10)	−.298 (9)	−.096
Right	.214 (93)	−.075 (3)	.070
Average	.160	−.187	−.013

Note. Data from Kimura (1961a). Sample size in parentheses.

dominant hemisphere, handedness has an independent effect of about half the magnitude of the speech lateralization effect. Left-handers with left-hemispheric speech are less right-ear dominant than their right-handed counterparts, and those few right-handers with right-hemispheric speech are likewise less left-ear dominant than left-handers with right-hemispheric speech.

Two hypotheses are available to account for these data. One is that individuals with speech lateralization on the same side as their dominant hand are less well lateralized than those whose dominant hand is opposite to their speech hemisphere. This is a plausible theory that would be readily acceptable to many, though there are few data to support it. Alternatively, one might argue that the performance on the dichotic listening task is affected by attentional variables that relate to handedness but not to hemispheric specialization (Bryden, 1978). If this is the case, it would imply that some components of performance might be related to handedness per se and that the comparison of handedness groups is not a wholly satisfactory way to demonstrate that performance on a particular task is related to the pattern of cerebral organization. If one could develop an adequate means for separating these two components, it would open up the possibility of determining what aspects of behavior were influenced by handedness in its own right.

The preceding pages have been concerned with the relation between handedness and speech lateralization. Although it is generally conceded that the right hemisphere is specialized for visuospatial abilities in much the same way as the left hemisphere is specialized for language, there has been remarkably little investigation of the relation of handedness to the functions of the minor hemisphere. However, Hécaen *et al.* (1981) have reported on the incidence of spatial disorders as a function of unilateral brain damage. They find, in fact, that spatial disorders are more likely to follow upon right-hemispheric damage but that both sex

Table 10.8
Incidence of Spatial Disorders following Unilateral Brain Injury (%)

	Side of lesion	
	Left hemisphere	Right hemisphere
Right-handers	22.9	51.7
Left-handers	45.3	53.7

Note. Data from Hécaen (1981) and Hécaen, DeAgostini, and Monzon-Montes (1981).

and familial history of sinistrality affect this relationship. Data from this study (Hécaen, 1981) are shown in Tables 10.8 and 10.9. Applying the same logic as was used with the aphasia data (Segalowitz & Bryden, forthcoming; Table 10.5) leads to an estimate of 69.3% right-hemispheric spatial representation in right-handers, and both increased bilateral representation and reduced right-hemispheric representation in left-handers. This analysis, however, ignores the influences of sex and familial sinistrality, assumes no bilaterality in right-handers, and makes a number of other simplifying assumptions about the equivalence of lesions in the two hemispheres. At best, it should be considered a preliminary estimate of the distribution of hemispheric dominance for spatial function.

It is worth noting that the dependence of visuospatial function on the right hemisphere is not nearly so extreme as that of speech on the left hemisphere. This suggests that it is inappropriate to assume that there is necessarily a complementarity of specialization—that is, to assume that simply because an individual shows speech lateralized to one hemi-

Table 10.9
Incidence of Left, Right, and Bilateral Representation of Spatial Abilities (%)

	Lateralization of spatial abilities		
	Left	Bilateral	Right
Right-handers	30.7	—	69.3
Left-handers	28.1	29.3	42.6

Note. Figures derived from Table 10.8.

sphere that he or she will necessarily have spatial processes lateralized to the opposite hemisphere. In fact, the data from the study of Hécaen *et al.* (1981) suggest that the representation of verbal and spatial processes are statistically independent of one another. Therefore, while many right-handers will manifest complementary specialization on a chance basis, it cannot be assumed that left-handers will. This suggests that it might be fruitful to investigate the differences between those who show complementary specialization and those who do not (cf. Bryden, 1979b; McGlone & Davidson, 1973).

Eye Dominance

In addition to having a dominant hand, most people also have a dominant eye—an eye they prefer to use in situations in which they can use only one. Because it is recognized that manifest handedness can be influenced by societal pressures, and many people who use the right hand report they were forced to do so in childhood, there are some who would argue that eye dominance is a more appropriate measure of an underlying lateralization than is handedness. Eye dominance is not such an obvious characteristic as handedness, and it is subject to relatively minimal environmental pressure. Such an argument has led to the popularization of the notion that one should be concerned about individuals who show mixed hand–eye dominance—that is, those whose dominant eye is contralateral to their preferred hand (Delacato, 1966).

Such an idea implies that there is normally an association between handedness and eyedness, and that we can agree on a measure of eyedness. A wide variety of different measures have been suggested for assessing eye dominance. These include the preferred eye for sighting monocular instruments, such as telescopes or microscopes; the dominant eye in rivalry situations; the eye with the best acuity; the controlling or lead eye during reading; and the eye that is most difficult to wink (Ogle, 1962; Porac & Coren, 1976). Many of the measures that have been suggested have subsequently proven to be unreliable (Porac & Coren, 1976), while other tests may measure a diversity of factors. Crovitz (1961), for example, showed that sighting dominance and acuity dominance were essentially unrelated—that is, the eye used in a monocular sighting task was not necessarily the eye exhibiting the best visual acuity. More recently, Coren and Kaplan (1973) investigated the interrelation of a variety of different measures of eye dominance using a factor analytic approach. They concluded that there are three basic types of eye dominance: sighting dominance, acuity dominance, and sensory dominance, as measured by binocular rivalry tasks. Of the three, it is usually sighting dominance that is invoked as a measure of some underlying lateralization. The Miles test is perhaps the best measure of sighting dominance (Miles, 1930). Acuity dominance can too obviously be affected by minor abberations of one eye, while sensory dominance has been relatively rarely investigated. In fact, Crider (1944) and Porac and Coren (1976) have argued that sighting dominance is the only truly significant form of eye dominance.

In a survey of a number of studies of sighting dominance, Porac and Coren (1976) indicate that approximately 67% of the population show a right-eye sighting dominance. With sensitive measures, very few are classified as having no sighting dominance, so most of the remainder are left-eyed. Clearly, there is a far lower incidence of right-eyedness than of right-handedness, although there remains a significant dextral bias. Data on nearly 1000 undergraduates collected at the University of Waterloo, using Crovitz and Zener's (1962) group test of sighting dominance, indicate that right-eyedness is somewhat more prevalent (70%) in right-handers than in left-handers (50%) (see also Bryden, 1973). However, other studies have failed to find any relationship between handedness and sighting dominance (e.g., Gronwall & Sampson, 1971; Porac & Coren, 1975). Porac and Coren (1976) conclude that there is little evidence to indicate that sighting dominance measures a factor associated with handedness.

We have already seen that there is only a weak association between handedness and speech lateralization. Despite the poor correlation between handedness and sighting dominance, then, it remains possible that sighting dominance is much more closely related to speech lateralization than is handedness. Unfortunately, the direct studies of speech lateralization using the sodium amytal procedure have not investigated eye dominance. However, if eye dominance were closely related to hemispheric lateralization, one would expect to find that it would be a better predictor of asymmetries in perceptual laterality tasks, such as dichotic listening or visual hemifield presentation, than is handedness. Although there are reports of a sighting dominance effect on some visual laterality tasks (Bryden, 1973), these effects are not uniform across all tasks, nor are all studies in agreement (cf. T. Hayashi & Bryden, 1967). It might be interesting to examine the relation between sighting dominance and lateralization on a dichotic listening task. Here, sighting dominance could not have a peripheral sensory effect, and any relation observed would be a truer assessment of the relation between sighting dominance and cerebral hemispheric specialization.

The emphasis on relating sighting dominance to cerebral asymmetry through visual procedures may have, in fact, produced some artifactual findings. While we can force virtually everyone to show left- or right-eye sighting dominance, most of us have at least reasonably good binocular integration in the binocular tachistoscopic situation normally used to assess laterality. However, some people are amblyopic or monocular suppressors and typically use only one eye even though both are functional. Such individuals will be classified as sighting dominant for one eye and will in fact use only that one eye in the visual test situation. If there are significant differences between nasal and temporal hemi-retinae (Overton & Weiner, 1966), this will tend to influence the magnitude of the laterality effect observed in these functionally "one-eyed" individuals. It may very well be that the conflicting data on the relation between sighting dominance and cerebral lateralization are due to the varying incidence of these monocular suppressors.

In conclusion, sighting dominance seems to be a stable phenomenon that exhibits a clear dextral bias. There is, however, little evidence to indicate that it is closely related to either handedness or to cerebral lateralization. While it remains an interesting phenomenon to study in its own right, there is little reason to be concerned about the dire consequences of mixed hand–eye dominance. Further, sighting dominance has certainly not provided us with a satisfactory measure of functional lateralization.

Other Lateralities

Lateral dominance of both foot and ear have also been suggested as measures of an underlying lateralization that would be less subject to environmental influence. Although the dominant foot, as used in kicking, is often measured and does seem to show a right bias, Raczkowski *et al.* (1974) indicate that questions about footedness have low reliability and validity.

Earedness is usually defined in a way analogous to eye dominance, as the ear used when only one can be used, as in using the telephone. This is almost certainly affected by the dominant hand, since one wishes to leave the writing hand free, and by the construction of many office telephones with a left shoulder rest. There is little evidence that this form of ear dominance is related to any other type of laterality (Coren & Porac, 1980a, 1980b; Porac & Coren, 1979).

Conclusions

The very fact that the vast majority of people are right-handed and an equally vast majority show a left-hemispheric specialization for speech has led many researchers to assume that the two phenomena are interrelated. For many years, it was assumed that speech was represented in the right hemisphere of the left-handed. More recent work has indicated that this is not the case and that the association between handedness and speech lateralization is a weak one, although it is true that left-handers show a higher incidence of right-hemispheric speech than do right-handers. Attempts to predict just which left-handers have right-hemispheric speech have examined such variables as strength of handedness, familial history of sinistrality, and writing posture, and have led to inconsistent and inconclusive results.

Nevertheless, handedness remains an important variable in the study of lateralized behavior in the normal. On the average, left-handers are far more likely to have right-hemispheric speech than are right-handers. Earlier, we have argued that the demonstration of a consistent laterality effect is not sufficient to show that a behavior is related to the differential functioning of the two hemispheres. Comparison of the performance of left-handers and right-handers remains as a technique for making the argument that a particular behavior is related to hemispheric asymmetry more tenable. One must, however, remain aware of the possibility that there are specific effects of handedness, such as an attentional bias toward the dominant side.

This chapter has also examined the reliability and validity of various measures of handedness. It is clear that many items that have been used to classify people as left-handed are quite unsatisfactory. At present, the most satisfactory measure of handedness would involve a short preference inventory (see Table 10.3) and a performance test involving tapping speed.

Attempts to assess cerebral lateralization by means of motor tasks using eyedness or footedness have proven to be even less satisfactory than the classification of people according to handedness. In part, this is due to a lack of adequate data, and further research in this area is justified.

11

Genetics of Laterality

The fact that so many clinicians and researchers consider it important to collect information about the familial history of sinistrality from their patients and subjects (e.g., Hécaen *et al.*, 1981; Hécaen & Sauguet, 1971; Zurif & Bryden, 1969) suggests that these investigators consider cerebral lateralization to have a heritable component. Indeed, it is difficult to imagine how various aspects of lateralization could be so consistent in all cultures and across all ages without being at least in part genetically determined. On the other hand, it is equally difficult to imagine how a gene can have a lateralized effect—how it would be, for example, that an enzyme might have as its target one side rather than the other of an otherwise fundamentally symmetric organism. This dilemma has led to a great deal of debate about the biological basis of lateralization (cf. Dimond & Blizard, 1977). The present chapter is concerned with evidence for a genetic basis for hemispheric asymmetry and other lateralized phenomena.

The Genetics of Cerebral Asymmetry

Despite the willingness of many clinicians to assume a genetic basis for cerebral lateralization, there are virtually no data that bear directly on this point. Clinical studies of cerebral function deal with various forms of head injury—epilepsy, stroke, gunshot wound, and the like—and it is rare for several members of a single family to present themselves for study. When one thinks of the population with which one is dealing, it is not so surprising that there are no genetic studies. The few data that we have come from investigations in which cerebral asymmetry in normals has been assessed by dichotic listening performance.

Bryden (1975) administered both stop consonant pairs and lists of digits for dichotic free recall to 49 families in which he was able to test both parents and at least two children. He found significant mother–son and mother–child correlations for the digit recall task, although there was also a negative intraclass correlation between siblings. With the stop consonant pairs, the mother–son correlation remained, but there was also a genetically inexplicable mother–father correlation. There was also some tendency for these correlations to be stronger in the 19 families that showed some evidence of familial left-handedness. M. Schwartz (1979) replicated this study on a somewhat larger sample and also found a significant mother–child correlation, in the absence of the embarrassing father–mother correlation.

The results of these two studies are sufficiently complex that no simple conclusions can be drawn. Furthermore, the most impressive correlations arise from the digit recall data, and it has earlier been pointed out that this procedure is highly contaminated by strategy effects and attentional biases that may be quite unrelated to hemispheric asymmetry. However, both studies provide evidence for a mother–child correlation. As shall be seen in subsequent sections, the existence of such a correlation is consistent with some genetic models, but also with models emphasizing prenatal nongenetic factors and environmental determinants.

Springer and Searleman (1978) have approached the genetics of cerebral laterality through a study of twins, using a dichotic stop consonant task. They found a negative correlation (−.34) between laterality measures for monozygotic twins and a small positive one (+.09) for dizygotic twins. Not wishing to completely abandon a genetic argument, they argue for a mirror-imaging mechanism that would lead monozygotic pairs to show a greater percentage of shared variance than dizygotic pairs. A simple genetic model, of course, would lead one to expect a significant positive correlation in monozygotic pairs. The mirror-imaging mechanism is suggested by the negative correlation. In addition, Springer and Searleman (1978) found a much higher correlation between total correct scores for monozygotic twins than for dizygotic twins. Whether this indicates anything more than a heritable attentional auditory discrimination component is not clear.

The one remaining study of the genetics of cerebral lateralization is that of Carter-Saltzman (1979). She employed both dichotic and tachistoscopic tasks as measures of cerebral lateralization, as well as a variety of measures of cognitive ability. She found evidence for a relation between cognitive performance and cerebral asymmetry that was affected by the familial history of the subject. Like many other studies, this work implicates the family pedigree but does not provide sufficient information for us to see how the various factors interact.

The few studies that have attempted to examine the heritability of cerebral asymmetry directly have provided us with only a few suggestive hints. The Springer and Searleman (1978) work would really be more relevant to the understanding of twinning rather than to the genetics of lateralization. The Bryden (1975) and M. Schwartz (1979) data provide us with some evidence for a mother–child correlation, but this is consistent with several models. To obtain further ideas about the genetics of cerebral laterality, it is necessary to examine the various models that have been developed to account for the distribution of handedness.

The Genetics of Handedness

It may seem rather strange to turn to genetic studies of handedness after having argued that handedness is only a poor correlate of cerebral asymmetry (see Chapter 10). However, ideas and models that are appropriate to one lateralized phenomenon may well have applicability to the other. Further, there is some dispute as to whether any gene can have a lateralized effect, and if a viable genetic model of handedness can be produced, then a genetic model of cerebral lateralization will also be admissable. It is too extreme, however, to say that the demonstration of a genetic effect for handedness requires one to accept a genetic basis for cerebral lateralization (Levy, 1976).

Before examining the various theories that have been proposed, it is well to let the reader examine the data concerning handedness in families and to discuss some of the problems that vex the researcher. There is really no wholly satisfactory study of handedness in families. The problems associated with the measurement of handedness have already been discussed. Family studies of handedness invariably violate one or more of the caveats presented in Chapter 10. They rely on self-report as a means of assessing handedness; the questionnaires are not standardized; they accept statements by the subjects about the handedness of relatives; the criteria for considering a person to be left-handed vary from study to study; and so on. Nevertheless, it is rare for theorists to obtain new data. It is a much more common practice to reanalyze the data from one or more of the reasonably careful large-scale studies, such as those of Chamberlain (1928), Rife (1940), and Annett (1973). Table

Table 11.1
Incidence of Left-handed Offspring as a Function of Parental Handedness (%)

Parental handedness	Annett (1973)	Rife (1940)	Chamberlain (1928)	Bryden (1979)	Sum
Total N	7476	2178	7724	18,260	35,638
R father/R mother	6875	1993	7225	16,097	32,190
N left-handed	669	151	308	1,609	2,837
% left-handed	9.7	7.6	4.3	10.0	8.8
L father/R mother	308	99	168	1,238	1,813
N left-handed	43	18	26	210	297
% left-handed	14.0	18.2	15.5	16.9	16.4
R father/L mother	288	49	137	822	1,296
N left-handed	82	16	27	159	284
% left-handed	28.5	32.7	19.7	19.3	21.9
L father/L mother	133[a]	11	100[b]	103	347
N left-handed	46	6	46	25	123
% left-handed	34.6	54.5	46.0	24.3	35.4

[a]Includes 128 children of families in which both parents are left-handed writers drawn from a special press and radio appeal.
[b]Includes additional subjects from special appeal.

11.1 presents a summary of these studies, as well as some data collected by Bryden (1979c). This table illustrates the major findings observed in most studies of handedness in families: Left-handed parents are rather more likely to produce left-handed offspring than are right-handed parents; the incidence of left-handedness is somewhat higher when the mother is left-handed than when the father is; left-handedness occurs fairly often when both parents are right-handed; and even when both parents are left-handed, the incidence of left-handedness is no more than 50%. It should be evident that no elementary genetic model will account for these data. However, the data in Table 11.1 do suggest that left-handedness is more likely if one has a left-handed parent. Annett (1973) has computed estimates of broad heritability from these data, and Bryden has carried out similar computations on his own data. Table 11.2 shows these various estimates of heritability. In all samples, the association between mothers and daughters reaches statistical significance. In addition, there are signs of an association between fathers and daughters and between mothers and sons in three of the five samples. These figures suggest a greater influence of mothers than of fathers, and that daughters are more influenced by their parents than are sons.

Estimates of broad heritability are no more than measures of association; they do not demonstrate that a particular characteristic is genetically determined. Some of the effects shown in Table 11.2 may, for example, be due to environmental influences in the home. Before leaping to an environmental conclusion, however, note that the vast majority of left-handed children have two right-handed parents.

One other problem for biological theories of handedness arises from twin data. A simple genetic model would predict that monozygotic twin pairs would have the same handedness; however, discordant twin pairs are relatively common. Carter-Saltzman, Scarr-Salapatek, Barker, and Katz (1976), for example, present data indicating that about 23% of monozygotic twin pairs and 21% of dizygotic twin pairs manifest discordant handedness. This discordance has led many theorists to argue for a concept of mirror imaging in twins (Newman, 1928), whereas others have concluded from the data that handedness is nongenetic in origin (Collins, 1970; Morgan & Corballis, 1978).

Any theory of the origins of handedness will have to deal with these data on handedness in families and in twins. At present, there seem to be four generally plausible classes of models, involving genetic factors to varying degrees. These include fully genetic models, partially genetic models, developmental gradient models, and environmental models. Let us examine each of these possibilities.

Table 11.2
Estimates of Heritability from Various Studies[a]

| | Chamberlain (1928) | Rife (1940) | Annett (1973) | | Bryden (1979c) | Median |
			Main sample	Parents only		
Males						
Fathers	40*	35	17	26	10	26
Mothers	49*	21	57*	−2	35*	35
Brothers	—	—	20	—	27*	23
Sisters	—	—	21	—	32*	27
Females						
Fathers	29	72*	4	56*	34*	34
Mothers	65*	81*	51*	103*	39*	65
Brothers	—	—	16	—	1	9
Sisters	—	—	44*	—	38*	41

[a]Except for Bryden (1979c), estimates of heritability are taken from Annett (1973). Unavailable data are expressed by dashes.
*$p < .05$.

Genetic Determination of Handedness

Over the years, there have been a number of attempts to account for the distribution of handedness by genetic mechanisms. Most of these have been rejected as being too simplistic. Trankell (1955), for example, argued that handedness was due to a simple recessive for which there is incomplete expression. Such a theory cannot account for the consistent sex differences and, in postulating incomplete expression of the recessive, really does no more than to move the focus of the problem to the mechanisms for the incomplete expression.

More recently, Levy and Nagylaki (1972) have proposed a model that has commanded somewhat greater attention. They postulate that two genes are involved: one (*Ll*) determines which hemisphere is dominant for language, while the other (*Cc*) determines whether hand control is contralateral or ipsilateral to the language-dominant hemisphere. *L* and *C* are the dominant alleles, while *l* and *c* are recessive. This model, then, attempts to account for the distribution both of handedness and of language lateralization, and provides a mechanism for the two to be imperfectly correlated. According to this model, the genotypes *LLCC*, *LLCc*, *LlCC*, and *LlCc* will be right-handed and have left-hemispheric speech. *llCC* and *llCc* will be left-handed and have right-hemispheric speech, while *LLcc* and *Llcc* will be left-handed and have left-hemispheric speech. Finally, *llcc* will be right-handed, with right-hemispheric speech (see Figure 11.1).

Levy and Nagylaki (1972) fitted their model to Rife's (1940) data on handedness in families and found very good agreement when the frequency of the dominant allele *C* was approximately .75 and that of L approximately .77. In fitting these data, they assumed that the incidence of left-hemispheric speech in sinistrals was 53%, deriving this figure from a study of left-handed aphasics by Goodglass and Quadfasel (1954). As indicated in Chapter 10, current data suggest that this is a somewhat low estimate, and the specific gene frequencies will change if this parameter is altered. Nevertheless, the basic thrust of the model remains unchanged.

Levy and Nagylaki (1972) have argued that their model can account for the distribution of both handedness and language lateralization, and for the relation between the two, as well as for the different recovery rates from aphasia in dextrals and sinistrals. They further suggest that one phenotypic manifestation of ipsilateral hand control consists of writing in an "inverted" posture, and Levy and Reid (1978) have presented data to indicate that writing posture can be used to classify left-handers as to speech lateralization. As indicated earlier, however, other investi-

LEVY–NAGYLAKI MODEL OF HANDEDNESS

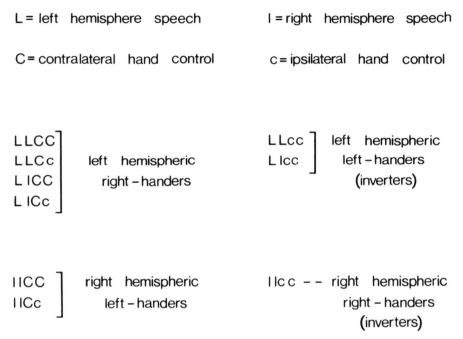

L = left hemisphere speech   l = right hemisphere speech

C = contralateral hand control   c = ipsilateral hand control

LLCC ⎤
LLCc ⎥ left hemispheric
L lCC ⎥ right – handers
L lCc ⎦

LLcc ⎤ left hemispheric
L lcc ⎦ left – handers
         (inverters)

llCC ⎤ right hemispheric
llCc ⎦ left – handers

llc c – – right hemispheric
         right – handers
         (inverters)

Figure 11.1. Levy–Nagylaki two-gene model of handedness, where L and C are dominant alleles and l and c recessives.

gators have not found writing posture to be so effective a predictor of speech lateralization. The point is not crucial for the model. It indicates only that writing posture is not solely a manifestation of ipsilateral hand control.

In developing their model, Levy and Nagylaki (1972) have completely ignored the twin data, arguing for mirror imaging in some twins. Indeed, Boklage (1977) has argued that twinning itself is an abnormality of symmetry and that the twin data should not be considered as crucial to a general model of laterality but should be dealt with separately.

Levy and Nagylaki have also not considered any sex differences in handedness or in cerebral lateralization, considering both effects to be tenuous at best. However, as shown earlier, sex effects are quite prevalent in family studies of handedness. Hudson (1975) commented on this point and contended that the model does not fit Annett's (1973) data. Levy (1977) countered this by arguing that Rife's (1940) data do not show a sex difference and that they provide the only truly suitable data for testing the theory since individuals who showed any sign of left-handedness were classified as sinistrals. She contends that Annett's (1973) data contain many instances of genotypic left-handers being classified as dextrals, citing the grossly different incidences in parents and children as evidence.

The Levy–Nagylaki model illustrates one way in which a genetic model can be fit to the basic data on handedness and breeding ratios. In addition, it explicitly relates handedness and cerebral lateralization and provides a number of testable predictions. Criticisms of it have tended to focus on the choice of data for fitting, the mechanism by which a gene can express a lateralized effect, and the investigators' decision to ignore the twin data. Levy (1976) has, in response, mustered the data supporting a genetic argument.

Genetic–Environmental Interaction

Annett (1972, 1978) has also developed a model for the genetics of handedness. Her model makes provisions for a considerable environmental influence on expressed handedness. In effect, she postulates a single gene with two alleles (*Rr*) to determine the presence or absence of a "right shift." *RR* and *Rr* genotypes will possess the right shift, but *rr* genotypes will not (see Figure 11.2). The environment interacts with the genotype to produce a normal distribution of skills centered at the appropriate mean. Thus, right-shift individuals will have a mean that favors the right hand, but environmental pressures are sufficient that a few of them will exhibit left-handedness. By her argument, *R* also controls speech lateralization, and *RR* and *Rr* genotypes are left-hemispheric for speech. Thus, the few who become environmentally left-handed will be included among the left-hemispheric sinistrals.

In the *rr* genotype, both handedness and speech lateralization are determined randomly by environmental factors acting both pre- and postnatally. Thus, among *rr* individuals, half will be right-handed and half left-handed, half will be right-hemispheric for speech and half left-hemispheric. The Annett model can also account for the frequent discordance of handedness in twins by postulating a high frequency of the *rr* genotype in twins.

ANNETT MODEL OF HANDEDNESS

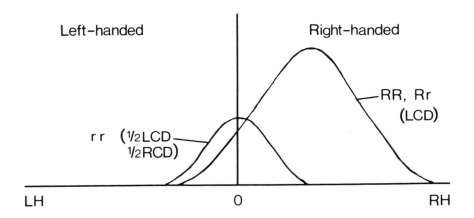

Differences in manual dexterity

Figure 11.2. The Annett model of handedness. Those not possessing the right-shift factor have scores normally distributed about a mean of 0, with half being left dominant for speech and half right dominant. Of those who possess the right-shift factor, all will be left-dominant for speech, but a few at the tail of the distribution will show a left-hand superiority.

Levy (1977) has argued that the Annett model leads to no testable predictions. Indeed, although the model provides a decent fit to most data, it is difficult to see how it could be tested. Morgan (1977) has suggested that the model might well be reversed, to postulate a gene for left-handedness rather than one for right-handedness. Certainly, one would expect environmental influences to have a right bias, rather than the random effect Annett (1978) postulates.

Laterality Arising from a Maturational Gradient

Morgan and Corballis (1978) have argued that there is no evidence that genes can specifically encode any left–right asymmetry and there-fore that neither handedness nor cerebral lateralization can be under direct genetic control. Genetic factors can, however, determine the degree of asymmetry that will be manifest, or even whether or not an asymmetry is expressed. Arguing from this viewpoint, Corballis and Morgan (1978) suggest that both handedness and cerebral lateralization are manifestations of a left-to-right maturational gradient, generally favoring early or more rapid development on the left than on the right. They suggest that, if the leading side is damaged or restricted in growth, the polarity will be reversed and development will proceed from right to left. By this argument, left-hemispheric speech representation and right-handedness would be the normal state, and, in fact, the right hemisphere would develop its functions by default. Disturbance or damage in early embryological development would lead to a reversal of the gradient, and a reversal of both handedness and speech lateralization. Decoupling of handedness and speech would occur only when damage was at a critical stage of development and, since handedness develops later than the neural basis for language, would almost invariably produce left-handers who are left-hemispheric for speech.

Corballis and Morgan (1978) present data in support of the notion of a left-to-right maturational gradient that is coded in the spatial structure of the oocyte rather than in the genes. According to their view, any genetic influence is on the degree of lateralization expressed, not on its direction.

Laterality Arising from Perinatal Brain Damage

In many pathological groups, especially epileptics and mental retardates, the incidence of left-handedness is significantly higher than in the general population (Satz, 1972). Satz has suggested that the increase in left-handedness is due to damage to the left hemisphere producing a mild hypofunction of the contralateral hand, thus leading the child to switch to the opposite hand for manual activities. Assuming side of early brain damage to be randomly distributed, this model also requires that some individuals who would normally be left-handed have suffered right-hemispheric brain damage and have become pathological right-handers. Because the incidence of left-handedness is so small in the general population, such cases of pathological right-handedness would be much less frequent than instances of pathological left-handedness, and the shift in the targeted pathological group would be toward a greater incidence of left-handedness. Satz and his colleagues have reported good support for this model (Satz, 1972, 1973; Satz, Baymur, & Van der Vlugt, 1979; Silva & Satz, 1979).

This argument can be taken to an extreme by arguing that all cases of left-handedness are pathological in origin. Bakan (1971) and Bakan *et al.* (1973) have reported that the incidence of birth stress (Caesarian section, prematurity, Rh incompatibility, breech birth, etc.) is about twice as high among left-handed undergraduates as among their right-handed counterparts. They suggest that left-handedness is the result of left-hemispheric cerebral anoxia following birth stress. M. Schwartz (1977), however, was not able to replicate the Bakan *et al.* (1973) study. Further, Liederman and Kinsbourne (1980) have shown a relation between parental handedness and neonatal head turning. This provides strong support for at least genetic involvement in lateralization.

Bakan's position seems to be a relatively strong view of the origins of left-handedness, considering it as a "benign form of brain damage." While it is clear that some left-handers are pathological in the sense of having become left-handed because of very mild early brain damage, there is little evidence to suggest that *all* left-handers fit this model. It would be interesting, however, to segregate left-handers with birth stress from other left-handers in a familial study of handedness. Perhaps one of the reasons for the low heritability values observed in family studies is that many pathological left-handers have been included, and their data obscure any familial relationship.

Inheritance of Degree of Laterality

As in so many of the topics we have discussed, no final answer is immediately evident. To test the various models described in the preceding pages, we need somewhat more detailed evidence about handedness in families. In particular, we need continuous, rather than dichotomous, data on both hand preference and hand performance, and we need to observe the performance of all subjects, rather than relying on our students to tell us about their parents. Bryden has been engaged in just such a project, and preliminary data are now available (Bryden, 1979c).

The first step was to develop a simple performance test. Subjects were asked to make dots in a series of small circles as rapidly as possible, first with one hand and then with the other. The score for each hand was the number of circles filled in 20 sec. This task was given as a group

test to introductory psychology classes. It has high split-half reliability
and correlates highly with scores on a shortened version of the Oldfield
questionnaire (Bryden, 1977; Tapley & Bryden, 1980).

Currently, data are being obtained from family units on this tapping
test, the shortened form of the Oldfield handedness inventory, and the
Miles test of sighting dominance. Student volunteers have been trained
to administer this battery and have obtained data from their extended
families.

The results of this testing are, at the moment, highly preliminary, but
they contain some interesting points. Let us begin by looking at the data
from the tapping test, broken down by sex into the four possible parent–child pairings. Correlations between parent-and child on this test
are negligible, as one might expect from the very small effect of parental
handedness we saw earlier. The tapping scores, which are usually expressed as negative values to indicate left-hand superiority and as positive scores to indicate right-hand superiority, were then reentered as
absolute value measures. The results of this manipulation are shown in
the right-hand column of Table 11.3: Three of the correlations increase to
statistical significance. In other words, there is some evidence that
strongly handed parents produce strongly handed offspring, without
determining whether or not these offspring are to be left-handed or
right-handed (see also Coren & Porac, 1980b).

The same approach was then applied to the data from the hand
preference inventory, with basically similar results (see Table 11.4). Parent–child correlations are small, whereas correlations based on the absolute values are higher and significant in the case of father–son and
mother–daughter relations. Canonical correlation indicates that a com-

Table 11.3
Familial Resemblance in Tapping Scores

	N	True values	Absolute values
Father–Son	51	.277**	.247*
Father–Daughter	77	.079	.232**
Mother–Son	66	.065	.103
Mother–Daughter	93	−.016	.244***
Parent–Child	287	.058	.202***

$^{*}p < .10.$
$^{**}p < .05.$
$^{***}p < .01.$

Table 11.4
Familial Resemblance in Hand Preferences Scores

	N	True values	Absolute values
Father–Son	51	.087	.359*
Father–Daughter	77	−.134	.115
Mother–Son	66	−.062	.088
Mother–Daughter	93	.007	.326*
Parent–Child	287	−.030	.208**

$*p < .01.$
$**p < .001.$

bination of the absolute performance and preference measures in the parents can predict the absolute measures in the children much better than the directional measures can predict one another.

It is true that there is a relatively small sample here and that like-sex correlations are higher than cross-sex correlations. One might argue that this is evidence for a sex-role influence. However, if one accepts the correlations at face value, they provide the beginnings for a model for the origins of handedness and lateral specialization. Such a model is based on the assumption that it is the degree of lateralization that has a genetic basis, and not the direction of lateralization (cf. Collins, 1977). For the sake of argument, let us assume that about 20% of the population are strongly lateralized and that the remaining 80% are weakly lateralized. At outset, or at conception, about half of each group will tend to become left lateralized and half right lateralized (see Figure 11.3). During embryological development, the bias toward a left-to-right developmental gradient postulated by Corballis and Morgan (1978) affects this distribution, by pushing some 50% of the "weak left" subjects over to "weak right." Thus, at birth, the distribution includes about 10% strong left and 10% strong right, and about 20% weak left and 60% weak right. These figures have been chosen quite arbitrarily, but they reflect the observation that the distribution of neonatal differences in brain size is about 30:70 and the observation that about 70% of the population is right-eyed.

At birth, the many perinatal trauma, such as forceps or breech delivery, Caesarians, and brief anoxia, enter the picture. These do not change the overall distribution, but they do shift particular individuals from one category to another. Those instances of right-hemispheric speech lateral-

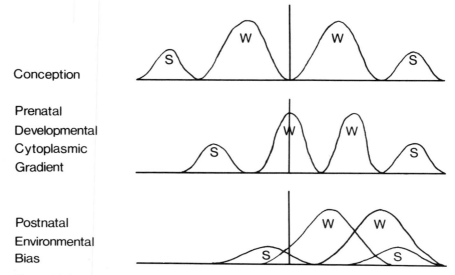

Figure 11.3. Hypothetical shifts in handedness shown by two populations, one exhibiting strong (S) laterality, and the other weak (W) laterality. At conception, a random bias to left or right is assigned to each group. The left-to-right developmental gradient results in a shift of all groups toward the right during prenatal development. Environmental pressures force all W subjects to the right, but S subjects resist environmental pressures and are less influenced. At the end, virtually all W subjects show a right-hand preference, while the S subjects are almost evenly divided between left- and right-handedness.

ization in right-handers, for instance, are probably instances of birth difficulty, according to the scenario being developed here.

After birth, the environmental pressure of what is essentially a right-handed world begins to take effect. The development of language and manual dexterity interact with one another to ensure that handedness and speech lateralization will agree in the majority of cases. Environmental pressure pushes the majority of the 20% "weak left" subjects over to the right side, and only those whose environment is left-handed or minimally biased remain left-handed (perhaps to become the left-hemispheric left-handers). On the other hand, only very strong environmental pressure will convert any of the 10% "strong left" individuals into right-handers. Ultimately, we end up with the distribution of handedness shown in Figure 11.3.

It should be reiterated that this is only a word picture of a very preliminary model. However, it does offer some interesting potential. The assumption that it is strength of handedness rather than direction that is genetically determined would be more acceptable to many geneticists, who have difficulty in imagining how a gene can have an asymmetric target, and, coupled with the notion of nongenetic pressures toward right-handedness, can be fit to the data on handedness in families. Because it is the postulated "strongly lateralized" subjects who make up the vast majority of left-handers, left-handedness appears to run in families. In fact, it is only strong lateralization that runs in families, and half of these genotypes turn out to be left-handed. (As an aside, it should be pointed out that this model makes left-handers "strong" only in the genetic sense; they are not phenotypically more lateralized than right-handers because of environmental pressures. In fact, left-handers are typically less lateralized than right-handers.)

As a further point, this model can cope with the twin data, in that it is no longer an embarrassment to have so many monozygotic twins of opposite handedness. In addition, it recognizes both environmental pressures and local perinatal disturbances.

Perhaps the biggest problem at the moment is getting the distribution of handedness and speech lateralization to come out right. The correlation between these two variables in the population, however, is only about .05: They are almost independent functions. Perhaps independent factors influence their distribution.

Finally, the genetic aspect of this model is fundamentally the same as that proposed by Annett (1978): In effect, the model is built on Morgan's (1977) suggestion that it is left-handedness, not right-handedness, that is genetically determined. However, in this model, "weak" subjects are heavily influenced by their environment and correspond in frequency to Annett's right-shift subjects; "strong" subjects are relatively uninfluenced by the environment, but correspond in frequency to Annett's subjects lacking the right-shift factor. While using different labels, the above model corresponds to Annett's (1978) version in many ways.

The Evolution of Laterality

In the absence of any wholly convincing genetic model for left-handedness or for cerebral organization, it may be quite pointless to engage in any speculations on the evolution of laterality. Unfortunately, the fossil record does not preserve information about the behavior of protohominids, nor does it tell us about the functional properties of the brain. Despite the obstacles, however, a few comments on the possible evolution of laterality are in order.

Humans have been predominately right-handed for a long time, and left-handedness has stubbornly remained with us for just as long. As mentioned earlier, Coren and Porac (1977) have noted no significant change in the incidence of left-handedness as portrayed in works of art over the past 10 millennia, and certainly left-handers were not uncommon in biblical times (Judges 20:15–16). Although there seems to be a somewhat variable expression of left-handedness, it does occur in all cultures (Dawson, 1977), with some 2% of the population resisting all cultural pressure to become right-handed and with about 12% being the maximum incidence of left-handedness.

We can say less about the history of cerebral organization, but again it is the left hemisphere that is specialized for verbal processes in some 95% of the population, regardless of culture or language.

Perhaps the fact that most of us are right-handed and left-brained for speech has led to the general assumption that the two must have something to do with one another. The relation between handedness and speech lateralization is a relatively weak one, however, and one problem in the present speculations will be in showing how the two can be decoupled. At present, one promising notion is Levy's (1972) suggestion that cerebral organization and ipsilateral/contralateral hand control are independently determined. Furthermore, it should be remembered that speech and spatial processes seem to be independently lateralized and thus have somewhat different origins.

Why are we unilateral for speech? Probably because bilateral speech control would have such a disruptive effect on the timing necessary to control the speech articulators (Jones, 1966). Bilateral speech would lead to a population of stutterers.

Why are we unimanual? Probably because of unimanual tools and the fact that a consistent way of using tools permits greater skill and efficiency.

Given unilaterality for both speech and hand use, why does that unilaterality take the form that it does? There is no obvious answer to that: We seem to have become right-handed through random accident, and as far as is evident, the world might just as well have become left-handed and right-hemispheric for speech. Once a right bias was established, however, manual control and speech control, emanating as they do from adjacent areas of the brain, almost certainly supported one another. In fact, there is much to be said for the argument that speech lateralization grew out of initial gestural communication with the preferred right hand (Kimura, 1979).

If there is any evolutionary pressure, it is much more likely to have been on handedness than on speech lateralization. Maynard Smith

(1976) has applied cost–benefit analysis to evolutionary theory, and his work suggests one reason why left-handedness remains with us. Maynard Smith has shown that a characteristic will reach equilibrium frequency in the population when the benefits of possessing the characteristic are balanced by the costs of having it. There may well be both costs and benefits associated with being left-handed. The costs are obvious, in terms of inefficient tool use because the tools are uncomfortable and in terms of social ostracism for being different. The benefits lie largely in "surprisal" during hand-to-hand combat, as any dextral who first encounters a left-handed tennis player can attest: The left-hander can attack where one is not expecting it. Perhaps the balance between these costs and benefits is sufficient to keep left-handedness at a low frequency, but to prevent it from dying out.

If one takes the alternative view of the biology of laterality—namely, that it is degree of lateralization and not direction that is inherited—the problem becomes rather different. The problem is not one of determining why one reaches a particular balance between strong lateralization and weak lateralization, since there are undoubtedly costs and benefits associated with each, but one of accounting for the bias that makes most of us left-hemispheric for speech and right-handed. Earlier, it was necessary to postulate a left–right gradient of development. At the moment, there seems to be no good reason for this gradient to be left-to-right rather than right-to-left, other than to observe that this is the way humans are made.

12

The Development of
Cerebral Lateralization

Questions about the developmental course of cerebral lateralization are important for a variety of reasons. If we understand the developmental changes that take place in cerebral lateralization, we are clearly in a far better position to understand its nature and its origins. Furthermore, a number of studies have reported evidence indicating that lateral specialization is abnormal in certain pathological groups, such as poor readers or the congenitally deaf. One frequent interpretation of these data has been in terms of maturational lag (e.g., Bender, 1958). For such an interpretation to be valid, one must show that there *are* developmental changes to be delayed.

In his very influential book on the biology of language, Lenneberg (1967) argued that language functions became increasingly lateralized to the left hemisphere throughout childhood, reaching the adult stage only at puberty. Lenneberg based his arguments largely on data summarized by Basser (1962), who had found that dysphasias were much more prevalent following right-hemispheric damage in children than in adults. Children also showed a fairly complete recovery from left-hemispheric aphasias, in marked contrast to adults. In a more recent review of the literature, Krashen (1973) suggests that, while lateralization does change developmentally, it is fully complete by age 5.

The most obvious alternative view is that lateralization does not change developmentally but is complete at birth. A number of studies have found evidence for lateralization in newborns (e.g., Molfese, Freeman, & Palermo, 1975), and anatomical differences between the hemispheres have been found in infants (Wade, Clark, & Hamm, 1975). The fact that lateralization can be observed in the neonate leads many investigators to argue that there are no systematic developmental changes in lateral specialization (e.g., Kinsbourne & Hiscock, 1977).

At the same time, one must recognize that the tasks employed to measure lateralization in the neonate are quite different from those used in adults, or even in older children. One simply cannot ask infants what words they heard in a dichotic listening task. A child's abilities change as he or she grows older, and these changes in cognitive capacity may be reflected in performance differences on the tasks used to assess cerebral lateralization. Witelson (1977), for instance, has argued that developmental changes in performance on behavioral tasks intended to assess cerebral specialization are more likely to be due to changes in the cognitive repertoire of the subject, rather than to changes in hemispheric specialization per se.

Studies of Early Brain Damage

Basser's (1962) early review indicated that 35% of his cases with early childhood aphasia and unilateral damage had lesions in the right hemisphere. This is in sharp contrast to the figure of 1–3% expected in adults. Hécaen (1976) also observed an elevated incidence of dysphasia following unilateral right-hemispheric damage in young children, although he cites a number of other studies in which the incidence of right-hemispheric dysphasias has not been particularly pronounced. Kinsbourne and Hiscock (1977) surveyed the reports of early childhood aphasia in a large children's hospital. They found no difference in the incidence of right-hemispheric damage as a function of age, but 14% of their 58 cases had right-hemispheric damage.

Lenneberg (1967) selected puberty as the critical time for the full establishment of left-hemispheric language functions, whereas Krashen (1973) argued for an earlier time, at about 5 or 6. In fact, there are remarkably few data available to distinguish between these two views. Basser (1962) reported on virtually no cases between 6 and puberty, and so Lenneberg's decision to place the critical time point at puberty is little more than an educated guess. Likewise, Hécaen's (1976) series contains no instances of unilateral right-hemispheric damage between ages 6 and 12.

However, several general conclusions do appear warranted. The incidence of aphasic disturbances following unilateral right-hemispheric brain damage is much higher in children than it is in adults. This is true in the Kinsbourne and Hiscock (1977) data and in four of the five studies cited by Hécaen (1976). If one must select a critical period, Krashen's

(1973) view of age 6 has more support than Lenneberg's (1967) argument for puberty. In the Basser (1962), Kinsbourne and Hiscock (1977), and Hécaen (1976) data, aphasia follows unilateral left-hemispheric damage in 40 cases, and unilateral right-hemispheric damage in 13 cases (24.5%), among those children age 6 or younger. Estimating figures from Hécaen's Table 1 (1976, p. 118), the incidence of right-hemispheric lesions in older childhood aphasics is about 4.4%, whereas that in adult aphasics is about 2%. In some sense, then, the involvement of the right hemisphere in language processes is more evident in young children than in older children or in adults. One cannot take this, however, as unequivocal evidence that cerebral specialization develops: There are too few cases, the criteria for the diagnosis of aphasia vary, and the etiology often leaves open the possibility of undetected damage in the opposite hemisphere. Before we can reach any final conclusions about the development of cerebral specialization, we must look at other sources of evidence.

One such source comes from the few cases of individuals who have had one entire cerebral hemisphere removed at an early age (Dennis & Whitaker, 1977). Although such hemidecorticates are rare, existing evidence suggests that those with early left-hemisphere removal show deficits in complex verbal skills when compared to those with early right-hemisphere removal. Conversely, left-hemidecorticates are better at spatial skills than are right-hemidecorticates (Dennis & Kohn, 1975; Kohn & Dennis, 1974a). These findings would suggest that the two hemispheres are not totally interchangeable. In some way, the left hemisphere is prewired in such a fashion that it can develop language skills better than the right, and the right hemisphere is prewired to acquire spatial skills. This tendency for the left hemisphere to be a better substrate for language development is in agreement with the observation that language disturbances are more likely to follow upon left-hemispheric damage than right, even in very young children (Basser, 1962; Hécaen, 1976; Kinsbourne & Hiscock, 1977).

In addition to the clinical data, there are a number of studies reporting anatomical differences between the hemispheres in infant brains. In general, these studies show that the planum temporale, a region that encompasses the posterior speech areas, is larger on the left than on the right (Wada *et al.*, 1975; Witelson & Pallie, 1973). Similar findings have been reported for adult brains (e.g., Geschwind & Levitsky, 1968; Rubens, 1977). It should be pointed out, however, that the left temporal planum is the larger in only about 60–70% of the cases, while left-hemispheric speech representation is found in a much higher percentage of adults. Furthermore, there is not yet any evidence indicating that a larger left temporal planum makes it any more likely that speech will ultimately be represented in the left hemisphere.

The clinical and anatomical data point to the existence at birth of a left-hemispheric site for speech representation. At the same time, there is evidence that speech is much more vulnerable to right-hemispheric damage in early childhood than it is in adulthood. Moscovitch (1977) has offered two speculations to account for the apparent anomaly. One possibility is that language systems, being poorly developed in preschool children, are vulnerable to many different types of cerebral insult and that right-hemispheric damage produces enough diffuse disturbance to generate dysphasic symptoms. Another possibility is that early language is more sensorimotor and concrete in nature, and thus more likely to involve structures in the right hemisphere as well as those in the left.

A Behavioral Study

Perhaps the classic behavioral study of the development of language lateralization is that of Kimura (1963). In this study, Kimura applied her dichotic listening procedure (see Chapter 3) to the study of normal children, ranging in age from 4 to 9 years. She reported significant right-ear superiorities in all groups except the 7- and 9-year-old girls. These findings suggested that left-hemispheric speech representation had fully developed by age 4.

The Kimura study, however, is not without its difficulties. Subjects were given 10 trials each with one pair, two pairs, and three pairs of digits. The scores reported are the total number of correct items summed across the 30 trials. Thus, the three-pair trials represent 50% of the maximum score on each ear, while the single-pair trials contribute only 17% of the final score. Furthermore, the procedure called for a free recall of as many of the digits as could be remembered. We have already seen how the free-recall procedure can be heavily influenced by attentional biases and how memory factors can be very important with lists of items. Finally, Kimura indicates that the 4 year olds were very hard to test and that two were unable to complete the series. Nevertheless, the data from these two subjects are apparently included in her test of the right-ear effect (Kimura, 1963, Table 1, p. 900).

Another curiosity that appears in Kimura's data has often been misinterpreted. The mean right-ear effect for the 4 year olds is 13.1 digits, whereas that for the 9 year olds is only 2.7 digits. At times, this has led to the argument that the right-ear effect is actually decreasing with age, and therefore presumably language is becoming less lateralized. What actually is occurring, however, is that overall accuracy is increasing with age. Because of a ceiling effect, the absolute magnitude of the right-ear effect is decreasing. If one expresses the laterality effect in terms of a laterality coefficient that takes the overall level of accuracy into account, one finds that the magnitude of the laterality effect remains approximately constant over the age range tested (see Chapter 2).

Despite these problems, the findings of the Kimura (1964) study have stood the test of time remarkably well. While there have been occasional reports of an increase with age in the dichotic right-ear effect, the vast majority of studies using the procedure have found no developmental changes in lateralization (Witelson, 1977).

Other Dichotic Listening Studies

Since Kimura's initial study (1963), a large number of developmental studies of dichotic listening performance have been carried out with verbal material. A review covering the majority of these studies has been published by Witelson (1977). In these studies, two general approaches have been followed. Some investigators have followed Kimura's lead and presented lists of numbers or words for free recall. Others have employed single pairs of items, usually using the currently popular set of six stop consonant–vowel syllables.

The studies of C. Knox and Kimura (1970), Schulman-Galambos (1977), and Bryden and Allard (1981) are fairly typical of the studies employing dichotic lists. None showed any age-related change in the right-ear effect, with children ranging in age from 5 years (kindergarten) to 11 years. Two notable exceptions are the studies of Inglis and Sykes (1967), who failed to find any right-ear effect at most age levels between 5 and 10, and Satz, Bakker, Teunissen, Goebel, and Van der Vlugt (1975), who found a clear age-related trend, with the right-ear effect being observed only after age 9.

Although Bever (1971) reports finding a right-ear superiority as early as 2½ years, most of the other failures to find a right-ear effect with dichotic lists have been with very young children (e.g., Geffner & Hochberg, 1971; Kinsbourne & Hiscock, 1977; Nagafuchi, 1970). Whether or not one should attach any significance to this is uncertain. A "failure" to obtain a right-ear effect usually indicates that the *t* test on the left and right ear means was not significant for the particular age group in question. Rarely is there a significant age by ear interaction. The comparisons that have been made are often on small sample sizes, and very young children are notoriously variable in their performance. It is entirely possible that error variance has swamped statistical significance. Certainly, if the earlier arguments (see Chapter 3) about experimental effects such as attentional biases are correct, one would expect considerable variability in young children that would be quite unrelated to language lateralization.

Berlin, Hughes, Lowe-Bell, and Berlin (1973) carried out a fairly large-scale study of dichotic performance with single consonant–vowel pairs, and their results are typical of experiments of this sort. They observed a large right-ear effect, with no age-related changes in its magnitude. Ingram (1975a) has found a right-ear effect for single pairs of similar-sounding words as early as age 3. Using a nonnutritive sucking procedure, Entus (1977) was able to observe a right-ear effect in infants of 1½–3 months, with single-pair material. About the only exception to this general finding is a study by Bryden and Allard (1978) that has failed to be replicated (Bryden & Allard, 1981).

However, even single-pair material is subject to response biases and memory effects. If one asks children to identify both items, accuracy on the second response given is at or barely above chance level. Including second-response data, then, does little more than to introduce noise. However, asking for only one response leaves it up to the subject as to what attentional strategy to adopt.

Several studies attempting to control for these attentional variables have been published. Bryden and Allard (1981), for example, asked children to attend to one ear and report only the item heard at that ear. With this procedure, they found a strong right-ear effect with no age-related changes.

Hiscock and Kinsbourne (1977) presented dichotic pairs, employing the digits 1–6. Subjects were preschool children aged 3, 4, and 5 years. In one condition, the subjects were instructed to monitor one ear and report only the number heard at that ear; in another condition, the cue as to which ear to report was given after the pair had been presented. Hiscock and Kinsbourne found right-ear effects in both conditions at all three age levels. However, Hiscock and Kinsbourne also found that intrusion errors from the right ear were far more common than intrusions from the left ear. While their data clearly show no age-related trends, the right-ear superiority could have emerged from either perceptual or attentional factors. Their study does not clearly demonstrate the existence of a right-ear effect in the absence of attentional biases.

Geffen (1978) presented lists of numbers varying in length from one to four pairs. She precued her subjects to report only the items from a specified ear. Subjects were aged 6, 8, and 10. All groups showed a right-ear effect, and there were no age-related trends in laterality. However, the right-ear effect did increase with longer lists and with later serial position in the four-item lists. Geffen suggests that the number of items in acoustic memory is one determinant of the magnitude of the laterality effect.

In another study, Geffen (1976) employed a signal detection procedure with single pairs of words, using subjects aged 5, 7, and 11. Subjects listened to lists of 120 paired monosyllabic words, presented at a rate of 1 pair per sec. Of the 240 words presented, 40 were instances of a particular target word, 40 were "noise" words that shared two phonemes in common with the target word, and the remaining 160 were irrelevant words with either one or no phonemes in common with the target word. In the dichotic condition, words heard on one ear were spoken in a male voice and words heard on the other ear were spoken in a female voice. Subjects were to indicate the presence of the target word on the right ear by pressing a response key with the right hand and the presence of a target word on the left ear by signaling with the left hand. In a binaural control condition, subjects heard identical inputs at the two ears and were to signal the target word in the male voice with one hand and in the female voice with the other hand.

The procedure permitted Geffen to determine a hit rate for each ear in the dichotic condition and for each voice in the binaural condition. By tabulating responses to the noise words, a false alarm rate could also be determined for each condition. From these figures, a measure of stimulus detectability (d') was calculated. In the binaural condition, subjects were more accurate responding with the right hand than with the left (see Table 12.1). In the dichotic condition, the superiority of responding to the right ear was even larger. Although d' increased with age, there were no interactions of ear or hand with age.

Although subjects were free to deploy their attention in any way they chose, measures of bias indicated no significant laterality effects. It would thus seem that subjects were successful in attending equally to left and right channels.

Geffen concludes that there are no significant age-related changes in dichotic verbal lateralization and thus that left-hemispheric specialization for language is fixed by age 5. In this, she is in general agreement with the vast majority of studies in the literature. However, there are potential difficulties in interpreting the results of her study. Performance on the binaural condition indicates that subjects are more accurate when responding with the right hand than when responding with

Table 12.1

Comparison of Dichotic and Binaural Detection Measures in Children

	Binaural			Dichotic			
Age	Left hand	Right hand	Difference	Left ear and hand	Right ear and hand	Difference	Dichotic–binaural difference
5 years	.71	1.14	.43	.70	1.41	.71	.28
7 years	1.12	1.22	.10	1.04	1.85	.81	.71
11 years	1.59	1.73	.14	1.75	2.77	1.02	.88

Note. Data from Geffen (1976).

the left hand (see Table 12.1). This manual asymmetry is slightly greater for the youngest group. Because subjects in the dichotic condition responded to right-ear targets with the right hand and to left-ear targets with the left hand, some of the dichotic effect will be due to the manual asymmetry. Geffen considers this effect minor, on the grounds that the lateral difference is significantly greater in the dichotic condition than in the binaural condition. However, if one considers the manual asymmetry to be a component of the dichotic left–right difference, then one might argue that the true perceptual difference is best measured by the difference between the dichotic effect and the binaural effect. These values are shown in the last column of Table 12.1: They increase steadily with increasing age. Geffen's failure to obtain a side by age by condition interaction in her analysis suggests that the trend is not statistically significant, but it would seem unjustified to ignore it completely, considering that only 12 subjects were tested at each age level.

By far the most common behavioral technique for testing the hypothesis that language processes become more fully lateralized in the left hemisphere with increasing age has been the dichotic listening procedure. The vast majority of such studies find no age-related effects on dichotic lateralization. The few studies that do find age-related effects employ procedures that permit the subject to adopt a biased attentional strategy, and they may indicate nothing more than changes in attentional bias with age. It is difficult to resist the conclusion that there are no systematic changes in the dichotic right-ear effect with age.

Several problems remain. Of the studies reviewed, very few have even attempted to control possible differences in strategy or attentional bias. Even in those that have, one gets the impression that the questions could have been better formulated or the data better analyzed. If the trend observed in Geffen's (1976) data (see Table 12.1) is at all real, there remains some possibility that a carefully designed study would reveal some age-related trend.

Furthermore, virtually all the dichotic listening experiments have involved fairly elementary speech recognition tasks, and as such they are concerned more with the detection and identification of phonemes than with any higher order language processes. It remains possible that semantic and syntactic processes do not become lateralized until puberty. One way to test this notion would be to modify Geffen's (1976) signal detection paradigm by requiring subjects to indicate words within a particular semantic category, rather than a single target word. This would ensure that higher order language processes were involved. One might expect to find an even more robust right-ear effect than is observed with a phoneme discrimination, and the difference between the two tasks might change with age.

At the present time, however, the dichotic listening literature points to the conclusion that language processes are lateralized to the left hemisphere at birth and do not change with increasing age.

Verbal Tachistoscopic Studies

The earliest developmental studies of visual-field differences in tachistoscopic recognition predated any concern with hemispheric asymmetry. Forgays (1953), for example, presented English words to the left or right of fixation and found that a right-visual-field superiority did not emerge until about age 12. Very similar findings have been reported by Miller and Turner (1973) and by Reitsma (1975). In all these experiments, familiar words were displayed horizontally and presented unilaterally in one visual field or the other.

Any assessment of verbal tachistoscopic studies of lateralization becomes inextricably entangled in the argument as to whether visual-field differences are the result of a superior left-hemispheric processing of verbal material or of directional scanning processes resulting from the fact that we read from left to right. In developmental studies, this problem becomes even more acute, because older children will necessarily be more fluent readers than younger ones. The problems of interpreting tachistoscopic studies of lateralization have already been considered in Chapters 2 and 4: In her review, Witelson (1977) argues that these difficulties are so severe as to make the studies virtually meaningless. She points out, for instance, that the Miller and Turner (1973) and Reitsma (1975) studies involve almost identical procedures and obtain almost identical results, yet Miller and Turner conclude that they have shown an age-related change in scanning, whereas Reitsma concludes that he has shown an age-related change in left-hemispheric language representation.

Moving to vertically displayed material does not provide a particularly satisfactory solution to the problem. Bryden (1970) noted that the sequential constraints in the language were not as effective for vertically arranged letter sequences as for horizontally arranged ones. Thus, words presented vertically would not be expected to have the same properties as words arranged horizontally, and any generalization from vertically presented words to horizontal ones would be questionable. One might employ single letters (Bryden, 1965), but even with this type of material, the right-visual-field effect may depend on the familiarity with the alphabet (Bryden & Allard, 1976).

One possible way of countering potential scanning effects is to use subjects who have learned to scan verbal material in directions other than from left to right. Hebrew, Arabic, and Urdu are among the common languages that are written and read from right to left, and Chinese is scanned from top to bottom.

Carmon, Nachshon, and Starinsky (1976) have taken advantage of this fact in a developmental study of visual-field differences in Israeli children. They presented Israeli schoolchildren varying in age from 6 to 12 years with single Hebrew letters, two- and four-letter Hebrew words (read from right to left), and two- and four-digit numbers (read from left to right). Materials were presented horizontally, and both unilaterally and bilaterally with order of report controlled.

Carmon et al. (1976) found a significant right-visual-field superiority for all types of material except the single letters. They argue that scanning effects must be minimal, since both Hebrew words and Arabic numerals produced a right-visual-field superiority, although they are scanned in different directions. Their data also showed a developmental trend, in that the older children showed a right-visual-field superiority for both words and numbers in both unilateral and bilateral conditions, whereas the younger children showed the right-field effect only with two-letter words presented bilaterally. Carmon et al. argue that there are developmental changes in the nature of left-hemispheric specialization and that the left hemisphere becomes increasingly involved in the sequential processing required for the identification of words and numbers. One might also argue that the typical word recognition experiment involves a greater semantic component than the dichotic listening experiments discussed earlier and that the Carmon results provide some support for contention that complex verbal processes become increasingly lateralized with age.

Tomlinson-Keasey, Kelly, and Burton (1978) also found evidence for an age-related change in lateralization for verbal material. They presented a single word or picture briefly in one visual field and, after a 2-sec interval, followed it with a second item that was either the same or different in the same visual field. They found a right-visual-field superiority for matching verbal stimuli in adults and in Grade 7 students, but not in Grade 3 students. Word matching is an odd choice for a task to maximally engage left-hemispheric language mechanisms, although the 2-sec intertrial interval may have prevented the possibility of a simple physical matching of the two stimuli (Posner, Boies, Eichelman & Taylor, 1969). However, the problems of scanning and fixation control are sufficiently severe as to make interpretation of this study difficult.

It is a frequent finding in verbal tachistoscopic studies that young children do not show clear laterality effects, whereas older ones manifest a right-visual-field superiority. How such data should be interpreted is far from clear. As children grow older, we expect them to become more familiar with the language, more knowledgeable about its structure and sequential constraints, and better able to control their eye movements and fixation. All these factors should have an influence on performance on a tachistoscopic word recognition task. The data of Carmon *et al.* (1976) would suggest that there may very well be developmental trends in lateralization over and above this, but a single study is not much of a foundation upon which to build a strong argument. The studies that have been done to date are simply not good enough to permit any firm conclusions.

Nonverbal Studies

As indicated earlier, the behavioral techniques for assessing cerebral lateralization are more robust when verbal materials are used. For this reason, most of the developmental studies have concentrated on the language processing skills of the left hemisphere. Despite the problems associated with such research, the preceding pages have provided some indication that language processes are lateralized to the left hemisphere even in very young children. But what of the right hemisphere?

Milner (1974) has used the term *complementary specialization* to refer to the distinctive functional specialization of the two hemispheres. One might well ask how best to interpret this concept. At its simplest, a complementary specialization implies that if the left hemisphere is specialized for language, the right hemisphere will be specialized for nonverbal processes, and vice versa. In a developmental context, however, rather different interpretations are possible. Perhaps one hemisphere acquires its peculiar specialization because the homologous areas of the other hemisphere are already committed to some other function. By this argument, specialization of one hemisphere lags behind that of the other. Since very early learning is largely sensorimotor, one might expect the lateral specialization of the right hemisphere to precede that of the left. Alternatively, since the functions usually attributed to the right hemisphere are relatively complex, one might argue that right-hemispheric development would follow after the development of the left. Certainly, the evidence for early functional specialization for language in the left hemisphere would leave no room for right-hemisphere functions to develop any earlier. (Furthermore, Chapter 10 indicates that the notion of hemispheric complementarity may be statistical rather than causal.)

In fact, there are so few behavioral studies of right-hemispheric lateralization in children that it is almost impossible to reach any firm conclusions. Knox and Kimura (1970) found a left-ear superiority for the recognition of dichotically presented environmental sounds, with no age-related change in lateralization between 5 and 8 years. Witelson (1977) cites two other auditory studies, one of which failed to find any ear difference and the other of which found it only with boys. Since left-ear effects are so notoriously unstable, one cannot put much weight on a failure to find a left-ear effect unless the same materials and procedure have been used successfully with adults.

Visually, Marcel and Rajan (1975) found a significant left-field superiority for face recognition in 7–9-year-old children, but again there were no age-related effects. Witelson (1976a) also found a left-field superiority for making same–different judgments on pairs of human figures, with no age effects between 6 and 13 years. In contrast, Diamond and Carey (1977) failed to find a left-field superiority for face recognition in children aged 9 and 10, although they did observe it in older children and adults.

Witelson (1974, 1976b) has found a left-hand superiority for the dichhaptic recognition of meaningless shapes, without any age-related effects. In her later study, however, the left-hand effect was observed only in boys, and not in girls.

In studies with very young infants, Entus (1977) found a left-ear superiority for dichotically presented musical passages in the same subjects that showed a right-ear effect for verbal material. Her subjects were babies ranging in age from 22 to 140 days. They were trained to suck to a dichotic stimulus, and, following habituation, the stimulus to one ear was changed. This resulted in a recovery of sucking. Nearly 80% of Entus's subjects showed greater recovery when the left-ear stimulus was changed than when the right-ear stimulus was changed in her music condition, which involved hearing the note A played on different musical instruments.

The Entus study, showing a clear distinction between the responses to verbal and nonverbal stimuli, is fairly convincing evidence that some form of dissociable lateral specialization exists at birth (but see Vargha-Khadem & Corballis, 1979). Similar task differentiation in infants, some as young as 48 hr, has been shown for a number of electrophysiological measures (Barnet, Vicentini, & Campos, 1974; Gardiner & Walter, 1977; Molfese, Freeman, & Palermo, 1975). One cannot, however, be certain that the laterality effects observed in infants are of the same magnitude as those found in older children, since the procedures employed are so very different.

In summary, the developmental studies of right-hemispheric function are even more unsatisfactory than those of left-hemispheric function. Very little has been done to explore the possibility that more complex musical and spatial tasks might show relatively late lateralization. However, the existing data show very little in the way of age-related trends, and the existence of left-ear effects for nonverbal auditory signals in newborns makes the likelihood of a developmental change in right-hemispheric function unlikely.

Motor Asymmetries

In Chapter 10, we have seen that there is a relation between handedness and cerebral organization, albeit a small one. Many of the conceptualizations of the origins of cerebral asymmetry link speech lateralization closely to asymmetries in the control of limb movements (e.g., Kimura, 1978). A brief examination of the evidence for developmental changes in motor asymmetries may therefore shed some light on the development of cerebral specialization.

It is often claimed that clearly differentiated hand preference does not appear until 7 or 8 years of age (Gesell & Ames, 1947; Palmer, 1964). Gesell and Ames, for instance, reported that babies aged 4–5 months reached for objects at the midline with their left hand (see also Seth, 1973) and that other periods of left-hand preference or no preference could be found in the preschool years. In contrast, Annett (1970b) found both right-hand preference and right-hand superiority in a manual dexterity task in children as young as 3½ years.

Turkewitz and his colleagues have found that neonates show a distinct tendency to turn their head and neck toward the right upon lateral stimulation (Turkewitz, 1977; Turkewitz, Gordon, & Birch, 1965a, 1965b; Turkewitz, Moreau, & Birch, 1968).Viviani, Turkewitz, and Karp (1978) have reported a significant correlation (.41) between the direction of head turning observed in infancy and a measure of lateral consistency taken at age 7 years. Unfortunately, Viviani *et al.* did not use a simple measure of hand preference but confounded it with an eye dominance measure. Eye dominance is not highly correlated with handedness and may be a dimension of lateral asymmetry quite unrelated to either handedness or cerebral lateralization (Porac & Coren, 1976, 1979). However, Viviani *et al.* do indicate that the one child (of a sample of 22) who was clearly left-handed at age 7 also showed a left-side head turning tendency as a neonate. Thus, there are some reasons for believing that neonatal head turning behavior is correlated with subsequent hand preference. We might also mention that Viviani *et al.* report no correlation between neonatal head turning and dichotic listening performance at age 7. However, their measure of dichotic performance was one of bias, rather than one of perceptual asymmetry, and their data are quite meaningless in settling any issues about cerebral lateralization.

Caplan and Kinsbourne (1976) have found that babies (aged 1–4 months) hold on to objects with their right hand longer than with the left. As with the Turkewitz studies, this is evidence that very young children show a right-side bias in motor behavior.

It seems, then, that a right-side or right-hand superiority can be observed at virtually all ages. Right-handedness, in terms of hand strength, grip time, tapping speed, dexterity, or preference, has been observed in children of all ages. Any failure to find a differentiated handedness seems attributable more to the procedures employed and to testing children who have not yet developed the requisite skills than to the absence of a right bias in handedness.

Since handedness is not an especially good predictor of cerebral lateralization, the fact that handedness can be observed in young children may be quite irrelevant to any understanding of the development of functional lateralization. Relatively few studies have tried to make a direct link between manual performance and other cerebral asymmetries. However, Kinsbourne and McMurray (1975) have reported that speaking interferes more with right-hand finger tapping than with left-hand finger tapping in 5 year olds. This would suggest that overflow from speech centers was influencing performance and would imply left-hemispheric speech representation. Ingram (1975b) found a right-hand superiority in 3–5 year olds for hand strength, finger tapping, and gesturing during speech, but a left-hand superiority for copying hand positions. Again, the task differentiation is consonant with the notion that cerebral differentiation of function had already been achieved.

Conclusions

In virtually all areas of developmental investigation, there is evidence for cerebral specialization in the neonate. Although most of the studies that have investigated children of different ages leave something to be desired in terms of their procedure, there is remarkably little evidence for any age-related changes in lateralization. In many ways, the concept of a gradually developing cerebral lateralization seems more wish fulfillment than reality. At the same time, one must recognize that there is ample room for improvement in the quality of developmental studies of lateralization.

Let us attempt to summarize what is known about developmental issues in lateralization.

1. At least some aspects of phoneme processing are lateralized to the left hemisphere at a very early age, probably at birth. There is little evidence for any age-related changes in this aspect of speech processing.

2. The child brain is more plastic than the adult brain. Recovery from early brain damage is fairly complete, and the evidence suggests that homologous areas of the opposite hemisphere can take over functions that would normally be lateralized to the damaged hemisphere. One cannot help but be impressed with how successfully some infantile hemispherectomies have learned to cope with their impairment.

3. Right-hemisphere specialization for nonverbal functions also seems to be evident even in the neonate. The evidence on the development of right-hemispheric functions is sparse, but there is little compelling evidence for age-related trends. Failures to observe right-hemispheric effects are more likely to be due to poor procedure or to the changing cognitive capacity of the child than to a developing right-hemispheric lateralization of nonverbal function.

4. Evidence for a greater right-hemispheric involvement in language in young children is more likely a manifestation of the more disruptive effect of early brain damage than a true indication of right-hemisphere language (cf. Moscovitch, 1977).

5. Visual–verbal laterality measures do show an age-related increase. This is not so much due to the development of new capacities in the left hemisphere, as to the fact that visual symbols acquire language properties only through experience. Only when one acquires a linguistic encoding of visual symbols should we except to find any left-hemisphere relevant components in visual information processing.

6. Finally, many of the developmental studies that have shown lateral asymmetries have done so not because of hemispheric asymmetries in cerebral organization, but because of what we have termed *experimental effects*. For instance, if older children have learned to scan verbal material from left to right more efficiently than younger children, they will exhibit a bigger right-visual-field superiority for verbal material than will the younger children. This really has nothing at all to do with cerebral organization; it is simply a manifestation of a changing behavioral strategy.

In summary, the evidence would suggest that lateral cerebral specialization does not change developmentally. In general, it is the capacities of the child that change, and not the brain organization (cf. Witelson, 1977). An increasing right-visual-field effect for letters or words does not mean that the left hemisphere is developing new capacities, but rather that the child has finally learned that particular arbitrary symbols are language related and is using language-related mechanisms to encode them.

This view puts the studies that deal with some pathological condition in children, such as deafness or reading disability, in a rather different light. Evidence for abnormal perceptual lateralization in such children is not so much evidence that their brains are organized in a different way than are normal children's but evidence that they deal with the stimuli in a different way.

At the same time, one must not fail to recognize that neural pathology can more readily lead to changes in cerebral organization in children than in adults. Milner, Branch, and Rasmussen (1964), for instance, have shown that early brain damage often leads to a right-hemispheric representation of speech functions. Although similar effects permit some recovery from aphasia in adults (e.g., Pettit & Noll, 1979), the ease of interhemispheric transfer is not as great.

13

Introduction to
Individual Differences
in Cerebral Organization

Twenty years ago, it might have been argued that the development of noninvasive techniques for the assessment of cerebral lateralization would have its greatest benefit in the preoperative assessment of cerebral function in neurological patients. Were some advance knowledge available of how speech was represented in a particular patient, for example, the surgeon would know better what tissue could be safely removed. Over the years, it has become clear that the noninvasive techniques are not so precise that they add much specific information about the nature of cerebral organization, whereas neurological procedures to provide similar information have become increasingly more sophisticated and precise. One must look elsewhere if one is to find a justification for research on cerebral asymmetries in the normal brain. This chapter, and the ensuing three chapters, are concerned with the relation between brain lateralization and various aspects of behavior in normal subjects.

There are two major views as to how different patterns of cerebral lateralization might be related to other behaviors. We know that linguistic and integrative processes are lateralized to the left hemisphere and, to a lesser extent, spatial and holistic processes are lateralized to the right hemisphere in the vast majority of normal individuals. One possible inference from this knowledge is that the reversed pattern of cerebral localization is somehow inferior and that people with right-hemispheric speech lateralization will be impaired on measures of cognitive abilities. Although such a notion may be implicit in the long history of imputing all sorts of negative characteristics to left-handers (L. J. Harris, 1980), it seems rather implausible. There seems to be no obvious reason for the brain functioning any less adequately (or more adequately) because it is mirror reversed.

Another view is that degree of lateralization is important and that the behavioral consequences of having two hemispheres whose functions are clearly distinct are different from those of having some overlap of function. Thus, for example, Levy (1974) has suggested that, in individuals with bilateral speech, the encroachment of speech functions into the right hemisphere interferes with the normal spatial processing capacities of that hemisphere and leads to a deficit in spatial abilities. The view that degree of lateralization may be important seems logically more plausible than an emphasis on reversed lateralization, but there are many problems in providing an adequate assessment of the theory.

In speculating about the possible significance to behavior of degree of lateralization, two issues must be resolved. One is the question of complementarity. Some authors talk about the importance of "degree of lateralization," while others refer to "bilateral speech representation." To what extent are these the same? Does bilateral speech representation also imply bilaterality of representation for the functions normally associated with the right hemisphere? The evidence cited in Chapter 10 suggests that knowledge of speech lateralization does not aid in determining the hemisphere responsible for visuospatial activities. The other problem concerns the measurement of degree of lateralization. The behavioral techniques for assessing lateral asymmetry are heavily influenced by what has been termed *experimental effects*. If we administer, say, a dichotic listening test and obtain differences in the degree of the right-ear effect, how are these differences to be interpreted? If these differences represent nothing more than the influence of experimental effects unrelated to hemispheric asymmetry, then we are not measuring degree of lateralization. Even if we do succeed in controlling irrelevant experimental effects, one subject may use a more verbal strategy than another and thus generate a bigger right-ear effect. Evidence that women are less likely to show a left-visual-field superiority on certain spatial tasks (Kimura, 1969) has been taken as evidence for the use of a verbal strategy by women, rather than as evidence for bilateral representation of spatial functions. These problems will make it very difficult indeed to provide a clear answer concerning the functional significance of degree of lateralization.

Evidence concerning Reversed Lateralization

There appear to be no studies that have directly tested the notion that individuals with right-hemispheric speech or reversed laterality are any different from others in their cognitive abilities. The idea that reversed laterality is bad for you, however, is hinted at by various theories that have proposed that left-handers are less intelligent (L. J. Harris, 1980). Similar conceptualizations undoubtedly underlie the argument that people with crossed hand–eye dominance show intellectual deficits (Delacato, 1966). Since right-hemispheric speech is more prevalent in left-handers than in right-handers, one might expect to find that left-handers as a group show a deficit when compared to right-handers. Although there are periodic suggestions that this is, in fact, the case (e.g., Levy, 1969; Nebes, 1971), a review of the literature by Hardyck and Petrinovitch (1977) failed to find any compelling evidence that left-handedness was associated with deficits of any kind. There seem to be no very good reasons for believing that reversed asymmetry leads to any cognitive deficit.

An Experimental Approach to the Degree of Lateralization Question

The majority of the studies of perceptual asymmetry have employed right-handed subjects. In doing so, they have ensured that the majority of the variability in performance is associated with experimental effects rather than with differences in neurological organization. If one is interested in studying how lateralization influences performance, one should be maximizing neurological variability. One way of doing this is to investigate performance in left-handers, where cerebral organization is uncertain, rather than in right-handers, the vast majority of whom show left-hemispheric speech representation.

This approach was followed in a preliminary study reported by Bryden (1979b). The subjects for this experiment were 40 left-handed undergraduates, 20 men and 20 women. Each subject was given a battery of handedness tests, the verbal reasoning and space relations subtests of the Differential Aptitude Test, and four tests of perceptual asymmetry. Each of the four perceptual asymmetry tasks had been used before with normal right-handed samples, and each had generated the expected laterality effect. The tests chosen included both verbal and nonverbal measures, using both auditory and visual procedures.

The visual tests involved the tachistoscopic presentation of items in random order in either the left or the right visual field. Exposure durations were individually determined for each subject to ensure approximately 75% overall accuracy. In the verbal test, single letters were presented for identification. In the nonverbal test, a cartoon drawing of a face was exposed very briefly and subjects had to identify it from one of four alternatives.

The verbal auditory test involved the common dichotic pairing of the six stop consonant pairs /pa, da, ga, ba, ta, ka/. On half the trials, subjects were told to monitor the left ear and report only the item presented there, while on the other half of the trials, they monitored the right ear and reported that item. For the nonverbal auditory task, such simple environmental sounds as water running, birds singing, sirens, and motors were paired dichotically. An ordered report procedure was used, whereby subjects reported left-ear items first on half the trials and right-ear items first on the remaining half.

Performance on all four perceptual laterality measures was expressed in terms of a laterality index that indicates the observed lateral difference as a proportion of the maximum possible difference observable at that level of overall accuracy (Halwes, 1969). A more sensitive measure would have been the index proposed by Bryden and Sprott (1981; Chapter 2).

The relations between degree of lateral specialization and cognitive ability were examined by computing partial correlations of verbal ability with the absolute values of the laterality scores, holding spatial ability constant, and of spatial ability with laterality, holding verbal ability constant. In addition, a composite laterality score was determined by standardizing the laterality scores for each of the four perceptual tests and summing them. The results are shown in Table 13.1. While the correlations are generally low, the trend is for good cognitive performance to be

Table 13.1
Predicting Cognitive Measures from Absolute Laterality Measures

	Spatial		Verbal	
	M	F	M	F
Letters	−32*	12	1	−16
Faces	1	27	8	−14
Stops	−35*	−43**	−40**	19
Sounds	16	−13	23	−28
Composite	4	−19	−30*	3

*p < .10.
**p < .01.

Table 13.2
Cerebral Organization and Cognitive Skills

	Complementary	Noncomplementary
Males		
V > S	3	6
S > V	9	2
Females		
V > S	4	6
S > V	7	3
All[a]		
V > S	7	12
S > V	16	5

[a] $\chi^2 = 4.81$ (p < .05).
V = verbal.
S = spatial.

related to *low* absolute laterality scores, the opposite to what would be expected from the notion that poor lateralization leads to spatial–verbal interference and thus to poor performance.

A somewhat different way of examining the same issue involves classifying the subjects as to whether lateral specialization is complementary or mixed. Subjects with complementary specialization show opposite signs for the verbal and nonverbal measures of lateral asymmetry, whereas mixed or noncomplementary subjects have the same sign for both verbal and nonverbal scores. Table 13.2 shows that those subjects with complementary specialization tend to score better on the measure of spatial ability than on the verbal measure, whereas those with non-complementary specialization have a higher score on the verbal than on the spatial measure. There is thus some support here for Levy's (1974) notion that bilateral speech representation (as exemplified by non-complementary specialization) leads to poorer spatial performance.

For a variety of reasons, this study did not prove to be entirely successful. Most particularly, the various perceptual tests of lateralization were not selected with sufficient care. Thus, not only were there signs of considerable experimental effects, but also the reliability of the measures was not as high as would have been desired. Therefore, the results presented here are not exhibited with any great confidence. However, the basic plan of the study is representative of one approach that should be pursued if we are to discover the relation between perceptual lateralization and other forms of behavior.

Other Studies of Individual Differences in Patterns of Lateralization

Two other studies have attempted to provide an examination of the relevance of the pattern of cerebral asymmetry to performance. Mc-Glone and Davidson (1973) tested a large group of right- and left-handers on a dichotic listening task involving the presentation of lists of numbers, a dot enumeration task that had previously been shown to yield a left-visual-field effect (Kimura, 1967), and psychometric measures of spatial ability. They classified their subjects as to whether the perceptual tests indicated that verbal and spatial abilities were lateralized to the same or opposite hemispheres (as in the complementary–noncomplementary distinction of Table 13.2).

Of their subjects, 43 showed complementary lateralization for the dichotic and dots tests, while 23 showed superior performance on the same side for both tests. Those showing complementary lateralization obtained somewhat higher scores on a spatial relations test, although the effect did not reach statistical significance (cf. Bryden, 1979b). Furthermore, there was a strong trend, again not statistically significant, for those subjects showing reversed lateralization to perform poorly on the spatial relations test.

A second pertinent study has been carried out by Fennell, Satz, Van den Abell, Bowers, and Thomas (1978). They tested both high school and university students on a dichotic listening task involving presentation of three pairs of words, a similar visual paradigm involving sequentially presented letter pairs (Hines & Satz, 1971), the block design subtest of the Wechsler Adult Intelligence Scale (WAIS), and the visual–spatial subtest of the Primary Mental Abilities battery. They found little evidence that either right-hemispheric speech representation or bilateral speech representation, as assessed by the two perceptual tasks, was related to performance on either of the two spatial ability measures. Their Table 2 (p. 210), however, indicates a trend for those subjects who show bilaterality on the visual task to have the lowest mean scores on the spatial abilities measures. This pattern is not repeated with the dichotic measures.

As with the other studies (Bryden, 1979b; McGlone & Davidson, 1973), some scepticism must be expressed about the choice of perceptual tests to assess laterality. The Fennell et al. (1978) study employed two tasks that involved the retention of lists of material, with relatively little concern for attentional biases in the dichotic procedure or for scanning factors in the visual procedure. Again, the study points in the direction research must go, but the study itself leaves one unconvinced about the generality of the findings.

Although these studies exemplify an approach to the issue of relating cerebral lateralization to cognitive abilities, the results are sufficiently disappointing that nothing can be concluded at the present time. One of the problems is that many of the measures of perceptual laterality are notoriously unreliable; even the old standby of verbal dichotic listening does not have sufficiently high reliability to make it a good psychometric test (Blumstein *et al.*, 1975; Shankweiler & Studdert-Kennedy, 1975; Teng, 1981). Even when the laterality measures are reasonably reliable, the procedures may be so highly influenced by experimental effects unrelated to cerebral asymmetry that they fail to give a meaningful assessment of cerebral organization in a given individual. If one has a rubber yardstick and is not even really sure what one is measuring, it is not surprising that attempts to relate the measure to other variables are not terribly successful.

This really is but one more example of the general problem of using experimental procedures to investigate individual differences. Rather than employing an experimental procedure of questionable reliability and validity to constitute groups that differ in patterns of cerebral organization, a more profitable approach might be to look at the problems in reverse. Hunt, Lunneborg, and Lewis (1975) have investigated verbal performance skills by using psychometric measures to constitute groups of high- and low-verbal ability and then comparing the performance of these two groups on various experimental measures. There is no reason the same approach cannot be applied to the study of cerebral organization.

At least in the area of spatial ability, some fairly specific predictions can be made. Levy (1974) has argued that individuals with bilateral speech representation will do more poorly than average on measures of spatial ability because portions of the right hemisphere that would normally be reserved for spatial processing are involved in speech. A group of subjects with good spatial abilities would be expected to show signs of clear lateralization on, say, a verbal dichotic listening test, whereas a group of subjects with poor spatial ability would show a reduced laterality effect. It is not clear what one would predict for nonverbal measures of lateralization, but differences between good and poor spatial subjects might well emerge.

Hunt *et al.* (1975) did not include measures of lateralization in their study of verbal ability, but one might logically expect to find that good verbal abilities were associated with clear lateralization of verbal function. Bilateral control of speech production can lead to severe stuttering (Jones, 1966); bilateral control of comprehension might also be expected to lead to deficits in verbal skills.

Unfortunately, this approach has rarely been applied to ask questions about the relevance of patterns of cerebral organization to basic verbal and spatial abilities. However, there are examples of the logic in the study of musical abilities and in personality research.

Bever and Chiarello (1974) reported that highly trained musicians showed a right-ear rather than a left-ear superiority on a complex auditory task. In their study, musically naive subjects exhibited the more commonly reported left-ear effect (Kimura, 1964). Bever and Chiarello suggest that the observed laterality effect is determined by the manner in which the stimuli are processed and that musical experience affects the way in which musical stimuli are processed. However, Gaede et al. (1978) found that performance was much more influenced by musical aptitude than by level of experience. They employed two monaural listening tasks, one in which subjects were required to discriminate the number of notes in a chord and another in which they were to remember a sequence of notes and identify which note had been changed. In general, subjects were better on the left ear in the chords test and on the right ear in the memory test. However, high-aptitude subjects (as measured by performance on the Drake Musical Aptitude Test, Drake, 1954) showed a much smaller difference in laterality between the two tasks than did low-aptitude subjects. Gaede et al. suggest that it is not experience that results in a shifting of musical processing from one hemisphere to the other, but that individuals with bilateral representation of musical processes have greater musical aptitude than those with unilateral specialization for music. Gordon (1980) has also failed to show a difference in laterality between skilled and unskilled musicians on a dichotic chords test. Rather, the professional musicians tended to show more extreme ear differences.

Another example of the group comparison method of studying cerebral organization developed from work in the 1950s relating personality to perception (R. W. Gardner, Holzman, Klein, Linton, & Spence, 1959). This group of researchers identified a variety of "cognitive styles," or ways of dealing with the world: One dimension of cognitive style is that of category width. Broad categorizers are individuals who classify a wide variety of similar objects or concepts together, paying little attention to detail or differences. Narrow categorizers, on the other hand, admit only a few members to any given category and attend to detail and to small differences.

Huang (1979) selected broad and narrow categorizers, using Pettigrew's (1958) Category Width Scale. In a verbal dichotic listening experiment, she found that narrow categorizers showed a significantly greater right-ear effect than did broad categorizers. Since narrow categorizers are considered to be more analytic and broad categorizers more integrative, she argues that narrow categorizers have greater dependence on left-hemispheric language processes. Huang (1979) also found that narrow categorizers were more likely to look toward the right during reflective thinking than were broad categorizers. To the extent that lateral eye movements are indicative of hemispheric activation (see Ehrlichman & Weinburger, 1978), this finding also supports the notion that narrow categorizers have greater reliance on left-hemispheric processes.

Huang's (1979) study also illustrates a problem that plagues virtually all research aimed at relating hemispheric asymmetry to their behavioral processes. Without better experimental procedures for measuring cerebral organization and without a full understanding of what it is these procedures measure and how performance on them can be influenced, it is impossible to tell whether narrow categorizers are more lateralized because they are more likely to use verbal strategies in dealing with incoming information or whether an initially strong lateralization of language functions to the left hemisphere has led them to become narrow categorizers. Similar comments might be made about almost any other attempt to show that one group is different from another in terms of lateralization.

In some cases, it is almost certain that differences in lateralization between groups result, not from different brain organizations leading to different behaviors, but from different behaviors leading to different ways of employing a constant underlying brain organization. Thus, studies of hemispheric asymmetry in alcoholics (e.g., Miglioli, Buchtel, Campanini, & DeRisio, 1979) and schizophrenics (e.g., R. E. Gur, 1979) seem to be addressed more to the issue of the information processing strategies of these groups than to any question about the way in which cerebral organization influences behavior.

Two further areas in which group comparisons on various measures of cerebral lateralization have become popular are those of sex-related differences and of language-related deficits in children. Neither area of research developed with any explicit formulation of the intent to deal with the behavioral consequences of differences in cerebral organization. In fact, in many cases the argument has been that one is dealing with different behavioral strategies rather than with any underlying differences in cerebral organization. Research in these areas, however, has become sufficiently voluminous that each warrants a chapter of its own.

Conclusions

The question of whether or not different patterns of cerebral organization have differing behavioral consequences is a critical one. The very fact that aphasias sometimes follow right-hemispheric damage makes it evident that there are differences in brain organization, and behavior is certainly dependent on the organization and action of the brain. If different cerebral organizations do not have any meaningful behavioral consequences, one of the primary justifications for expending so much effort to understand hemispheric specialization in the normal brain becomes an empty one.

Despite the importance of the problem, one can feel little but disappointment in the attempts that have been made to investigate it. Remarkably few studies have been carried out that attempt to relate cerebral lateralization to basic cognitive processes. Of those that have, the measures of cerebral organization are sufficiently influenced by experimental effects that the classification of subjects must remain open to question. Further, the studies do not yet permit us to determine whether one is really dealing with differences in cerebral organization or simply with differences in strategy. At the present time, the research justifies no firm conclusions one way or the other, but leaves only a feeling that further research is needed.

14

Sex Differences
in Laterality

One topic that has generated immense interest in the past decade, both in academic circles and in the popular media, is that of sex-related differences in behavior and their possible biological origins. *Psychology Today* (October 1978) devoted an issue to the topic, and innumerable books and articles have appeared on the subject. Given the current fascination with hemispheric asymmetries, it should not be surprising that the literature on sex-related lateral asymmetries is also beginning to swell (see Bryden, 1979a; McGlone, 1980, for reviews).

In reviews of possible sex-related differences in cognitive ability, three areas are repeatedly mentioned as ones in which men and women differ (Maccoby & Jacklin, 1974; Sherman, 1978; Wittig & Petersen, 1979). In general, males are found to do better than females on measures of spatial ability and mathematical aptitude, whereas females excel over males in the area of verbal skills. Of these three areas, verbal skills are attributed to processes normally represented in the left hemisphere, whereas spatial skills are attributed to processes normally represented in the right hemisphere.

Although rarely conceived in this way, it is not difficult to imagine studies of sex-related differences in lateralization as being addressed to the question of how cerebral organization influences behavior. If men excel over women in spatial abilities, for example, and also show a difference in the pattern of cerebral lateralization, then perhaps the differences in hemispheric specialization produce the differences in spatial abilities. At the same time, much of this book has been concerned with the influence of experimental effects on measured laterality. In considering the literature on sex-related differences in lateralization, one must not lose sight of the possibility that they arise through experimental effects and are indicative of the fact that men and women perform the same task in different ways.

Different theorists have linked sex-related differences in cognitive ability to notions of hemispheric asymmetry in different ways. Buffery and Gray (1972), for example, conclude that females are *more* lateralized than males. They argue that the early acquisition of language in females is indicative of an earlier specialization of the left hemisphere for speech. As a result of this earlier development in females, both speech processes and spatial skills become more completely lateralized in females and remain bilaterally represented in males. This argument assumes that it is beneficial to have language processes lateralized in one hemisphere but detrimental to have unilateral representation of spatial ability. Furthermore, the argument is based on the assumption of a gradually developing hemispheric specialization, an assumption that is not well founded (see Chapter 12).

An alternative view (e.g., Levy 1972, 1974) is that bilateral representation of speech encroaches on the normally spatial right hemisphere, leading to poorer performance on spatial tasks. Levy argues that women are relatively poor spatially because they are more likely to have bilateral speech representation. By this argument, the female is *less* lateralized than the male. As will become evident, the data provide more support for this view than for the notion that women are more lateralized.

Studies of Perceptual Asymmetry in Adults

Perhaps the most common procedure for investigating perceptual asymmetry is the verbal dichotic listening procedure originally developed by Kimura (1961a, 1961b). In earlier chapters, we have seen that this procedure is very robust in producing a right-ear advantage. At the same time, a variety of experimental effects that may be unrelated to cerebral lateralization can affect the magnitude of the ear effect observed.

In particular, the use of free recall with dichotically presented lists of items permits a wide variety of experimental effects to intrude. Nevertheless, it remains a popular procedure, and many of the studies reporting data on men and women separately have employed such a procedure. Briggs and Nebes (1976) found a slightly larger right-ear effect for men than for women, although the difference was not statistically significant. However, accuracy on their task was in excess of 90%, and a ceiling effect may very well have occurred. Carr (1969) also found no sex-related differences for the free recall of three pairs of items, but his sample was small, and again a ceiling effect may have occurred. With lists of four pairs of numbers, Bryden (1965) found no sex-related differences in a sample of 10 right-handed men and 10 right-handed women. Sex-related differences were also not observed for lists of numbers in a reanalysis of Bryden's (1975) data presented by Bryden (1979c).

Greater right-ear effects for males can be found for list material in the data presented by Bryden (1966), where 75% of the men but only 58% of the women showed greater accuracy on the right ear. Almost identical figures were observed by McGlone and Davidson (1973). However, a trend toward a bigger right-ear effect for women appears in the data of Demarest and Demarest (1979). Studies of the free recall of dichotic lists, then, generally show either no sex-related differences or greater laterality effects in males.

Studies employing single pairs of dichotic material do not provide the same opportunity for reorganization of the material in memory and are less subject to other biasing factors than are free-recall studies. They may therefore provide a somewhat more sensitive test of the hypothesis of sex-related differences in lateralization. One of the largest such studies is that of Lake and Bryden (1976). Subjects were presented pairs of consonant–vowel (CV) syllables dichotically and asked to report the items they were sure they had heard. The study involved both left- and right-handers, but it is difficult to know what to expect in left-handers, and we shall be concerned here only with the data from the right-handers. Among men, 94% showed a right-ear effect, whereas only 67% of the women did, a highly significant difference. Furthermore, men showed an average right-ear superiority of 4.31 items, whereas women averaged only a 1.47 item difference. Thus, men were more likely both to show a right-ear effect and to show a larger effect than did women.

Harshman, Remington, and Krashen (1975) have reanalyzed three dichotic studies using CV pairs—one of their own and those of Van Lancker and Fromkin (1973) and Ryan and McNeil (1974). All studies show slight sex-related differences favoring the males. When combined, they yield a statistically significant difference between the sexes, with men showing a larger right-ear effect.

Bryden (1975, as reported in Bryden, 1979c) did not observe sex-related differences for single CV pairs in his study of dichotic listening in families. This seems to be the one failure to find a greater right-ear effect in men among the studies involving CV pairs and permitting the subjects freedom to deploy attention as they chose.

In a monitoring study, Piazza (1980) reports similar results with right-handed subjects. Unfortunately, it is not possible to determine whether or not the sex-related difference is significant for her right-handers, since her design and analysis also incorporate factors of handedness and familial sinistrality.

However, Bryden *et al.* (1980) reported no sex-related differences in two studies designed to control attentional bias by instructing subjects to alternately attend to one ear or the other. It should be noted that monitoring procedures such as those employed by Piazza (1980) and Bryden *et al.* (1980) have been criticized by Harshman *et al.* (1975). They point out that such procedures require the subject both to identify the item and to localize it correctly in space. When they reanalyzed a set of data that required a similar response, they found sex-related differences when localization was ignored, but not when only correctly localized responses were scored. Ultimately, however, some control over attentional processes must be employed to be certain that the task measures language lateralization and not attentional bias.

In summary, verbal dichotic studies of sex-related differences are about evenly divided between those that show no sex-related effects and those that show a greater degree of lateralization for the males. Studies involving lists of words do not show very clear sex-related differences, whereas those involving single pairs of CV syllables are almost unanimous in showing greater lateralization in the males. Too few studies involving monitoring procedures have been done to make any firm statements about this procedure, although Piazza's (1980) data do point in the direction of a sex-related difference.

The only data concerning sex-related differences for nonverbal auditory material appear in Piazza's (1980) study. In her main study, in which subjects were tested on a variety of different measures of lateralization, an environmental sounds condition was included. In this test, subjects heard dichotic pairs of familiar sounds, such as a bell ringing or a man singing. They were instructed to attend to one ear and to report only the sound that had been heard at that ear. In this monitoring task, right-handed men showed only a weak left-ear advantage, whereas right-handed women were significantly more accurate on the left ear. However, no specific test was made of the difference between men and women.

In a supplemental experiment, Piazza (1980) employed a dichotic melodies tape, following the procedure first employed by Kimura (1964). Following the dichotic presentation of a pair of melodies, subjects heard four monaurally presented melodies: Of these, two corresponded to the melodies that had been presented dichotically and two were foils. The results were virtually identical to those obtained with environmental sounds and a monitoring procedure. Women showed a significant left-ear superiority, whereas men showed a small but insignificant left-ear advantage.

Piazza's (1980) two studies are consistent in indicating that nonverbal auditory lateralization is greater in women than in men. These findings contrast with the verbal auditory studies, where the trend is for men to show greater lateralization, and suggest that earlier conclusions that males are generally more lateralized (Bryden, 1979a; Harshman & Remington, 1975) may have to be modified.

Studies of visual lateralization employing verbal stimuli or verbal tasks have involved a diversity of experimental procedures. Like the verbal dichotic listening studies, however, the majority have indicated greater right-visual-field effects in men than in women.

Hannay and Malone (1976) presented a single word to one visual field and had their subjects look at a second test word (either the same or different) after delay intervals of 0, 5, and 10 sec. They found a greater right-visual-field superiority in males at all delay intervals, with the maximum sex-related difference occurring at a 5-sec delay. However, Hannay and Boyer (1978) were not able to replicate these findings. In addition, using bilateral presentation of words, Piazza (1980) found only a very slightly greater right-field effect in men than in women.

Kail and Siegel (1978) presented four numbers, appearing in random positions of a 3×3 matrix, using a unilateral presentation procedure. Men showed a significant right-visual-field superiority in recalling the digits, whereas the women did not.

Sex-related differences were also reported by Bradshaw, Gates, and Nettleton (1977). They employed a lexical decision task, in which words or nonwords were presented randomly to the left and right visual fields, and subjects were required to indicate whether or not the stimulus was a real word. Men were slower than women, and they showed a right-visual-field superiority, whereas women did not. In a subsequent series of experiments, Bradshaw and Gates (1978) extended this work. In a replication of their original study using a lexical decision task, they again found that men showed a clear and consistent right-visual-field superiority. In contrast, women were slightly better on the left in the earlier trials, shifting to a right-visual-field effect only after considerable experience in the experimental situation. In a second experiment, subjects were shown either pronounceable nonwords or homophones of real words; they were required to make a manual response to indicate whether the stimulus sounded like a real word or not. The majority of the men (9 out of 12) produced faster responses in the right visual field, whereas the majority of women (9 out of 12) were faster for items in the left visual field. However, this difference did not reach statistical significance by analysis of variance. In a similar experiment using naming latency as a response, sex-related differences were rather smaller, and women did not show any tendency toward a left-visual-field superiority. In general, then, Bradshaw and Gates (1978) found women to show a small left-visual-field superiority when they had to indicate whether a target was a real word or sounded like a real word and a right-visual-field effect when the task involved naming the word. In contrast, men showed a right-visual-field superiority on all tasks. Bradshaw and Gates (1978) suggest that women have a greater degree of bilateral representation of language processes. They postulate that this right-hemispheric language center operates at a largely lexical level and has invaded space otherwise reserved for visuospatial processing.

McKeever and Jackson (1979) also reported reduced right-visual-field superiorities in women, especially in the first half of the experimental session, in an experiment involving object naming latencies. When latencies to naming colors were recorded, a right-visual-field superiority was obtained, but the sex-related difference almost completely disappeared. McKeever and Jackson (1979) suggest that object identification has a sufficient spatial component to involve right-hemispheric mechanisms in women, while color naming avoids the possibility of spatial confusion.

In contrast to studies involving complex language-related materials, such as words or pictures of familiar objects, the sex-related difference does not seem to occur in the recognition of single letters (Bradshaw, Bradley, & Patterson, 1976; Bryden & Allard, 1976). In fact, the reverse trend, with women showing a larger right-visual-field superiority, was found by Bryden (1965).

In general, the verbal studies of lateralization using tachistoscopic procedures show a greater right-visual-field effect for men than for women. In order to obtain this sex-related effect, one must move beyond very elementary language-related tasks, such as naming colors or single letters. With more complex tasks, there remain some inconsistencies. For instance, McKeever and Jackson (1979) find a sex-related effect for object naming, while it is when a naming response is required that Bradshaw and Gates (1978) find that their sex-related effects disappear. Furthermore, one must remember that even the lexical decision task employed by Bradshaw and Gates (1978) may involve directional scanning processes that affect the magnitude of the laterality effect without necessarily implying any differences in cerebral organization.

The majority of studies investigating sex-related differences in nonverbal visual laterality effects have employed dot localization or line orientation tasks. Kimura (1969) presented a single dot randomly in the left or right visual field and asked subjects to indicate where this dot was located with respect to the fixation point. In her initial experiment, she found that men were more accurate in the left visual field, whereas women were more accurate in the right visual field. Her second experiment employed the exposure duration at which the dots were correctly localized, rather than accuracy of localization, as the dependent measure. Again, men were better on the left, whereas women showed no significant visual-field effects. In two further experiments, a circular frame rather than a rectangular one was used as a response card and to determine the location of the dots in the exposure field. In one of these experiments, sex-related differences were not mentioned; in the other, a slightly larger left-field effect was obtained for women than for men.

Bryden (1976a, 1976b) has extended Kimura's work by combining the dot localization task with a simultaneous detection task. In these experiments, a dot actually appeared on only two-thirds of the trials. Subjects were required to localize the dot on a response card if they detected it or to say "no" if no dot was present. In none of the four experiments reported in Bryden (1976a) are there any significant sex-related differences. However, in a subsequent paper (Bryden, 1976b), data are included from two further studies of dot localization. When the data from all six studies are combined, 65% of the men and 57% of the women show a left-visual-field effect for dot localization. While the difference is not statistically significant, it is in the same direction as that found by Kimura (1969) in her first two experiments.

A further investigation of dot detection has been published by Davidoff (1977). He found that men were more accurate in detecting a dot presented in the left visual field, whereas no visual-field effects were obtained for women. This study involves detection, rather than localization. Bryden (1976a) did not find similar sex-related differences in detection, although women were rather more likely to give left-visual-field responses when no dot had been presented.

McGlone and Davidson (1973) used an enumeration task, in which subjects were required to estimate the number of dots present in one visual field or the other. They indicate that the vast majority of men are more accurate in the left visual field, whereas women show no consistent field differences. Because their sample included a very large number of left-handers, it is impossible to determine scores for right-handers alone.

Walter, Bryden, and Allard (1976) found sex-related effects for a line detection task. In this experiment, a faint line embedded in visual noise appeared in the left or right visual field, and subjects were required to detect its presence. Men showed a clear left-visual-field superiority, whereas women were just as likely to do better in the right visual field as in the left. Although the study involved only eight subjects of each sex, the interaction of sex with visual field was highly significant. However, Piazza (1980) indicates that she found no visual-field differences or sex-related effects for a task involving discrimination of line orientation.

In most cases, any sex-related differences found with nonverbal visual tasks have been in the direction of men showing left-field effects and women not. It has been very difficult to obtain stable right-hemispheric effects with many of these tasks, however, and the interpretation of sex-related differences remains uncertain. While it is possible that women are less lateralized for spatial functions than men are, it is equally possible that they are more likely to use verbal strategies to perform the tasks set them.

Table 14.1 sets out a general summary of the evidence for sex-related differences on perceptual asymmetry tasks involving adult subjects. While the evidence in any one of the cells is not totally compelling, some general conclusions do seem justified. There is certainly no support in the data for Buffery and Gray's (1972) hypothesis that women are *more* lateralized than men. Rather, the general picture supports the view that males are more lateralized (Bryden, 1979a). This is much more clearly the case for the verbal measures than for the nonverbal ones. As indicated earlier, perceptual measures of supposed right-hemispheric effects are not as strong or consistent as measures of left-hemispheric function. Any evidence for sex-related differences suffers from this same lack of consistency; the studies that exist point in the direction of women being more lateralized for nonverbal auditory processes but less lateralized for visuospatial functions, but it is clearly premature to reach any firm conclusions. On the other hand, virtually every study that shows a sex-related difference for verbal processing, whether dichotic or tachistoscopic, indicates that men are more lateralized than women. While experimental effects certainly bias some of these studies, the convergence of different procedures adds credence to the conclusion that

Table 14.1
Summary of Adult Studies on Lateralization

	Auditory	Visual
Verbal	General trend for greater lateralization in *male,* especially with single-pair material	Greater lateralization in *male,* when task is complex language related
Nonverbal	Two studies showing greater lateralization in *females*	Weak trend to greater lateralization in *males*

men are indeed more lateralized. Thus, the adult literature provides at least reasonable support for Levy's (1974) contention that bilateral representation of language-related processes is more common in women than in men.

Studies with Children

It is important to deal separately with those studies on sex-related differences in children for a variety of reasons. Although Chapter 12 provides little support for the idea, the theory that lateralization is a maturational process and changes with age is a common one (Krashen, 1973; Lenneberg, 1967), and it is important not to bias the examination of sex-related differences by including data from subjects in whom lateralization processes were not yet complete. Perhaps more critically, cognitive abilities are developing throughout childhood, and children certainly have different capacities and may very well employ different strategies than do adults. Thus, children may perform differently than adults on the tasks intended to measure cerebral lateralization.

As with studies on adults, the majority of studies providing data on sex-related differences in children have employed some variant of the dichotic listening procedure. The first such study was carried out by Kimura (1963). She presented digit lists varying in length from one to three pairs and observed a right-ear superiority at all age levels from 4 to 9 years. While the laterality effect was not statistically significant in her 7- and 9-year-old girls, there are no clear signs of sex-related differences in her data. In a subsequent replication, Kimura (1967) found very similar results, but the failure to observe a significant right-ear effect appeared among the 5-year-old boys. The bulk of other dichotic studies using lists of items also show no consistent sex differences. No sign of sex-related differences appear in the studies of Geffner and Hochberg (1971), using two pairs of digits with 4–7 year olds; Knox and Kimura (1970), using digit lists with 5–8 year olds; and Satz *et al.* (1975) and Borowy and Goebel (1976), using lists with 5–11 year olds. Bryden (1970) found no overall sex-related difference among 152 right-handed children aged 7–11, although the difference in ear asymmetry between right- and left-handers was manifested earlier in girls than in boys. Nagafuchi (1970) found a greater right-ear effect in boys than in girls aged 3–5 years, but Dorman and Geffner (1974) observed a somewhat larger right-ear effect in 6-year-old girls.

On simple paired items, Knox and Kimura (1970) and Ingram (1975a) show no sex-related differences, although there is a slight trend for greater right-ear effects in Ingram's boys than in her girls (aged 3–5 years). Using CV pairs, Berlin *et al.* (1973) found no sex-related differences in children ranging from 5 to 13 years. In a compilation of several studies using CV pairs and involving 316 children, Bryden (1979a) reported a trend toward a higher incidence of the right-ear effect in girls as opposed to boys.

The dichotic verbal studies with children, therefore, show no very convincing signs of sex-related differences. Some studies show a greater lateralization in girls at some ages (Bryden, 1979a; Geffner & Hochberg, 1971; Kimura, 1967); others show greater lateralization for boys (Geffner & Dorman, 1976; Nagafuchi, 1970); the majority show no difference.

These results can be taken in a number of ways. In one sense, they weaken the adult data that show a greater laterality in males and suggest that there are no meaningful sex-related differences at all. It is worth noting that the developmental studies are almost always done on a broader sampling of the general population than the adult studies, which usually involve university undergraduates. On the other hand, the concern with strategy effects and attentional biases has not been as great in the developmental studies as in the adult studies (cf. Bryden, 1978), and therefore the developmental studies may not have provided a very good control over experimental effects. Finally, the cognitive capacities of children may not be sufficiently well developed for them to show the same patterns of lateralization that are observed with adults (Witelson, 1977).

Sex-related differences have been reported less frequently with other perceptual measures of hemispheric asymmetry employed with children. Knox and Kimura (1970) found that boys were better than girls at the recognition of environmental sounds and animal sounds, but there were no sex-related differences in the magnitude of the left-ear effect obtained with these materials. Young and Bion (1979) found a greater left-visual-field superiority for the enumeration of dots in boys than in girls. This greater lateralization in boys is in agreement with the slight trend found for visuospatial lateralization in adults.

The clearest evidence for sex-related differences in children comes from studies by Witelson (1974, 1976b) employing a nonverbal tactual analogue to dichotic listening. Witelson (1976b) had subjects palpate two hidden nonsense shapes simultaneously for 10 sec, using the index and middle fingers, and then select the correct shapes from among six alternatives presented visually. She administered this "dichhaptic stimulation" test to 200 boys and girls ranging in age from 6 to 13 years. She found that the boy's left-hand score was significantly higher than their right-hand score, whereas there were no differences between the hands for the girls. Although there was an improvement in overall accuracy with age, age did not interact with the hand effect: Boys were more accurate on the left hand at all ages, whereas girls did not show differences between hands at any age. Witelson (1976b) suggests that the right hemisphere is more specialized than the left for the processing of spatial information in boys, whereas spatial abilities are bilaterally represented in girls at least until adolescence. The clearer lateralization in boys for spatial processes is in agreement with the visual study of Young and Bion (1979) and with the trend in adults (see Table 14.1). However, Witelson's procedure gives ample opportunity for subjects to bias their attention to one hand or the other, and at present we have no information on how attentional or strategy factors may influence performance on the dichhaptic task.

In contrast to Witelson's findings, Ghent (1961) reports that a greater sensitivity to pressure on the left thumb, as opposed to the right, appears earlier in girls than in boys. Kimura (1963) reports a replication of the Ghent study, although the data are not presented in her paper. Kimura states that by age 9 girls show a superior pressure sensitivity on the left thumb, whereas boys do not. Pressure sensitivity, however, is not a spatial task, and if a spatial component is necessary to show a right-hemispheric superiority, Witelson (1976b) may have developed a better procedure for assessing it.

The studies of sex-related differences in lateralization with children only partially duplicate the pattern seen in adults (see Table 14.1). In adults, there is fairly strong evidence for a greater lateralization of language-related processes in males; this is not seen in the studies with children. On the other hand, there was weak evidence for a greater lateralization of spatial processes in adult males: Two developmental studies (Witelson, 1976b; Young & Bion, 1979) show this effect very clearly and add weight to the argument that spatial processes are bilaterally represented in females. The one developmental study of nonverbal auditory lateralization (Knox & Kimura, 1970) found no sex-related differences and contrasts with the single adult study showing greater lateralization in females (Piazza, 1980). If the developmental literature provides any modification of the conclusions from the adult literature, it is in the direction of indicating greater bilaterality for both language and spatial processes in females.

Effects of Brain Damage

Relatively little attention has been paid to sex-related differences in the clinical neuropsychological literature (but see McGlone, 1980). The vast majority of studies have involved relatively small samples, where sex-related differences are all but impossible to detect. The majority of the large-sample studies have involved war veterans and thus have investigated only male subjects. In recent years, however, evidence has been accumulating for sex-related differences in the effects of cerebral damage. Most of this work has contrasted the effects of cerebral damage on verbal and performance subtests of standard intelligence tests.

McGlone (1978) has shown a greater verbal IQ deficit in males with left-hemispheric lesions, relative to females with similar lesions and to subjects of either sex with right-hemispheric damage. Lansdell (1961, 1973) has also reported that males show a greater impairment than females on tests of verbal ability after damage to the left hemisphere. As is the case with normal perceptual studies, however, the sex-related differences are not always evident (e.g., Lansdell, 1968a; McGlone & Kertesz, 1973).

Males also exhibit some tendency toward greater deficit than do females on tests of performance IQ or visuospatial ability following right-hemispheric damage. McGlone and Kertesz (1973) have noted this pattern on a block design task, and Lansdell (1962, 1968b) has noted similar effects. Lansdell and Urbach (1965) have reported that the differing effects of right- and left-hemispheric damage are greater in men than in women. Similarly, McGlone (1978) has reported that the difference between verbal and performance IQ is affected by side of damage in men only, although she did not find a significant difference between men and women in performance IQ for either right- or left-hemispheric damage.

Inglis and Lawson (1981) have carried out a survey of published studies on the effects of unilateral brain damage on intelligence test performance. In some of the studies they reviewed, left-hemispheric damage selectively impaired verbal IQ and right-hemispheric damage affected performance IQ; in other studies, this interaction was not evident. Inglis and Lawson were able to show that the interaction with side of lesion was found in studies in which only male subjects were employed but did not occur when significant numbers of female subjects were included. Since none of the studies surveyed by Inglis and Lawson (1981) were designed to assess sex-related differences, their findings provide strong support for McGlone's (1980) contention that cognitive processes are less lateralized in the female than in the male.

Further support for this argument comes from data on the incidence of aphasia following unilateral brain damage published by Hécaen et al. (1981). Data from their right-handed subjects are shown in Table 14.2. Among men, aphasia follows upon left-hemispheric damage far more

Table 14.2
Sex Differences in the Incidence of Aphasia following Unilateral Brain Damage

| | Side of lesion | | | | | | Speech lateralization (%) | |
| | Left | | | Right | | | | |
	Aphasics	Total cases	%	Aphasics	Total cases	%	Left	Right
Men	23	43	53	1	30	3	95	5
Women	13	27	48	4	30	13	79	21

Note. Data from Hécaen, DeAgostini, and Monzon-Montes (1981).

often than after right-hemispheric damage. The incidence ratios suggest that about 95% of men have language represented in the left hemisphere, a figure in agreement with those presented in Chapter 10. In contrast, aphasia following right-hemispheric damage is far more prevalent in women, and the best estimate for left-hemispheric language representation is only 79%. Similar calculations on the incidence of spatial disorders (Hécaen, 1981; Hécaen *et al.*, 1981) also indicate that spatial processes are more likely to be right-hemispheric in men than in women. While these calculations are based on relatively few cases, they provide compelling evidence for the view that more men than women show the normal pattern of cerebral organization. They do not, however, indicate that men are any more lateralized than women. So far as the evidence goes, it indicates that the woman who is left-hemispheric for speech is just as lateralized as the left-hemispheric man: It is simply that there are proportionately fewer of them. Such an interpretation would be supported by the findings of Lake and Bryden (1976), who found no sex-related difference in the absolute value of dichotic ear effects, although a higher percentage of men showed a right-ear advantage.

Sex-Related Anatomical Differences

There has been a resurgence of interest in anatomical differences between the two cerebral hemispheres (e.g., Geschwind & Levitsky, 1968; Wada *et al.*, 1975; Witelson & Pallie, 1973). The studies indicate that the left temporal planum tends to be larger than the right. Wada *et al.* (1975) indicated that there is a trend for the left planum to be larger in adult males than in adult females and that more male infants than female infants show the reversed pattern of asymmetry. In contrast, Witelson and Pallie (1973) reported female infants tended to show slightly greater asymmetry. Wada (1976) reported that the temporal planum was larger on both sides in infant males than in infant females. This provides some evidence that the asymmetry of the temporal planum increases with age, and more so for males than for females. In addition, Wada reported that there was a trend for the left frontal operculum to be larger in infant females than in infant males—that is, the pattern indicated greater asymmetry in this region for females than for males.

This evidence must be considered to be suggestive at best. While there are certainly signs of sex-related differences in several studies, the small sample sizes and great variability preclude any statistical significance. Since these regions correspond closely to the classical "speech areas," it is logical to assume that anatomical asymmetry may lead to functional asymmetry. However, there is no direct evidence that such is the case. Furthermore, the distribution of asymmetry reported by Wada (1976) is not so extreme as usually given for speech lateralization. In 100 adult brains, he reports the left temporal planum was larger in 82, the right in 10; for 100 infant brains, the left planum was larger in 56, the right in 12. However, at least for adult brains, the sex-related difference is in the same direction as that indicated by the behavioral studies.

Conclusions

The literature on sex-related differences in lateralization is rife with inconsistencies. The procedures vary, the samples are often small, and extraneous effects can frequently obscure any possible differences. To a large extent, one's conclusions rest on the choice of which studies to emphasize and which to ignore. It is very tempting to agree with Fairweather's (1976) assessment of the situation and to argue that there are no convincing data for sex-related differences in cerebral lateralization. However, it is perhaps time to be brave and offer a somewhat more positive conclusion. Furthermore, it is also time to return to the original question of whether the study of sex-related differences in lateralization can tell us anything about how lateralization relates to normal behavior.

Of the two alternative speculations about sex-related differences in lateralization, there is virtually no support for Buffery and Gray's (1972) argument that women are more lateralized than men. The evidence instead provides support for Levy's (1974) contention that the male is more lateralized than the female. But one must grant that this evidence is not without its problems.

The support for the notion that women are less lateralized than men comes primarily from studies of verbal processing and of spatial processing. In fact, if there are any sex-related differences for nonverbal nonspatial functions, they lie in the direction of greater lateralization in the female (Ghent, 1961; Piazza, 1980).

The majority of the verbal dichotic listening studies that show any sex-related effects indicate a greater degree of lateralization in the male. The same is true for the verbal tachistoscopic studies. While these studies are almost all open to some criticism about uncontrolled experimental effects, the fact that basically the same pattern emerges from both auditory and visual studies makes the argument for a true sex-related difference more convincing. When one adds the signs of anatomical differences (Wada *et al.*, 1975) and of differences following brain damage (Hécaen *et al.*, 1981; McGlone, 1978), the cumulative impact is simply too much to dismiss as an artifact. Rather, this evidence points fairly strongly to a sex-related difference in the representation of language functions, with left-hemispheric representation of linguistic processes being less prevalent in the female than in the male.

The other area in which sex-related differences persistently show a greater lateralization in males than in females is that of spatial processing (e.g., Kimura, 1969; Witelson, 1976b; Young & Bion, 1979). While the present review suggests that sex-related differences are not so consistent in this area as in the verbal domain, they do appear in both visual and tactual modalities. There is not as strong supplementary evidence from anatomical or clinical studies for greater right-hemispheric lateralization of spatial processes in men, although Hécaen's (1981) data point in this direction. It is also true that the laterality effects measured in studies of perceptual asymmetry can be profoundly influenced by the way in which the subject approaches the task. This makes it very difficult to determine whether the sex-related differences in spatial lateralization are due to differences in brain organization or to differences in the way in which subjects perform the tasks. Women may tend to use verbal strategies to solve spatial problems and to encode spatial displays, and they may generate a reduced laterality effect, not because their right-hemisphere is any less "spatial," but because they use left-hemisphere processes to perform the task. On the basis of the evidence to date, this alternative seems at least reasonably plausible.

On the basis of these data, and especially those of Table 14.2, it may well be that men and women differ in the pattern of cerebral organization, rather than in the degree of lateralization. If we assume that hemi-

Table 14.3
Hypothetical Percentage Distribution of Sex Differences in Cerebral Organization

	Cerebral lateralization					
	Language		Spatial		Complementary	Noncomplementary
	L	R	L	R	(LR+RL)	(LL+RR)
Men	95	5	25	75	72.5	27.5
Women	80	20	40	60	56.0	44.0

spheric representation of linguistic and spatial functions are causally unrelated to one another, a rather interesting picture emerges. In general, men are more likely than women to have left-hemispheric representation of language and right-hemispheric representation of spatial processes. On a purely chance basis, then, men are more likely than women to show complementarity of specialization (see Table 14.3). If noncomplementarity—that is, primary dependence on the same hemisphere for both language and spatial processes—is detrimental to spatial ability, then sex-related differences in spatial ability could be a direct consequence of differences in patterns of cerebral organization (Bryden, 1979c; McGlone & Davidson, 1973).

15

Reading and Language-Related Deficits

If individuals vary in the extent to which language mechanisms are lateralized to one hemisphere, it becomes a plausible hypothesis that people with unilateral representation of language will find it easier to integrate diverse linguistic information and therefore will be linguistically superior to those whose language mechanisms are more bilaterally represented. This logic can be turned about, and it can be argued that individuals who show some form of language-related deficit should manifest signs of poorer cerebral lateralization than those who are more skilled at language. Thus, one way of investigating the question of whether different patterns of cerebral organization influence normal behavior would be to compare groups that differ in some language-related skill and see if there is any evidence for differences in cerebral organization.

This chapter is concerned with a variety of different studies that have followed this basic approach. These studies have all taken the form of isolating some group deficient in some language-related ability and postulating that the deficit may have occurred because of poor or incomplete cerebral lateralization. Virtually all the studies deal with children, and it is not uncommon to find the argument that cerebral lateralization has not yet developed. As indicated in Chapter 12, however, there is little evidence that cerebral organization changes developmentally. Rather, any changes in observed laterality seem to be more the result of changing cognitive capacities that permit children to perform more complex tasks. Thus, the reader should be skeptical about any evidence for a "developmental lag" in cerebral organization. It is more likely that any such evidence is simply a manifestation of a deficiency in carrying out certain cognitive operations. Nevertheless, it remains plausible that those individuals who are deficient in language-related skills have failed to develop normally because of an initially poor cerebral lateralization.

Many different types of dysfunction have been suspected of being related to poor cerebral lateralization. In the following pages, the emphasis will be on the evidence for differences in cerebral lateralization in poor readers. While other groups with specialized language problems, such as stutterers, the deaf, and second-language learners, have also been studied, the problems are essentially the same.

Reading

Because literacy is so important in our contemporary society, a vast amount of research and speculation has been addressed to the problem of how best to teach children to read (e.g., Chall, 1967), and much concern has been expressed about those children who show deficiencies in acquiring reading skills (e.g., Benton & Pearl, 1978; Knights & Bakker, 1976; Pirozzolo & Wittrock, 1981). Although some children who fail to learn to read adequately also show deficiencies in a wide variety of other skills, there remains a disturbingly high percentage of children who show a *specific developmental dyslexia*—the development of poor reading skills despite normal intelligence and the lack of any other obvious sensory or neurological impairment (Rutter, 1978).

The notion that specific developmental dyslexia arises from poor cerebral lateralization has enjoyed popularity for a number of years. Orton (1928, 1937) argued that point-to-point interconnections between the two hemispheres implied that a visual pattern presented in the right visual field, for example, would not only be projected directly to the left visual cortex but also be represented in mirror-image form in the right visual cortex (see Figure 15.1). In order to read properly, Orton argued, one would have to suppress this unwanted mirror-image representation, and this would be possible only if one hemisphere were clearly the master. Orton felt that inconsistent use of the hands (mixed laterality) or consistent use of one hand and the opposite eye (crossed laterality) were both signs of a poorly established hemispheric specialization, and the precursor of subsequent reading disabilities.

Orton's specific arguments have not stood the test of time very well. There is little evidence that poor readers actually perceive visual stimuli in mirror-image orientation, nor do they make an abnormal number of letter or word reversals (Liberman, Shankweiler, Orlando, Harris & Berti, 1971; but see Corballis & Beale, 1976, for a resurrection of some of

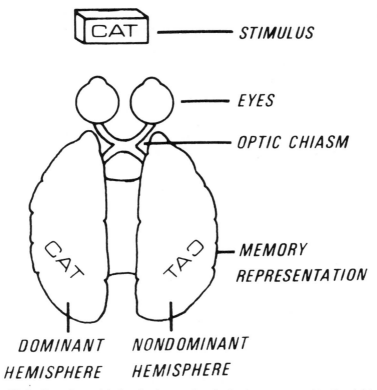

Figure 15.1. Orton's model showing how a visual stimulus presented to the right visual field would be represented by a mirror-image representation in the nondominant hemisphere. [From Corballis, M. C. The left-right problem in psychology. *Canadian Psychologist*, 1974, *15*, p. 25. Copyright (1974) Canadian Psychological Association. Reprinted by permission.]

Orton's ideas). Likewise, sighting dominance has not been shown to be clearly related to cerebral lateralization (Porac & Coren, 1976), and thus Orton's criterion of mixed hand–eye dominance as a sign of incomplete cerebral lateralization has little empirical support. Nevertheless, Orton's work has had considerable influence and does provide an impetus for investigating the relation of cerebral lateralization to specific developmental dyslexia.

The development of dichotic listening and tachistoscopic procedures for assessing cerebral lateralization made it possible to attempt a somewhat different test of Orton's (1937) hypothesis that incomplete cerebral lateralization was related to reading disability. If Orton's notions were correct, one should expect to find that poor readers would be less likely than good readers to show evidence of clear lateralization for language. This general approach has been used with various dichotic procedures, tachistoscopic techniques, and somatosensory techniques. Much of the literature in this area has been critically assessed by Satz (1976) and Naylor (1980), and this chapter will not attempt to duplicate these treatments. Rather, the aim here will be to provide a general feeling about the success of this work.

One of the biggest difficulties in assessing this work is the diversity of criteria that have been employed in selecting subjects. Some investigators have worked with clinic populations and thus have chosen severely retarded readers; others have used school populations and therefore less severely deficient readers. More seriously, some studies have defined their groups solely in terms of reading retardation and have thus confounded specific developmental dyslexia with general intellectual impairment, while others have been concerned with poor readers of normal intelligence. Furthermore, the particular tasks used to measure lateralization have often left the subject free to develop varying strategies that would affect the magnitude of the laterality effect. All these problems should be kept in mind in the ensuing discussion.

Reading and Dichotic Listening

Many of the studies have followed Kimura's (1961a, 1961b) initial procedure of presenting simultaneous lists of items to each ear, with a free recall of those items remembered. Thus, Bryden (1970) tested 90 schoolchildren in Grades 2–6 with two- and three-pair dichotic lists of numbers. Children were also given group reading tests (Gates–MacGinitie) and intelligence tests (Otis). Those whose reading scores fell below their IQ scores were classed as "relatively poor readers." This is obviously a very weak criterion, although it does make some attempt to identify specific developmental dyslexics rather than those with a more general intellectual deficit. Bryden's (1970) results failed to show any clearly evident differences between good and poor readers in terms of the frequency or magnitude of a right-ear superiority. In part, this was due to the fact that 10 of the 90 subjects were left-handed, and no very clear predictions could be made about their performance. It was noted that, among boys, the poor readers were much more likely than the good readers to have an ear superiority opposite to their handedness: Right-handers showed a left-ear advantage, whereas left-handers showed a right-ear advantage. The girls showed a similar trend, but much reduced in magnitude. At best, this study can be described as providing a hint that there might be a relation between reading ability and dichotic listening performance. At about the same time, Satz and Sparrow (1970) found no significant difference in right-ear superiority between good and poor readers, although again a higher incidence of left-ear superiority was seen in the poor readers.

Many other studies using lists of numbers or words have failed to find significant differences in the size of the right-ear effect between normal and dyslexic groups (e.g., Abigail & Johnson, 1976; McKeever & VanDeventer, 1975; Witelson, 1976a; Yeni-Komshian, Isenberg, & Goldberg, 1975). Witelson and Rabinovitch (1972) did suggest that poor readers drawn from a learning disability clinic failed to show the normal right-ear effect, and Thomson (1976) reported that dyslexic children of unspecified age did not show the normal right-ear effect for the recall of lists of two or four pairs of words. Likewise, Leong (1976) found a larger right-ear effect in normals than in dyslexics.

Major series of investigations of performance on dichotic lists and the relation to reading ability have been carried out in Holland by Bakker and his colleagues and in Florida by Satz and his colleagues (Bakker, Teunissen, & Bosch, 1976; Satz, 1976). Both Bakker and Satz argue that there is a relation between developmental dyslexia and dichotic lateralization only among older dyslexics (aged 10–12). Their argument, derived from Satz and Sparrow (1970), is that there is a maturational lag in the development of speech lateralization among dyslexic children. This theory, of course, presumes that speech processes become more completely lateralized with increasing age. Our own assessment of the developmental literature suggests that performance on dichotic lists changes with age and that signs of increasing lateralization are more likely to be signs of changing attentional and memory strategies (see Chapter 12). Furthermore, the data for good and poor readers shown by Satz (1976, pp. 282–283) seem to indicate that there is a reduced right-ear effect in their poor readers at all ages from 5½ years to 12 years.

With single-pairs of CV syllables, such as the stop consonant set popularized by Studdert-Kennedy and Shankweiler (1970), differences between normal and dyslexic children have been reported less frequently. For instance, Mercure and Warren (1978) found significant right-ear effects for both adequate and inadequate Grade 3 readers. A detailed analysis of the particular phonetic contrasts suggested that adequate readers may have a stronger lateralization in that they are better able to resist the effects of an unvoiced sound to the left ear. In general, the unvoiced member of a pair was better identified than the voiced member, but the good readers were able to overcome this effect when the unvoiced syllable was presented to the left ear. The selection of subjects in this study leaves something to be desired, however, and replication is necessary before the findings are accepted as conclusive.

Another study involving CV pairs was carried out by Springer and Eisenson (1977). They found evidence to indicate that poor readers showed the same laterality effect as normals, but those with expressive or receptive language problems as well as reading impairment manifested very small laterality effects. The study, however, involves only 10 dyslexics, 5 of whom also showed language impairments.

Some support for the notion that it is language impairment, and not specific reading disability, that is related to reduced dichotic laterality is seen in a study by Pettit and Helms (1979). They found virtually no right-ear advantage in subjects (aged 6–9 years) who were classified as subnormal by the Illinois Test of Psycholinguistic Ability, using lists of three pairs of numbers or of animal names. In contrast, both normals and children with articulatory disorders showed large right-ear effects.

Relatively few of the dichotic studies with dyslexic children have made any serious attempt to control the various strategies that subjects might adopt for performing the task. Leong (1976) did score his free-recall data according to whether the subject recalled the right ear first or the left ear first. Thus, the means in the analysis represent the performance that would have been observed had each subject initiated recall with left- and right-ear items equally often. Leong reports that disabled readers performed significantly worse in terms of right-ear superiority than their counterparts matched for age, sex, and general intelligence. In contrast to this finding, Yeni-Komshian *et al.* (1975) found no difference in ear asymmetry between normal and dyslexic children when order of recall was controlled by instruction.

Although there are frequent hints that dyslexic children may show a reduced ear asymmetry on dichotic listening tasks, there are enough problems and inconsistencies to thwart any attempt to reach a simple conclusion. Satz and Sparrow (1970) have taken a developmental lag position: They argue that dyslexic children have not shown the normal development of speech lateralization and that their reading difficulties arise from this poor lateralization. This general view is supported by Bakker *et al.* (1976), Leong (1976), and Satz (1976), among others.

According to the model, young children have poorly established cerebral lateralization, and so there should be no clear relation between ear asymmetry and reading ability; only in older children should the relation be observed. Here, normal children have well-established cerebral lateralization, whereas dyslexics are lateralized like their younger normal counterparts. The studies in the Dutch and Florida series cited by

Bakker *et al.* (1976) and by Satz (1976) often report patterns consistent with this notion, and Leong (1976) supports the developmental lag view, although his subjects average only age 9:3. Other similar studies fail to find any difference between normals and poor readers at age 10 or older (e.g., McKeever & VanDeventer, 1975; Witelson, 1976a). It is also rather difficult to accept a theory that postulates a developmental lag in the establishment of cerebral lateralization when one can find so little convincing evidence that there are any systematic changes in cerebral lateralization with age (see Chapter 12). Satz and Bakker are among the few who find any evidence for systematic age-related trends in lateralization assessed through dichotic listening (e.g., Satz *et al.*, 1975). One is tempted to conclude that any trend toward an increasing right-ear effect in normals is due to the procedure employed rather than to any increased lateralization for speech. By this view, the differences between dyslexics and normals could be attributed to differences in the way the two groups handle the task, rather than to differences in cerebral lateralization.

An alternative view is that one might expect to find a difference between normals and dyslexics in the early stages of reading acquisition, rather than in the late stages. Bilateral representation of speech might lead to poor habits during early reading and to a failure to recognize reading as primarily a language-related process, thus resulting in a deficiency. In contrast, the reading performance of older children is affected by a sufficiently wide variety of different factors that any relation between cerebral lateralization and poor reading might be swamped. Again, however, there are few data to support this view. Bryden (1970), Satz (1976), and Witelson (1976a) also show very slight trends to a reduced ear asymmetry in their younger children (ages 5–8 years), but the effects are not large enough to be compelling.

Many researchers have attempted to classify disabled readers into different types: Frequently a distinction is made between those with language-related problems and those with visuospatial problems (e.g., Boder, 1970, 1973; Kinsbourne & Warrington, 1963). As an auditory task, the dichotic listening procedure may be sensitive to the lateralization of processes intimately related to speech comprehension. One might expect, then, that poor speech lateralization would lead to deficiencies not only in reading but also in language. Thus, not all poor readers would show weak lateralization, but only those who also manifested some deficiencies in expressive or receptive language. Although there seem to be no studies that have employed the dichotic listening procedures with different types of poor readers, such as Boder's (1970, 1973) *dysphonetics* and *dyseidetics*, some evidence that poor auditory lateralization is related to language disorders, rather than to all forms of reading disability, can be found in Springer and Eisenson's (1977) data. They reported a reduced right-ear superiority only in those dyslexics who also showed expressive or receptive language problems. However, their study involved only 10 dyslexic children and is clearly in need of replication and extension.

Reading and Visual Laterality

Because reading involves visual material, many researchers have chosen to study lateralization in poor readers through visual techniques rather than through auditory ones. For instance, Marcel, Katz, and Smith (1974) presented single words, horizontally displayed, to either the left or right visual field. They used good and poor readers of approximately 8 years of age, with no control for general intelligence. They found that right-visual-field superiority observed with normal readers was much attenuated in the poor readers. Marcel *et al.* (1974) were quite aware of other possible interpretations of their data and discussed quite extensively the possibility that the groups differ in terms of eye movements, the deployment of attention, and scanning. Although they rejected each of these alternatives in favor of a cerebral lateralization argument, their case is not entirely convincing. With a similar paradigm, normal subjects will identify disconnected letter strings better in the right than in the left visual field. With such a procedure, the serial position curves are quite different on the left and right. The curve for the left visual field tends to show peaks at both extremities, whereas that for the right visual field drops sharply as one progresses to the right. In other words, partial identification encompasses quite different letters in the left and right visual fields. Since normal readers are more familiar with the language than are poor readers, it may very well be that their strategies of guessing from partial information are quite different from those of poor readers and that these guessing strategies are particularly advantageous for the type of partial information that is obtained from right-visual-field presentations. Despite these objections, it is worth noting that the basic findings have been replicated (Marcel & Rajan, 1975).

Greater lateralization for words presented visually has also been found by Kershner (1977). He used a bilateral presentation procedure, employing a fixation control item. Subjects were 10-year-old children: 12 high-IQ gifted readers, 11 good readers, and 10 poor readers (at least 2 years retarded in reading). Both gifted and good readers showed a large right-visual-field superiority; the poor readers showed a reduced one. Once again, however, the use of horizontally displayed words makes it possible that the overall right-visual-field superiority is influenced not only by cerebral lateralization but also by directional scanning factors (M. J. White, 1973). Poor readers may have different strategies of scanning and encoding words, and this difference may contribute significantly to the observed difference in the right-visual-field superiority.

Essentially the same procedure has been employed by McKeever and Huling (1970) and by McKeever and VanDeventer (1975) with adolescent dyslexic subjects. In neither case did the overall right-visual-field superiority differ for normals and dyslexics.

A rather different technique for ensuring fixation was employed by Yeni-Komshian *et al.* (1975). They presented vertically oriented words serially, with the first, third, and fifth words lateralized to one side, and the second and fourth words centered at fixation. Their poor readers (mean age: 12:8) showed a *larger* right-visual-field superiority on this test than did their good readers, largely because accuracy in the left visual field was much lower for poor readers than for good readers. Yeni-Komshian *et al.* suggest that right-hemispheric processing is degraded in poor readers or that interhemispheric transmission is poor. Similar effects were obtained with Arabic numerals as stimuli, although the overall right-visual-field effect was not significant. This task requires a constant shifting of attention from center to periphery, with the pattern differing for left- and right-visual-field presentations. The poor readers seem to have some specific difficulty with the left-center-left-center-left sequence required for good performance in the left visual field. It remains unclear to what extent performance was determined by experimental factors rather than by cerebral organization.

A further study showing a greater right-visual-field superiority for poor readers was reported by K. Gross, Rothenberg, Schottenfeld, and Drake (1978). They measured duration thresholds for lateralized presentations of the letters *A,N,O,* and *S,* in subjects ranging from 10 to 13½ years. Normal subjects showed only a very small right-visual-field superiority, whereas poor readers exhibited a large one. In the normal group, reading scores with age partialled out correlated negatively with the difference in threshold between the visual fields ($r = -.48$). Thus, relatively poor normal readers showed the biggest right-visual-field superiority. This was not true for the poor readers, although the absolute magnitude of the lateral difference tended to correlate with reading improvement scores.

There are a number of problems with the K. Gross *et al.* (1978) study. Presentation was monocular, with the dominant eye being used by all subjects. Thus, differences between temporal and nasal hemiretinae confound visual-field differences. Furthermore, duration thresholds were very much shorter for normals (12.6 msec) than for poor readers (52.7 msec). The clear right-visual-field effect for the poor readers may simply be because greater precision of measurement was possible at the longer exposure durations or because the longer exposure durations permitted a more detailed analysis of the stimulus. Of 11 normal subjects showing a visual-field difference, 9 showed lower thresholds on the right. Precisely the same figures are seen for the 11 right-handed poor readers.

A few studies have turned away from verbal material and have investigated differences between good and poor readers on lateralized face recognition tasks. Marcel and Rajan (1975) found no differences in an overall left-visual-field superiority between good and poor readers, but Witelson (1976a) reported a significant left-visual-field effect for normal boys, but not for dyslexic boys. Although the dyslexics did not show a left-visual-field superiority for face recognition, the interaction of group with visual field was not significant in Witelson's study.

Pirozzolo and Rayner (1979) have made a serious attempt to solve the problems encountered in studies such as those reviewed here (see also Pirozzolo, 1979). They selected a group of poor readers whose deficits were primarily language related (Boder, 1973) and compared them to normal readers on both verbal and nonverbal tasks. Both normal and disabled readers were more accurate in the left visual field on a face recognition task, but the normal readers showed a significantly greater right-visual-field superiority on word recognition than did the disabled readers. Furthermore, a relatively high percentage of the errors made by the poor readers in the right visual field were phonetic rather than visual confusions. The interaction of visual field and error type within the poor reader group suggests that the results are not simply a consequence of impaired reading ability in the poor readers. However, the study involved only nine poor readers. Extension of this work is clearly in order.

In summary, the literature on visual laterality and reading disability is rife with inconsistencies. Some of the verbal studies report decreased right-visual-field effects in poor readers (e.g., Marcel *et al.*, 1974; Pirozzolo & Rayner, 1979), others increased laterality effects (e.g., Yeni-Komshian *et al.*, 1975), still others no difference (e.g., McKeever & Huling, 1970). The nonverbal studies are inconsistent, although some slight trend exists for a reduced left-visual-field effect in dyslexics (Witelson, 1976a).

Since reading involves the analysis and decoding of visual stimuli, and good and poor readers necessarily differ in their abilities to perform the requisite tasks, it seems almost self-defeating to investigate laterality differences between normals and dyslexics using tasks that involve the visual presentation of words. While it is unquestionably true that some of the right-visual-field superiority that is observed on such tasks is due to the left-hemispheric superiority at language processing, it is equally true that the specific magnitude of the laterality effect observed can be profoundly influenced by experimental factors related to reading skill. So long as this is the case, we can never be certain that any difference in laterality between normals and dyslexics is not simply a function of the fact that the two groups process words differently. Since good reading also involves the development of good scanning patterns and good eye movement control, for instance, even a move to nonverbal material does not eliminate the possibility that observed laterality differences are more a function of differences in the way the two groups process visual information than of any potential difference in the way various functions are represented in the two cerebral hemispheres (see also Young & Ellis, 1981).

Reading and Somatosensory Laterality

The most detailed study of somatosensory lateralization and reading ability has been carried out by Witelson (1976a). She tested 85 right-handed dyslexic boys, ranging in age from 6 to 14 years and with an average reading lag of 2.6 years. Normal readers were 156 right-handed boys of the same age range and of normal intelligence. Included in her tests were both verbal and nonverbal measures of somatosensory lateralization, as well as dichotic listening and face recognition tests that have been mentioned earlier.

As a nonverbal task, subjects were required to feel two different nonsense shapes simultaneously for 10 sec, one with each hand. They were then required to select these two shapes from a visual display of six. Ten trials were administered, and the accuracy on each hand analyzed. This task was given to 100 normals and 49 of the dyslexics. On this task, left-hand scores are significantly higher than right-hand scores. In addition, Witelson (1976a) reports a highly significant interaction between reading group and hand, with the dyslexic children showing a slight right-hand superiority. Although no higher-order interactions are reported, Witelson's data (1976a, pp. 242–243) indicate that a left-hand superiority rather comparable to that found in normal readers is seen in dyslexic children aged 6–9 years, whereas a right-hand superiority is found in dyslexics aged 10–14 years. Thus, the two reading groups seem to differ significantly only after age 10. This is reminiscent of Satz's (1976) argument that reading should be related to lateralization only in older children, when normal lateralization had failed to develop. Witelson's (1976a) data, however, do not fit a hypothesis of a maturational lag in cerebral lateralization: One would have to postulate that a perfectly normal cerebral lateralization in younger dyslexics had suddenly reversed itself after age 10.

Witelson (1976a) herself suggests that right-hemisphere spatial processing is deficient in the dyslexics and that there is a greater involvement of the left hemisphere in spatial activity in this group. This involvement of the left hemisphere in spatial processing would presumably detract from language-related skills normally dependent on the left hemisphere. Again, Witelson's procedure does not provide any control over the way in which subjects distribute their attention during the 10-sec trial. Rather than providing definitive evidence about hemispheric specialization, Witelson may only have discovered that normal and dyslexic children have different attentional strategies.

Witelson (1976a) also tested some of her children on a verbal somatosensory task. In this task, two different block letters were presented simultaneously, one to each hand, for 2 sec and followed by a second pair of letters presented in the same way. Subjects were then to identify the letters they had felt. This procedure is analogous to a two-pair dichotic list with free recall, although the rate of presentation is much slower and opportunities for attentional bias and reorganization in memory are that much greater. Witelson (1976a) reported data on 28 normal boys and 46 dyslexics on this task. Normal boys were more accurate on the right hand, whereas dyslexics were better on the left hand, yielding a highly significant hand by reading group interaction. As with the nonverbal task, however, younger dyslexics did not differ from the normal boys (Witelson, 1976a, p. 249). Witelson sees these findings as support for the idea that dyslexic boys have a bilateral representation of spatial abilities and that this interferes with normal left-hemispheric verbal processes. The data are suggestive, but there are too many uncontrolled experimental effects to be certain that the differences between the two groups lie in cerebral organization.

Reading and Handedness

There has been a long history of studies attempting to relate reading disability to handedness. Although there are occasional reports that left-handers are poor readers, Hardyck and Petrinovitch's (1977) careful survey of the literature found little evidence to support this contention and many more studies that found no difference between handedness groups. The relation between handedness and cerebral organization is so weak that it would be very difficult to interpret a difference between left- and right-handers in terms of differences in cerebral organization.

One brief report may provide an interesting link between laterality and learning disability. N. H. Schwartz and Dean (1978) have found that parent's handedness, but not subject's handedness, can be used to discriminate between normal and learning-disabled children. Left-handed parents produce children with learning disabilities (and presumably reading problems) more often than right-handed parents do. Although this may be indicative of no more than an increased incidence of birth trauma and subsequent brain damage in the offspring of left-handed parents, the fact that parental laterality is as good a predictor of group membership as maternal laterality would suggest that other factors are relevant. The relation of reading disability to parent's lateralization deserves further investigation with better subject populations and different measures of lateralization.

Speculations on Reading and Lateralization

Despite a variety of methodological problems that make it quite unclear whether one is dealing with different strategies of information processing or different patterns of cerebral organization, the notion that specific developmental dyslexics show reduced lateralization for both verbal and spatial material runs through the literature. With verbal material, this pattern is seen in dichotic and somatosensory studies, as well as in some of the visual experiments. While the present treatment has tended to minimize the importance of the visual studies because poor readers are almost certainly deficient in many aspects of visual information processing, the fact that the same pattern recurs in different sensory modalities makes it more credible.

Because there is so much contamination of cerebral asymmetries by experimental effects, it would obviously be foolish to argue that a relation between reading disability and laterality had been demonstrated. Nevertheless, enough evidence points in this direction to justify further, more careful, experimentation.

It seems unwarranted to think that all instances of reading disability are alike or that all have the same etiology. Some progress has been made in classifying dyslexic children into different categories. Boder

(1970, 1973), for instance, has distinguished between *dysphonetic* readers, who make many language-based errors, and *dyseidetic* readers, who make errors that are more visually based. A somewhat similar distinction has been made by Kinsbourne and Warrington (1963). It would seem equally unwarranted to argue that all cases of reading disability are instances of incomplete cerebral lateralization. Rather, it would seem that problems of cerebral organization would be but one possible antecedent of poor reading. Certainly, Satz (1976) did not find dichotic listening lateralization to be a particularly valuable predictor of subsequent reading performance in his longitudinal study of reading ability. One direction for further research would be to investigate cerebral lateralization in different diagnostic categories of reading disability. The data presented by Springer and Eisenson (1977) and Pirozzolo and Rayner (1979), for instance, suggest that incomplete lateralization is associated with reading disability only in conjunction with language disorders. Thus, perhaps it is only dysphonetic subjects who show abnormal patterns of lateralization.

In general, this research suggests some relation between diffuse cortical representation and deficits in reading or language-related skills. However, this relation has not been shown to be sufficiently strong to be diagnostic or predictive. Some children with perfectly normal functional lateralization become poor readers, whereas other children with poorly lateralized verbal and/or spatial processes overcome this difficulty and become quite skilled at reading and language.

Laterality and Other Language-Related Deficits

A number of studies of perceptual asymmetry have been conducted on deaf children. Most early-deaf children show severe language impairment and very rarely learn to read at the normal level. Because they have not engaged in normal linguistic activity, one might argue that any initial bias for lateralizing language processes to the left hemisphere would be lost and that early-deaf or congenitally deaf children would not show the usual left-hemispheric lateralization of verbal processes.

Most studies of the deaf have, in fact, supported this notion. Reduced laterality effects have been found with words, pictures, and drawings of American Sign Language positions (Manning, Goble, Markman, & LaBreche, 1977; McKeever, Hoemann, Florian, & VanDeventer, 1976; Phippard, 1977). A left-visual-field superiority for the matching of two successively presented words or pictures has been observed by Kelly and Tomlinson-Keasey (1977), but it is not clear to what extent this task involves anything more than simple physical stimulus matching even when words are used as stimuli (cf. Cohen, 1972).

In a study that predates the current enthusiasm for perceptual measures of cerebral lateralization, Gottlieb, Doran, and Whitley (1964) found that deaf high school students who were both right-handed and right-eyed were superior in speech and language skills to those deaf children who showed mixed hand–sighting dominance. In view of the difficulty of showing a relation between sighting dominance and any measure of cerebral lateralization, the significance of this finding is rather obscure, although Gottlieb *et al.* do suggest that poor functional lateralization is associated with difficulties in language acquisition. Gottlieb *et al.* also find that the incidence of right-eye sighting dominance is much reduced among their deaf sample. It is difficult even to guess at the reasons for this.

As with the studies of reading disability, visual laterality does not seem to be the best approach to the investigation of cerebral lateralization in the deaf. The deaf are notoriously poor readers, and to the extent that performance on visual tasks depends on skills acquired and/or perfected in learning to read, there will be differences in visual processing between the hearing and the deaf. These differences may account for all the differences between groups in measured laterality. It would seem to us important to verify the visual studies with somatosensory procedures, using variations on some of the techniques developed by Witelson (1976b) and Nachshon and Carmon (1975).

Gibson and Bryden (1982) have made a start in this direction, using a dichhaptic laterality procedure (see Chapter 5). Although their 10-year-old hearing subjects showed a right-hand superiority for letters and a left-hand superiority for unfamiliar shapes, deaf children tended to show the reverse pattern, with a marked left-hand superiority for the letters and no significant hand difference for the shapes. While this is suggestive of a deviant cerebral organization in the deaf, it is also possible that the deaf children treated the tactually presented letters as nonverbal material.

To the extent that the idea of a reduced lateralization for language in the congenitally deaf can be accepted, however, these studies are important. They suggest that an initial bias to a left-hemispheric specialization for language can disappear or be distorted if early language experience is abnormal. Such a view is also supported by the abnormal pattern of lateralization exhibited by Genie, an adolescent girl deprived of language experience and kept in isolation for many years (Curtiss, 1977; Fromkin, Krashen, Curtiss, Rigler, & Rigler, 1974). This interpretation is reminiscent of the effect Hubel and Wiesel's (1963) data on orientation-specific cells in the cortex of young kittens had on Hebb's (1949) theory of perceptual learning: It is not that left-hemispheric language special-ization develops with age but that it may be lost if early language experi-ence does not provide an adequate opportunity for use.

Yet another area in which it has been suggested that cerebral organiza-tion is important is that of second-language learning. Albert and Obler (1978), for example, suggest that learning a second language may result not only in reduced lateralization for the second language but also in less dependence on left-hemispheric systems for the primary language. In support of this, they cite studies by Hamers and Lambert (1977) and Walters and Zatorre (1978) indicating that bilinguals show less of a right-visual-field effect for word recognition than do monolinguals. An alterna-tive view is that it is only the second language that involves right-hemispheric mechanisms, and then perhaps only in early stages of language acquisition (Silverberg, Bentin, Gaziel, Obler, & Albert, 1979). Unfortunately, it is difficult to separate cerebral organization from the effects of reading skills and other experimental variables in this type of research (Vaid & Genesee, 1980).

Before we close this section, the studies of cerebral lateralization and stuttering also deserve brief mention. It is clear (Jones, 1966) that severe stuttering can be produced by bilateral representation of speech produc-tion. In Jones's cases, stuttering was alleviated by surgical removal of right-hemispheric speech areas. However, attempts to show that all stuttering is the result of abnormal speech representation have not been entirely successful. While some studies have shown stutterers to be different from normals in dichotic listening performance (Rosenfield & Goodglass, 1980), others have failed to find group differences (Brady & Berson, 1975).

So What Does It Mean?

There has been little to indicate that the "normal" case of left-hemi-spheric language processing and right-hemispheric spatial and integra-tive systems is any better or any worse than the reverse organization. The situation with respect to bilateral representation of function is some-what different. Despite unreliable measuring instruments, a plethora of experimental effects that contaminate the results, various methodologi-cal absurdities, and frequent instances of contradictory evidence, one theme continues to recur. That is the notion that bilateral representation of function is associated with deficit. With poor readers, with the deaf, and with female spatial abilities, there are signs that poor performance is associated with weak lateralization or bilateral representation. The generality fails for verbal skills in women, where women seem to be less lateralized but show better verbal skills than men.

This review has indicated that one can hardly take the case for an association between deficit and poor lateralization as proven. Nevertheless, the present evidence is sufficiently convergent to indicate that it is a plausible working hypothesis. At present, there is an urgent need for research that is more sensitive to the contaminating effects of the experimental procedures. Only then will we have a clear answer to the question of whether bilaterality is a burden. In the preceding chapters, some indications of the directions this research might take have been offered.

The bulk of the evidence also indicates that bilateral functional representation is not simply a lag in the normal maturation of cerebral asymmetries. Rather, it may sometimes be acquired through the lack of the appropriate experience, as we suggested was the case for the congenitally deaf, and may in part be simply a result of the biological organization of the brain. Hints that it is degree of lateralization and not direction of lateralization that is genetically determined (Bryden, 1979c; Collins, 1977) raise the possibility that bilateral functional representation may be genetically determined.

16

Control of
the Active Hemisphere

The preceding three chapters have been concerned with one of the major issues of individual differences in laterality research: Do individual variations in the pattern of cerebral lateralization have any consequences for normal behavior? This chapter deals with a second major aspect of individual differences in laterality: To what extent can one control the use of one hemisphere rather than the other?

Early discussions of functional lateralization (e.g., Kimura, 1966, 1967) emphasized the point that different laterality effects were obtained with different types of material. At least implicitly, these papers presented the view that one made use of the hemisphere that was most adequately specialized for the demands of the task being performed. Thus, the left hemisphere (normally) would be involved when the task was a verbal one, and the right hemisphere would be involved if the task were spatial or musical. In effect, this view is one of a fixed lateralization that a person can do little to change.

Almost at the opposite pole is the view expressed by the enthusiasts for conjugate lateral eye movement research (e.g., Bakan, 1969). Many investigators have found consistent individual differences in the direction of lateral eye movements made to reflective questions (e.g., Bakan, 1969; Bakan & Strayer, 1973; M. E. Day, 1964): Some people habitually look toward the left, others toward the right. It has been postulated that people who look to the left are activating their right hemispheres (Bakan, 1969) and therefore are giving primacy to the modes of thought for which the right hemisphere is specialized. Thus, left-lookers should be more spatial and holistic and less verbal in their thinking. Conversely, people who consistently look to the right are thought to be activating their left hemispheres and therefore to be more verbal in their thought. By this view, one is either a left-hemispheric person or a right-hemispheric person, and one's hemispheric preference overrides the particular task being performed and pervades all of one's behavior. Taken to the extreme, this view has been used to explain the differences between Western and Oriental philosophies and the communication gap between generations (Ornstein, 1972).

Intermediate between these two views is a situationalism that sees the use of a given hemisphere as being controlled by an interaction between the task and the individual. One version of this has been presented by Kinsbourne (1970, 1973, 1975a). Kinsbourne has argued that ongoing verbal thought serves to activate the left hemisphere, thus leading to superior performance on the right side. Conversely, spatial thought serves to prime the right hemisphere. The particular hemisphere that is activated can be determined by the task, by experimental manipulation of concurrent activities, or by the biases of the subject. By this argument, laterality effects depend not only on the task but also on the context in which the task is performed. Furthermore, the subject has some personal control over which hemisphere is primed through the selection of appropriate priming activities. The critical questions concern when such priming effects occur and to what extent they are under personal control.

Lateral Eye Movements and Hemisphericity

Bakan's (1969) suggestion that the direction of lateral eye movements to reflective questions was related to an individual's preference for using one hemisphere has stimulated a great deal of research. Much of this work has been critically assessed by Ehrlichman and Weinberger (1978), and only a general overview will be presented here.

Although varying criteria have been used for classifying individuals as left-movers or right-movers, there is general agreement that many individuals are consistent in their direction of gaze. One common criterion is to consider a person consistent if 70% of the scoreable movements are in one direction. This criterion has been used by R. E. Gur and Gur (1975), G. H. Tucker and Suib (1978), and Paradowski, Brucker, Zaretsky, and Alba (1978), among others. In these three studies, 117 of 134 subjects, or 87%, could be classified as consistent. Ehrlichman and Weinberger (1978) estimate the incidence of "bidirectional" movers as somewhat higher than this incidence of 13%. Measurement of lateral eye movement patterns has also been shown to be fairly reliable, with test–retest values around .75–.80 frequently reported (Bakan & Strayer,

1973; Ehrlichman, Weiner, & Baker, 1974; G. H. Tucker & Suib, 1978; but see Templer, Goldstein, & Penick, 1972, for a low value).

While sex differences are often not reported, Beveridge and Hicks (1976) and M. E. Day (1964) show evidence that men are more likely to be right-movers and women more likely to be left-movers. If one is to relate lateral eye movement phenomena to hemispheric asymmetry, this finding seems counterintuitive. Women, who are notoriously poor at spatial tasks, are left-movers, supposedly indicating a preference for the right (spatial) hemisphere. Conversely, the less verbally fluent male is the one who shows the left-hemispheric (verbal) bias.

If the differences between left-movers and right-movers are due to a differential use of one hemisphere rather than the other, one would expect to find right-movers better on verbal tasks while left-movers excelled on spatial tasks. Evidence on this point is rather equivocal. Tucker and Suib (1978) reported that left-movers were much better on the Block Design and Object Assembly subtests of the Wechsler Adult Intelligence Scale, whereas right-movers excelled on the Vocabulary and Verbal Information subtests. Similar effects were not obtained by Hiscock (1977b), and Galin and Ornstein (1974) failed to find a difference in eye movement pattern between lawyers (high verbal) and ceramicists (high spatial).

One of the few studies that has attempted to provide a direct link between lateral eye movements and other measures more clearly related to cerebral organization is that of Nielsen and Sorensen (1976). They found that left-movers exhibit a smaller right-ear advantage on a dichotic listening task than do right-movers. However, a similar study attempted at the University of Waterloo found little evidence for any relation between preferred direction of gaze and dichotic lateralization (Davies & Bryden, 1980).

Bakan's (1969) original study reported that left-movers were more hypnotically susceptible than right-movers and less scientifically oriented in their choice of major field. Since then, lateral eye movement behavior has been related to virtually everything from menstrual cramps and psychosomatic symptoms (R. E. Gur & Gur, 1975) to political leanings (Ashton & Dwyer, 1975). Very few of the personality correlates of lateral eye movement behavior have any obvious connection with hemispheric asymmetry, however, and we must concur with Ehrlichman and Weinberger's (1978) conclusion that, while such correlates may exist, they do little to support the contention that people have a preferred hemisphere.

The evidence that people consistently use one hemisphere rather than another in all situations is very weak, and the position is almost certainly too extreme. The use of lateral eye movements as a technique for assessing a postulated hemisphericity is highly questionable. There seems to be little direct evidence to support the view that left-movers are consistently right-hemispheric and vice versa. Nevertheless, there are enough hints at a relation between cerebral asymmetry and individual differences in eye movement pattern (e.g., Nielsen & Sorensen, 1976; Tucker & Suib, 1978) that further research could be profitable.

Eye Movements and Cerebral Organization

A somewhat different approach to lateral eye movement phenomena has been advanced by Kinsbourne (1972). He observed that people tended to move their eyes to the right when asked a question that involved verbal thought, whereas they moved their eyes to the left when asked questions about spatial relations. Rather than emphasizing the overall consistency of individuals, Kinsbourne proposed that spatial thought activated the right hemisphere and thus led to a lateral eye movement in the opposite direction, to the left. Verbal thought, by this argument, has the opposite effect, activating the left hemisphere and inducing a right-eye movement.

Kinsbourne (1972) presented results to support this theory: Verbal questions elicited more right-eye movements and spatial questions elicited more left-eye movements. Furthermore, the distinction between spatial and verbal questions was considerably blurred in a group of left-handers, in whom hemispheric specialization would be much less consistent. This general finding has frequently been replicated (e.g., R. E. Gur, Gur, & Harris, 1975; Kocel, Galin, Ornstein, & Merrin, 1972), although a number of failures to observe such a question effect have been noted (Ehrlichman, 1977; Hiscock, 1977a). Ehrlichman and Weinberger (1978) have, in fact, concluded that there are as many failures to find differences in eye movement direction between spatial and verbal questions as there are successes.

It is clear, however, that many factors can influence the direction of lateral eye movements. R. E. Gur et al. (1975) have observed that distinctions between spatial and verbal questions are observed when the experimenter is seated behind the subject, but not when the experimenter faces the subject. They suggest that this latter situation is more anxiety producing and that subjects tend to fall back on a habitual bias to the left or right under these conditions. Furthermore, the specific questions are clearly critical to the effect: They must be of sufficient difficulty for the subject not to inhibit all eye movement, and they must be of an appropriate nature to activate left- or right-hemispheric mechanisms. Galin and Ornstein (1974), for example, included arithmetic questions in their verbal set in an initial experiment that failed to find a spatial–verbal distinction, but they subsequently found a question effect with a new set of items excluding arithmetic questions. Kinsbourne (1974a) has discussed some of the factors that may mitigate against observing a question effect. Despite Ehrlichman and Weinberger's (1978) rather pessimistic conclusions, there seems to be at least reasonably strong evidence for a question effect in lateral eye movement research.

One further verification of the link between lateral eye movements and the cognitive activation of the hemispheres would be obtained by showing that directing the gaze to one side facilitated the cognitive skills of the opposite hemisphere. Thus, one should expect to find that looking to the right improved performance on verbal tasks. Research of this sort is just beginning. Y. Gross, Franko, and Lewin (1978) presented subjects with a set of three words in which one word was synonymous with a second but rhymed with the third. Subjects were asked to listen to these words and choose the odd item. When looking to the left (priming the right hemisphere), subjects made significantly more rhyming choices than when looking to the right. In another study, a very weak effect of gaze direction on spatial relations and creativity measures was found for males only (Hines & Martindale, 1974). While neither of these studies represent a very strong test of the hypothesis that induced eye movements will have an effect on lateralized cognitive abilities, they do represent the initial steps in an area that will see much further research in the future.

The investigation of the question effect in lateral eye movement research has turned the main focus of this work away from the notion of a characteristic hemisphericity. Now it seems rather more likely that lateral eye movement techniques will become another way of assessing the differing capacities of the two hemispheres. Ultimately, it may prove to be a better tool for studying individual differences in cerebral organization than for examining which hemisphere is habitually used.

Controlling the Active Hemisphere

The experiments on lateral eye movements (Kinsbourne, 1972) represent but one component of a series of studies conducted by Kinsbourne in the process of developing an attentional model for perceptual laterality effects (Kinsbourne, 1970, 1973, 1974b, 1975a). In effect, Kinsbourne's argument is that verbal thought activates processes in the left hemisphere, and through spread of activation to adjacent cortical tissue, several effects can be observed: The frontal eye fields may be activated, inducing head and eye turning to the right; and other portions of the left hemisphere will be activated, making the left hemisphere more sensitive to incoming stimuli regardless of their nature. Activation of the left hemisphere also leads to a concurrent inhibition of the right. When the left hemisphere is active, there is also a bias to treat incoming information with systems that are appropriate to the left hemisphere, and verbal information will be given priority in processing.

Kinsbourne's views emphasize the interaction between the information presented and the task required. The notions have certain intuitive appeal. For example, if subjects engage in verbal thought during an experiment, the resulting activation of the left hemisphere will serve to reduce the effect observed in any supposedly right-hemispheric task and accentuate the laterality effect in left-hemispheric tasks. Nonverbal laterality effects are far less robust and consistent than verbal ones. The right-ear effect in dichotic listening, for example, is extremely strong, yet virtually every report of a left-sided superiority has its counterexample. By Kinsbourne's arguments, this would come about because subjects find it difficult to avoid verbalization or verbal thought during the experiment.

As one test of his hypothesis, Kinsbourne (1970) presented right-handed subjects with outline squares falling to the left or right of a central fixation point. Half of these squares had a gap in one side. In a control condition, accuracy in detecting the gap was the same in both left and right visual fields, but when subjects had to remember a list of six words during each trial, performance was significantly better in the right visual field. Kinsbourne argued that the verbal load had activated the left hemisphere, resulting in both an attentional bias to the right and a selective priming of information coming to the right visual field.

Two major predictions result from Kinsbourne's model. First, virtually any experimental task can be considered to be self-priming. Because a subject expects to carry out a particular task, he or she will be prepared to do so and will have activated the hemisphere appropriate to the task. By this argument, laterality effects should be much more pronounced when the subject knows what the task is to be. Randomly intermingling verbal and nonverbal tasks on the same experiment should lead to a marked decrease in laterality effects, since the subject would not know what to expect on any one trial. Second, concurrent activity should affect laterality: Verbal activity should increase left-hemisphere performance, whereas spatial thought should improve right-hemisphere performance.

Although Kinsbourne (1973, 1975a) has mustered an impressive array of experiments to support his theory, independent attempts to test the predictions of the model have not always been successful. Although laterality effects are sometime altered by mixed presentation of verbal and nonverbal material (e.g., Hellige, 1978), this is not always the case (Kallman, 1978). Furthermore, both Goodglass and Calderon (1977) and Ley and Bryden (1982) have found it possible to obtain both left- and right-hemispheric effects on the same trial.

Manipulations of concurrent activity have also not met with unequivocal success. Using a signal detection approach, Gardner and Branski (1976) found that neither verbal nor musical activity affected the laterality effect in a gap detection task. Boles (1979) also found no effect of concurrent activity on gap detection, even when he replicated the Kinsbourne procedure as closely as possible. Similarly, Allard and Bryden (1979) found no effects of concurrent activity on dot localization, and Goodglass, Shai, Rosen, and Oscar-Berman (1971) found only very limited support for Kinsbourne's model. Hellige *et al.* (1979) and Hellige and Cox (1976) have found complex effects of verbal memory load on lateralization, but these effects vary with the amount and type of material being held in memory and with the task being performed. Hellige *et al.* (1979) also failed to find any systematic effects of a nonverbal memory load, contrary to what would be expected from Kinsbourne's model.

The investigations of the effects of concurrent activity represent an attempt to activate one hemisphere and see how this activation affects measured laterality. One of the reasons for failure may be that the concurrent task does not have the desired effect. An example may be drawn from the experience of Bryden and colleagues in using a task suggested by Kinsbourne (1973). As a verbal task, subjects were asked to remember sentences of the form "The circle is to the right of the square and below the triangle." In spatial form, subjects were shown a diagram with geometric forms in the arrangement just described and asked to visualize it and hold it in memory for subsequent reproduction. In this experiment, verbally oriented subjects being tested under the spatial condition would simply describe the pattern to themselves verbally and remember that description. In contrast, spatially skilled subjects being tested under the verbal condition would visualize the relations described in the sentence and remember that. In other words, subjects distorted the task to make it spatial or verbal, as they preferred. Hellige *et al.*'s (1979) nonverbal manipulation was to require subjects to remember the location of random dots in 3 × 3, 4 × 4, and 5 × 5 matrices. Perhaps their subjects too found it possible to devise verbal strategies for encoding the dot locations, thus defeating the attempt to activate the right hemisphere.

Our objective in this section, however, is not so much to evaluate Kinsbourne's attentional model as to determine the extent to which individuals can control the hemisphere they are using. The work on concurrent activity indicates that we, as experimenters, have not been profoundly successful in controlling our subjects. Nevertheless, verbal memory loads do have fairly consistent effects on the laterality effects observed both with verbal material and with random shapes (Hellige, 1978; Hellige *et al.*, 1979). These effects do not involve simply the activation of the left hemisphere but also involve capacity effects and interference effects due to task similarity.

A number of studies indicate that laterality effects are determined not only by the material being processed but by the manner in which the material is processed. Thus, for example, Spellacy and Blumstein (1970) showed that dichotically presented vowel sounds showed a right-ear effect when they were included as part of a test involving speech sounds, but a left-ear effect when they were presented in the context of nonverbal sounds. Bryden's emphasis on strategy effects indicates that subjects have considerable personal control over the way in which they choose to process some types of material. This seems particularly evident with supposedly "spatial" tasks, in which subjects often use verbal encoding strategies and thus do not make full use of right-hemispheric mechanisms. Paivio's (1971, 1978) work on dual coding of verbal material would suggest that similar problems might occur with high-imagery verbal material, where it would be possible to use both verbal and visual codes to store the information. In fact, some evidence has been presented for different effects of high- and low-imagery words (Day, 1977; McFarland, McFarland, Bain, & Ashton, 1978), although imagery manipulations have not always been successful (cf. O'Neil, 1971).

These studies indicate that there are optional strategies open to subjects for dealing with at least some types of materials. To the extent that some strategies favor verbal or analytic processes that are dependent on left-hemispheric mechanisms, whereas others are dependent on spatial or holistic processes that are more right-hemispheric, there is subject control over which hemisphere is being most fully utilized.

At the same time, one should recognize that there are not competing left- and right-hemispheric strategies available for dealing with all tasks and all types of material. There seems to be no alternative to left-hemisphere processing for dealing with dichotically presented stop consonant–vowel syllables, for instance. Darwin, Howell, and Brady (1978) have found a right-ear superiority for such material even when the first formant is played to the left ear and the syllable is localized to the left, while the second and third formants, which cue the place of articulation, are played to the right ear. The fact that there are no viable optional strategies available may be one reason that dichotic listening and other verbal procedures provide such robust left-hemispheric effects. Likewise, the fact that optional strategies *are* available may be one reason for the inconsistency and frustration associated with the development of measures of right-hemispheric performance. The choice of tasks for which no optional strategies were available may be one reason why Goodglass and Calderon (1977) were able to obtain simultaneous right-ear superiority for speech and left-ear superiority for musical sequences.

Concurrent activity manipulations, then, may have little effect through selectively priming one hemisphere. Rather, they may serve more to guide the choice of processing strategies under conditions in which there is some choice. Thus, the overall effect of concurrent activity should be complex. If the concurrent activity is similar to the laterality task, one should expect to observe a decrement in performance because of structural interference. As the primary and concurrent tasks become more demanding, capacity interference will also occur. At the same time, concurrent tasks may serve to guide subjects to employ particular processing strategies.

This is not to deny that attentional biases such as those proposed by Kinsbourne (1975a) occur. In many experiments in which attentional bias was measured, Bryden has found evidence that subjects are biased to one side or the other (Bryden, 1963, 1976a; Bryden *et al.*, 1980). These biases, however, are variable and cannot be attributed to a single underlying factor, such as unilateral hemispheric activation. At the same time, the lateral eye movement data do suggest that biases to the right can be expected with verbal activity and to the left with spatial activity (Ehrlichman & Weinberger, 1978; Kinsbourne, 1972). It would seem reasonable to suggest that there are great individual differences in lateral bias. Some people seem highly sensitive to the tasks and exhibit biases characteristic of those tasks, whereas others are relatively insensitive to the task. Whether these differences relate to various hypothesized perceptual–personality dimensions, such as field dependence–independence (Witkin, Dyk, Faterson, Goodenough, & Karp, 1962), or to locus of control (Rotter, 1954) remain topics for further investigation.

The answer to the original question of whether people could control the hemisphere they use, then, is a qualified yes. On the one hand, there seems to be no particularly good reason for believing that the generalized use of one hemisphere provides a useful typology for characterizing individual differences. The description of societies, philosophies, and people as left-hemispheric or right-hemispheric is more metaphorical than scientific. On the other hand, there is clearly some optional control over the strategies that can be used to perform many of the tasks that are used in laterality research. Just what options are exercised and what effect they will have depends on an interaction of the tasks with the subject.

17

Some Final Words

It is clear that the two hemispheres of the human brain have rather different functional properties. Furthermore, some indication of these functional differences can be seen in the intact subject by examining behavioral and physiological indicators. At the same time, research on normal lateralization has proceeded so rapidly and with such enthusiasm that many extravagant claims have been made for the significance of such research. The goal of the preceding chapters has been to provide a more balanced view of research on lateralization.

Perhaps the most important point to emerge from this review is the observation that many factors other than cerebral asymmetry can affect performance on the tasks used to assess lateralization. That is, not only are there true laterality effects, but there are also what have been termed *experimental* or *strategy effects*. For laterality research to make a significant contribution to our understanding of brain function, it is essential that we understand and control these experimental effects.

Isolating Strategy Effects

Basically, one of the big problems comes from assuming that any observed laterality effect arises because of differences in cerebral lateralization. To the extent that experimental or strategy effects influence behavior on the lateralization task, this assumption will be unjustified. What can be done about this problem?

Consider first the case in which the experimental situation leads to some systematic bias in laterality. If, for example, it is easier to identify a word from an initial fragment than from a terminal one, and we display words horizontally to the left or right of fixation, then the words on the right will have an advantage over those on the left that has nothing to do with any postulated left-hemispheric superiority for processing words. If we test a group of subjects, their mean laterality effect, L_o, will be made up of two components, the true hemispheric asymmetry effect, L_t, and the biasing effect of the experimental procedure we have used, L_e. How can we show that there is a true hemispheric effect, L_t, that is not zero?

The best approach would be to obtain a second group of subjects for whom the function in question was known to be lateralized to the opposite hemisphere. In such individuals, the value of L_t would be opposite in sign, and thus the observed laterality effect would be equal to $L_e - L_t$ rather than $L_e + L_t$. Since there is rarely a direct measure of lateralization in the intact brain, this is perhaps a rather idealistic goal to have for research involving normal subjects, although the regional cerebral blood flow techniques hold promise. Failing this, it seems necessary to fall back on handedness. Despite all the problems, we do know that cerebral organization is much less predictable in left-handers than in right-handers. Thus, the mean value of L_t should be different in a left-handed group than in a right-handed group. Providing that we are willing to make the assumption that the experimental effects are the same in left-handers as in right-handers, a comparison of such groups will at least indicate whether or not there is a hemispheric asymmetry effect at all on a given task. While such comparisons have often been made (e.g., Bryden, 1965, 1973; McKeever & VanDeventer, 1977b; Piazza, 1980), the approach is not used as often as it should be.

Two additional comments are in order. The decomposition of L_o into L_e and L_t indicates that evidence for a nonzero value of L_t can be obtained from *any* comparison of two groups in which we can assume that cerebral organization differs but the experimental effects remain constant. However, this argument cannot be used to justify many of the group comparisons that are popular. To return to the example of word recognition, it would be rash to presume that normal readers and dyslexics, to give but one example, read in the same way. In a comparison between such groups, it is at least as likely that it is L_e that differs, and not L_t.

Second, the analysis of Kimura's (1961a) dichotic listening data in Chapter 10 indicated that handedness may have an effect quite distinct from cerebral speech lateralization. If this is true, it weakens the value of the comparison of left- and right-handers and makes it even more important to be able to isolate a subgroup of left-handers who are right-hemispheric for speech (or whose lateralization for visuospatial processing can be defined). It is for this reason that the variable of handwriting posture (Levy & Reid, 1976) was greeted with so much enthusiasm, though subsequent findings have not been so promising (e.g., Moscovitch & Smith, 1979). There are reasons to favor familial handedness as a variable for selecting those left-handers with right-hemispheric speech (cf. Hécaen & Sauguet, 1971; Zurif & Bryden, 1969). This, however, presumes a genetic model of handedness (see Chapter 11), and there are problems with such an assumption. However, the likelihood of a difference between groups in L_e is much less when comparing familial and nonfamilial left-handers than when comparing sinistrals and dextrals. Certainly, we need more studies of laterality effects in left-handers and a more comprehensive study of the genetics of lateralization.

Because L_e cannot be estimated for any single individual by this technique, the strategy of comparing sinistrals and dextrals will only tell us if there is a cerebral asymmetry component to our laterality task, and not whether a particular individual uses the left or right hemisphere for a given function. Even if we can assume no systematic bias in the laterality effect—that is, that the mean of L_e is zero—individual differences in attention and strategy may have their effect. These effects may not influence the overall mean, but they will have an effect on the variance of individual scores. As a result, the observed variance σ_o^2 will be a joint function of the variance of the true laterality measure σ_t^2 and variation due to experimental or strategy effects, σ_e^2.

There seem to be several ways of dealing with this problem. One is to understand the experimental procedure so fully that one can control or eliminate all idiosyncratic variation in strategy. In the dichotic listening task, for example, the evidence indicates that the deployment of attention, the organization of the response sequence, and the length of time items have to be held in memory all affect the accuracy of recall and therefore potentially affect the observed laterality. Bryden *et al.* (1980) tried to control for these effects by using only a single pair of items, instructing subjects to attend specifically to one ear and respond only to a single item. By so doing, they reduced the variance in the right-ear effect and made it more stable. Although the results are promising, the approach does presume that Bryden *et al.* were successful in identifying and controlling all the relevant experimental sources of variation in laterality, and that may be rather unlikely. It remains possible, for example, that subjects find it easier to attend exclusively to one ear than to the other.

An alternative approach is to dissociate different cerebral lateralization effects. If we can design our experiment so that experimental and strategy effects are the same for two different tasks, and if we can show different laterality effects for these tasks, then at least the relative measure of lateralization becomes independent of strategy effects (see Table 17.1). It is because of this relationship that the earlier chapters have emphasized those studies that have attempted to provide a dissociation of left- and right-hemispheric laterality effects.

One should note, however, that the logic of Table 17.1 works only if one can be assured that L_e is the same for both tasks. It is not sufficient, for instance, to demonstrate that a group of individuals shows a left-hemispheric effect on one task at one time and a right-hemispheric effect on a different task at a different time, since the contribution of experimental and strategy effects may be quite different in the two situations. Unfortunately, most of the studies showing a dissociation of laterality effects have been of this type, in which different conditions are presented in distinct blocks. Such experiments leave open the possibility that different strategies are used on the different tasks. The dichotic listening experiments of Goodglass and Calderon (1977) and Ley and Bryden (1982) and the visual physical and name matching experiments (e.g., Cohen, 1973; Geffen et al., 1972) are examples of experiments that have provided a simultaneous dissociation of left- and right-hemispheric effects.

The approaches of dissociating right- and left-hemispheric effects or of completely controlling experimental and strategy effects are also the only procedures that provide sufficient control to yield an adequate assessment of laterality in the individual. Even here, one should expect statistical error of measurement. As a result, studies that attempt to correlate laterality measures with one another, or with personality or other individual difference measures, are almost certainly doomed to failure if they concentrate on right-handed subjects. In a group of right-handers, virtually all subjects will be left-hemispheric for speech. Thus, even if one has controlled experimental effects, much of the variability in laterality scores will be due to error of measurement: The variance in cerebral organization will have been eliminated by the subject selection. To correlate laterality measures with other variables, one should attempt

Table 17.1
Dissociation of True and Experimental Laterality Effects

Verbal task	$LL_o = LL_t + L_e$
Nonverbal task	$LR_o = LR_t + L_e$
	$LL_o - LR_o = LL_t - LR_t$

to maximize variance attributable to differences in cerebral organization. In other words, if we want to relate individual differences in laterality to other variables, we should be studying groups of unselected subjects—or better yet, groups of left-handers, where neurological variance will be large relative to error variance—rather than groups of right-handers.

Relatively few studies meet the criteria advanced in this section. As a result, much of the existing work on lateralization must be viewed as both preliminary and speculative. The time is now ripe for a more systematic attack on the major issues that have been touched on in earlier chapters.

On Complementary Specialization

The idea that behavioral or physiological measures can be more directly linked to cerebral asymmetry by dissociating left- and right-hemispheric effects all but implies acceptance of the concept of complementary specialization. This concept refers to the idea that an individual's two cerebral hemispheres are functionally specialized for distinctively different processes. Certainly, the left hemisphere is specialized for language processes in the majority of individuals, and a left-hemispheric superiority is found for a wide variety of language-related tasks. Likewise, visuospatial and integrative processes seem to depend on the integrity of the right hemisphere. In the general sense that the left hemisphere is usually the language hemisphere and the right the integrative hemisphere, then, there is a complementary specialization.

How well does this concept hold up at the level of the individual? The majority of us are right-handed, and right-handers as a rule are left-hemispheric for speech and right-hemispheric for visuospatial and integrative processes. Therefore, by statistical chance alone, the majority of right-handers exhibit what can be called complementary specialization, with the two hemispheres subserving distinct functions.

What about left-handers? Here, the picture is not so clear. If there really were complementary specialization, those left-handers with right-hemispheric speech would be left-hemispheric for visuospatial processes. There is remarkably little information available on musical abilities or visuospatial abilities in left-handers, but what little there is does not support a notion of complementarity. In Hécaen and Sauguet's (1971) study of unilateral brain damage, for example, visuospatial deficits were no more likely to be associated with left-hemispheric damage in left-handers than in right-handers (see also Hécaen et al., 1981). With more indirect behavioral measures on normal subjects, both McGlone and Davidson (1973) and Bryden (1979b) found a high incidence of both verbal and nonverbal effects being lateralized to the same side. Furthermore, bilateral speech representation is a phenomenon often associated with left-handedness (Rasmussen & Milner, 1977; Satz, 1980). In fact, then, there is virtually no evidence for anything other than statistical complementarity (see also Chapter 14). The observation in an individual that one hemisphere is specialized for a particular function implies nothing about the functions of the other hemisphere in that individual.

This does not invalidate the dissociation technique. On a purely statistical basis, the vast majority of people, especially the right-handers, are left-hemispheric for analytic and linguistic functions and right-hemispheric for integrative and spatial functions. Furthermore, those individuals who do not have complementary specialization will produce small values of (LL − LR). They would be individuals who exhibit a true hemisphericity, in that one hemisphere is superior for both analytic and integrative functions. Such individuals certainly warrant investigation. One might find, for example, that there was a relation between complementary specialization and general verbal and/or spatial abilities.

If, in fact, there is only statistical complementarity, then the distribution of hemispheric specialization shown in Table 14.3 will hold. Among right-handed men, about 71% would be expected to show normal complementarity, about 1% reversed complementarity, and the remaining 28% would show a lack of complementarity because both spatial and verbal functions would be primarily dependent on processes in the same hemisphere. If a dissociation procedure was successful in cancelling the contribution of experimental effects, as suggested by Table 17.1, the resulting distribution of $(LL_t - LR_t)$ would be expected to look something like that shown in Figure 17.1. This curve was drawn on the assumption that there would be some residual error of measurement and indicates how difficult it would be to separate those individuals with complementary specialization (lying between 0 and +2), and those without complementarity (lying between −1 and +1). Of course, if error of measurement is reduced further, the separation of groups would become clearer, as in Figure 17.2. Even in the weaker case of Figure 17.1, the dissociation procedure would provide enough of a separation of complementary and noncomplementary categories to permit some hope of finding correlations with other variables.

The fact that hemispheric complementarity is quite probably statistical rather than causal suggests that it would be wise to add a third condition, one giving a baseline of no laterality effect, to dissociation studies. While it is often difficult to decide what an appropriate "no laterality" control would be, simple detection tasks might be a good choice (Bryden, 1976a; Moscovitch, 1979).

The argument that complementarity is only a statistical fact raises questions about the general integrity of hemispheric processes. Both music and visuospatial processes have been described as dependent on right-hemispheric function: Is there any reason to believe that both processes involve the same hemisphere in all individuals? Unfortunately, there are very few data on this point, since laterality researchers rarely

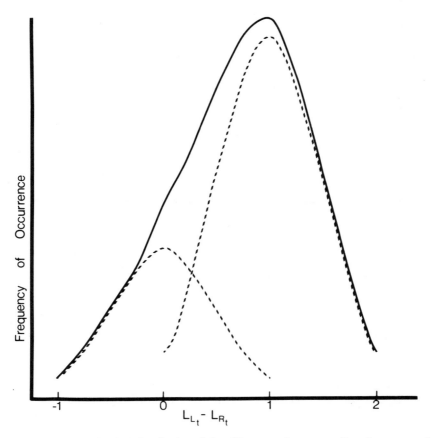

Figure 17.1. Hypothetical distribution of the differences between a "true" measure of verbal laterality (L_{L_T}) and a "true" measure of nonverbal laterality (L_{R_T}), and assuming a moderately large residual error of measurement. The smaller distribution on the left represents those with noncomplementary specialization; the larger one on the right, those with complementary specialization. Note how difficult it would be to classify those individuals with scores around zero.

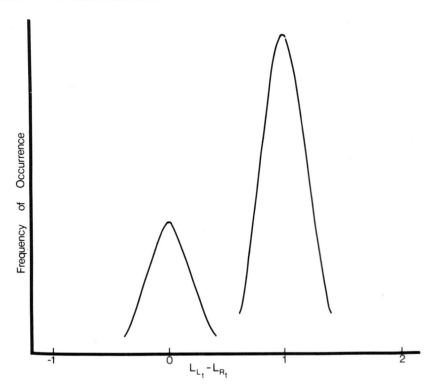

Figure 17.2. Hypothetical distribution of the differences between a "true" measure of verbal laterality and a "true" measure of nonverbal laterality, as in Figure 17.1, but with a small error of measurement. The smaller distribution represents those with non-complementary specialization; the larger, those with complementary specialization.

administer multiple tasks to the same subjects and those concerned with brain damage do not often report conditional probabilities. However, there is no reason to believe that the various functions of the right (or left) hemisphere could not be statistically dissociable. Ojemann and Mateer (1979), for instance, have noted that different portions of the left hemisphere are involved in phonetic and semantic processes (see Figure 17.3). It is conceivable that one could find some individuals with pho-netic processes lateralized to one hemisphere and semantic ones later-alized to the opposite hemisphere. Likewise, Zurif and Bryden (1969) found no correlation between dichotic and tachistoscopic verbal later-ality effects, suggesting the possibility that different aspects of these two tasks were separately lateralized. Again, this is a problem worthy of further research.

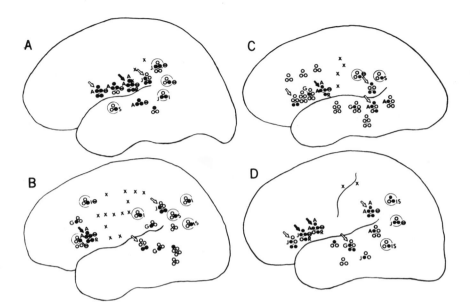

Figure 17.3. Sites where stimulation alters language functions in dominant hemispheres of four patients. Naming, reading, and short-term memory measured at each
site identified by a triangle of circles: naming performance, top; reading, lower left;
short-term memory, lower right. Filled circles indicate statistically significant ($p < .05$)
errors in that function during stimulation. Sites with two additional circles below a line
also had tests of phoneme identification (left) and orofacial movements (right). The
letter beside the filled circle identifies the type of error. Naming errors: *A*, arrests of
speech; no letter, inability to name but demonstrated ability to speak (anomia). Reading
errors: *A*, arrests, failure to read, or production of only a few words of the sentence; *J*,
jargon, reading fluent, but with frequent errors in individual words, including nouns; *G*,
grammatical errors, production of incorrect or deletion of syntactic elements. These
last two types of reading errors were not seen on control trials. Short-term verbal
memory errors: *I*, *S*, errors following stimulation during input or storage; θ, errors at the
time of retrieval. Orofacial movement errors: *R*, errors in repetition of the same movement; no letter, errors only on sequencing different movements. Phoneme identification
errors were not further classified. Arrows and large circles are sites included in the
major subdivisions of the language cortex. Filled arrow, final motor pathway for speech.
Open arrow, sequential motor–phoneme identification (SM–PI) system. Large circle,
memory system. X, sites of evoked motor or sensory responses identifying rolandic
cortex. (A) Male, verbal intelligence quotient (VIQ) = 98, stimulation at 5 mA between
peaks of biphasic pulses. (B) Female, VIQ = 90, 7 mA. (C) Female, VIQ = 98, 3 mA. (D)
Male, VIQ = 93, 8 mA. [From Ojemann, G. A., & Mateer, C. Human language cortex;
Localization of memory, syntax, and sequential motor-phoneme systems. *Science*,
1979, *205*, 1401–1403. Copyright (1979) by the American Association for the Advancement of Science.]

The Hemispheric Dichotomy

As indicated in Chapter 6, many different descriptions of the differing functions of the two hemispheres have been offered. The left hemisphere is often described as verbal, analytic, or concerned with fine spatial and temporal detail. The right hemisphere is considered to be involved in those things the left hemisphere is not: It is integrative, spatial, or concerned with gestalts. The difficulty with such descriptions is that they are often taken as theories of brain function, when they are in fact only convenient mnemonics. What are we to decide, for example, if we find evidence for left-hemispheric involvement in mental rotation (Ornstein et al., 1980)? Mental rotation tests are among the best predictors of spatial ability (McGee, 1979). Does the left-hemispheric alpha activation found by Ornstein et al. mean that these tests have suddenly become verbal or analytic, that they are less spatial than we thought, or that the dichotomy is not as clear-cut as we might have believed? Without some independent definition of what we mean by analytic, or spatial, or verbal, the argument becomes tautological.

This is not to say that the dichotomous descriptions of hemispheric function have no place. Certainly they help us keep in mind just what kind of laterality effects to expect. However, one must remember that the common dichotomies are aids to memory, rather than theories of hemispheric function.

There are numerous examples in which a simple verbal–nonverbal distinction fails. For example, Bryden and Allard (1976) found strong left-visual-field effects for single letters in uncommon typefaces. Likewise, many "nonverbal" tasks, such as those involving attention to serial order, show left-hemispheric superiority (Carmon & Nachshon, 1973; Halperin et al., 1973).

Perhaps the broadest mnemonic is the analytic–integrative distinction, although it often becomes difficult to decide a priori whether a task is analytic or integrative. Most of the tasks that have produced right-hemispheric effects can be conceived as broadly integrative: visuospatial tasks, music, environmental sounds, tactual shape recognition, emotion, face recognition, and the like. Likewise, most of the left-hemispheric tasks are broadly analytic. However, it becomes difficult to see just how much integration is involved in determining line orientation, and one must remember that fairly detailed attempts to specify the analytic–integrative dimension have not been wholly successful (e.g., Bradshaw, Gates, & Patterson, 1976).

Semmes (1968) has provided a strong argument in favor of the analytic–integrative dimension. She found, in studies of somatosensory deficit following unilateral head injury, that left-hemispheric damage led to severe deficits on specific tasks on the right hand, whereas right-hemispheric damage led to more general, but less severe, deficits that appeared on both hands. She suggested that cortical representation in the left hemisphere was focal, with specific regions of the cortex subserving relatively specific functions. In contrast, according to Semmes, representation in the right hemisphere was much more diffuse, with the regions subserving several functions overlapping in space (see Figure 17.4). Semmes points out that such a pattern of representation would lead the right hemisphere to be particularly efficient at integrating information across space, time, and sensory modality, and it is just such processes for which we have seen a right-hemispheric superiority. On the other hand, the more specific or focal representation of the left hemisphere would encourage attention to fine detail and good resolution of both temporal and spatial features—processes that can be loosely described as analytic.

If, however, the arguments advanced in the preceding section about complementary specialization being only a statistical phenomenon are valid, then the search for a unifying description of hemispheric asymme-

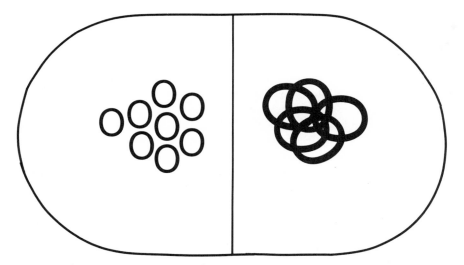

Figure 17.4. A schematic representation of Semmes's (1968) model. Functions in the left hemisphere are focally represented (small cirlces). A small lesion will destroy one function while leaving others intact. Functions in the right hemisphere are more diffusely localized (large circles). A small lesion will not destroy any single function, but will impair several different ones.

try may be a futile one. It may well be that different functions are localized to different hemispheres almost at random, with merely a bias toward localizing verbal functions in the left hemisphere and integrative functions in the right. Perhaps, for instance, chance variations in the cellular density in specific regions determine whether or not a particular function will be localized to one hemisphere or the other. Witelson's (1980) review of neuroanatomical asymmetries suggests that left–right differences exist at a variety of loci. Variation in asymmetry at different loci within the same individual would permit a decoupling of the many and diverse laterality effects that exist in the normal population. Thus, we may require not one theory of laterality, but many.

Two further comments are necessary. The laterality effects discussed in this book are perceptual and cognitive, rather than sensory. There is little evidence for lateral asymmetry in the early stages of sensory processing (Moscovitch, 1979). Furthermore, there must be some diffuse effects whereby a priming task can selectively activate a portion of one hemisphere and lead to an alteration of laterality effects (e.g., Ley, 1980b). However, models of this priming process (e.g., Kinsbourne & Hicks, 1978) have not proven to yield consistent predictions (cf. Cohen, 1979).

Where Are We Now?

The preceding chapters have provided a detailed review of many of the phenomena of lateral specialization in the normal brain. There are many other topics that have been touched on only briefly for reasons of space (e.g., bilingualism: Albert & Obler, 1978). In general, the book has been critical of the methods and approaches that have been used in the area and suggests that many of the effects that have been ascribed to lateral specialization are the by-products of the experimental procedures. At the same time, there is a core of information upon which to build. If nothing else, perhaps this review will serve to point future researchers in the direction of a broad and integrative theory of hemispheric specialization.

Despite the critical views presented here, many of the behavioral and physiological measures are, in fact, related to cerebral lateralization. The first problem for future researchers is to eliminate as much of the irrelevant variability due to experimental procedures as possible. Given some good techniques for assessing lateralization, the next step is to tackle the question of individual differences in cerebral lateralization. If it can be shown that such differences are related to performance on various cognitive tasks, then we have a potential tool for understanding at least some aspects of individual differences. In addition, such findings would make studies of abnormal lateralization in such groups as dyslexics, the deaf, schizophrenics, and second-language learners far more meaningful.

References

Abigail, E. R., & Johnson, E. G. Ear and hand dominance and their relationship with reading retardation. *Perceptual and Motor Skills*, 1976, 43, 1031–1036.

Albe-Fessard, D. Organization of somatic central projections. In W. D. Neff (Ed.), *Contributions to sensory physiology*. New York: Academic Press, 1967.

Albert, M. L., & Obler, L. K. *The bilingual brain*. New York: Academic Press, 1978.

Alema, G., Rosadini, A., & Rossi, G. F. Psychic reactions associated with intracarotid amytal injection and relation to brain damage. *Exerpta Medica*, 1961, 37, 154–155.

Alford, L. B. Localization of consciousness and emotion. *American Journal of Psychiatry*, 1933, 89, 789–799.

Allard, F., & Scott, B. L. Burst cues, transition cues, and hemispheric specialization with real speech sounds. *Quarterly Journal of Experimental Psychology*, 1975, 27, 487–497.

Allard, F., & Scott, B. L. Burst cues, transition cues, and hemispheric specialization with real speed sounds. *Quarterly Journal of Experimental Psychology*, 1975, 27, 487–497.

Andersen, P., & Andersson, S. A. *Physiological basis of the alpha rhythm*. New York: Appleton, 1968.

Anderson, A. L. The effect of laterality localization of focal brain lesions on the Wechsler-Bellevue subtests. *Journal of Clinical Psychology*, 1951, 7, 149–153.

Annett, M. The binomial distribution of right, mixed, and left handedness. *Quarterly Journal of Experimental Psychology*, 1967, 19, 327–333.

Annett, M. A classification of hand preference by association analysis. *British Journal of Psychology*, 1970, 61, 303–321. (a)

Annett, M. The growth of manual preference and speed. *British Journal of Psychology*, 1970, 61, 545–558. (b)

Annett, M. The distribution of manual asymmetry. *British Journal of Psychology*, 1972, 63, 343–358.

Annett, M. Handedness in families. *Annals of Human Genetics*, 1973, 37, 93–105.

Annett, M. Handedness in the children of two left-handed parents. *British Journal of Psychology*, 1974, 65, 129–131.

Annett, M. Hand preference and the laterality of cerebral speech. *Cortex*, 1975, 11, 305–328.

Annett, M. A coordination of hand preference and skill replicated. *British Journal of Psychology*, 1976, 67, 587–592.

Annett, M. *A single gene explanation of right and left handedness and brainedness.* Coventry, England: Lanchester Polytechnic, 1978.

Ashton, V. L., & Dwyer, J. H. The left: Lateral eye movements and ideology. *Perceptual and Motor Skills,* 1975, *41,* 248–250.

Attneave, F. Physical determinants of the judged complexity of shapes. *Journal of Experimental Psychology,* 1957, *53,* 221–227.

Axelrod, S., Noonan, M., & Atanacio, B. On the laterality of psychogenic somatic symptoms. *Journal of Nervous and Mental Disease,* 1980, *168,* 517–525.

Bakan, P. Hypnotizability, laterality of eye movement and functional brain asymmetry. *Perceptual and Motor Skills,* 1969, *28,* 927–932.

Bakan, P. Birth order and handedness. *Nature,* 1971, *229,* 195.

Bakan, P. Left-handedness and alcoholism. *Perceptual and Motor Skills,* 1973, *36,* 514.

Bakan, P., Dibb, G., & Reid, P. Handedness and birth stress. *Neuropsychologia,* 1973, *11,* 363–366.

Bakan, P., & Strayer, F. F. On reliability of conjugate lateral eye movements. *Perceptual and Motor Skills,* 1973, *36,* 429–430.

Bakker, D. J. Left–right differences in auditory perception of verbal and nonverbal material by children. *Quarterly Journal of Experimental Psychology,* 1967, *19,* 334–336.

Bakker, D. J., Teunissen, J., & Bosch, J. Development of laterality–reading patterns. In R. M. Knights & D. J. Bakker (Eds.), *The neuropsychology of learning disorders: Theoretical approaches.* Baltimore: University Park Press, 1976.

Barnet, A. B., Vicentini, M., & Campos, M. EEG sensory evoked responses (E.Rs) in early infancy malnutrition. *Neuroscience Abstracts* (No. 43). Fourth Annual Meeting of the Society for Neuroscience, St. Louis, Mississippi, 1974.

Barnsley, R. H., & Rabinovitch, M. S. Handedness: Proficiency versus stated preference. *Perceptual and Motor Skills,* 1970, *30,* 343–362.

Bartholomeus, B. Effects of task requirements on ear superiority for sung speech. *Cortex,* 1974, *10,* 215–223.

Barton, M. I., Goodglass, H., & Shai, A. The differential recognition of tachistoscopically presented English and Hebrew words in the right and left visual fields. *Perceptual and Motor Skills,* 1965, *21,* 431–437.

Bashore, T. R. Vocal and manual reaction time estimates of interhemispheric transmission time. *Psychological Bulletin,* 1981, *89,* 352–368.

Basser, L. S. Hemiplegia of early onset and the faculty of speech with special reference to the effects of hemispherectomy. *Brain,* 1962, *85,* 427–460.

Beaton, A. A. Hemispheric emotional asymmetry in a dichotic listening task. *Acta Psychologica,* 1979, *43,* 103–109.

Beaumont, G., & Mayes, A. Do task and sex differences influence the visual evoked potential? *Psychophysiology,* 1977, *14,* 545–550.

Bender, L. Problems in conceptualization and communication in children with developmental alexia. In P. H. Hock & J. Zubin (Eds.), *Psychopathology of communication.* New York: Grune & Stratton, 1958.

Benton, A. L. Disorders of spatial orientation. In P. Vinken & G. Bruyn (Eds.), *Handbook of clinical neurology* (Vol. 3): *Disorders of higher nervous activity.* Amsterdam: North-Holland, 1969.

Benton, A. L. The amusias. In M. Critchley & R. A. Henson (Eds.), *Music and the brain: Studies in the neurology of music.* Springfield, Ill.: Thomas, 1977.

Benton, A. L. Body schema disturbances: Finger agnosia and right–left disorientation. In K. M. Heilman & E. Valenstein (Eds.), *Clinical neuropsychology.* New York: Oxford Univ. Press, 1979.

Benton, A. L., Hannay, H. J., & Varney, N. R. Visual perception of line direction in patients with unilateral brain disease. *Neurology,* 1975, *25,* 907–910.

Benton, A. L., & Hécaen, H. Stereoscopic vision in patients with unilateral cerebral disease. *Neurology,* 1970, *20,* 1084–1088.

Benton, A. L., Levin, H. S., & Varney, N. R. Tactile perception of direction in normal subjects. *Neurology,* 1973, *23,* 1248–1250.

Benton, A. L., & Pearl, D. (Eds.). *Dyslexia: An appraisal of current knowledge.* New York: Oxford Univ. Press, 1978.

Benton, A. L., & VanAllen, M. W. Impairment in facial recognition in patients with cerebral disease. *Cortex,* 1968, *4,* 344–358.

Benton, A. L., Varney, N. R., & Hamsher, K. de S. Lateral differences in tactile directional perception. *Neuropsychologia,* 1978, *16,* 109–114.

Berent, S. Functional asymmetry of the human brain in the recognition of faces. *Neuropsychologia,* 1977, *15,* 829–831.

Berlin, C. I., Hughes, L. F., Lowe-Bell, S. S., & Berlin, H. L. Dichotic right ear advantage in children 5 to 13. *Cortex,* 1973, *9,* 393–401.

Berlin, C. I., & McNeal, M. R. Dichotic listening. In N. J. Lass (Ed.), *Contemporary issues in experimental phonetics.* New York: Academic Press, 1976.

Berlucchi, G., Brizzolara, D., Marzi, C. A., Rizzolatti, G., & Umilta, C. The role of stimulus discriminability and verbal codability in hemispheric specialization for visuospatial tasks. *Neuropsychologia,* 1979, *17,* 195–202.

Berlucchi, G., Crea, F., DiStefano, M., & Tassinari, G. Influence of spatial stimulus–response compatibility on reaction time of ipsilateral and contralateral hand to lateralized light stimuli. *Journal of Experimental Psychology: Human Perception and Performance,* 1977, *3,* 505–517.

Bever, T. G. The nature of cerebral dominance in speech behaviour of the child and adult. In R. Huxley & E. Ingram (Eds.), *Language acquisition: Models and methods.* New York: Academic Press, 1971.

Bever, T. G., & Chiarello, R. J. Cerebral dominance in musicians and nonmusicians. *Science,* 1974, *185,* 537–539.

Beveridge, R., & Hicks, R. A. Lateral eye movement, handedness and sex. *Perceptual and Motor Skills,* 1976, *42,* 466.

Blumstein, S., Goodglass, H., & Tartter, V. The reliability of ear advantage in dichotic listening. *Brain and Language,* 1975, *2,* 226–236.

Boder, E. Developmental dyslexia: A new diagnostic approach based on the identification of three subtypes. *Journal of School Health,* 1970, *40,* 289–290.

Boder, E. Developmental dyslexia: A diagnostic approach based on three atypical reading patterns. *Developmental Medicine and Child Neurology,* 1973, *15,* 663–687.

Bogen, J. E. The other side of the brain I: Dysgraphia and dyscopia following cerebral commissurotomy. *Bulletin of the Los Angeles Neurological Societies,* 1969, *34,* 73–105. (a)

Bogen, J. E. The other side of the brain II: An appositional mind. *Bulletin of the Los Angeles Neurological Societies,* 1969, *34,* 135–162. (b)

Bogen, J. E., & Gazzaniga, M. S. Cerebral commissurotomy in man: Minor hemisphere dominance for certain visuospatial functions. *Journal of Neurosurgery,* 1965, *23,* 394–399.

Boklage, C. E. Embryonic determination of brain programming asymmetry—a caution concerning the use of data on twins in genetic inferences about mental development. *Annals of the New York Academy of Sciences,* 1977, *299,* 306–308.

Boles, D. Laterally biased attention with concurrent verbal load: Multiple failures to replicate. *Neuropsychologia,* 1979, *17,* 353–362.

Borod, J. C., & Caron, H. S. Facedness and emotion related to lateral dominance, sex and expression type. *Neuropsychologia*, 1980, *18*, 237–241.

Borowy, T., & Goebel, R. Cerebral lateralization of speech: The effects of age, sex, race, and socioeconomic class. *Neuropsychologia*, 1976, *14*, 363–370.

Bradshaw, J. L., Bradley, D., & Patterson, K. The perception and identification of mirror-reversed patterns. *Quarterly Journal of Experimental Psychology*, 1976, *28*, 221–246.

Bradshaw, J. L., & Gates, E. A. Visual field differences in verbal tasks: Effects of task familiarity and sex of subject. *Brain and Language*, 1978, *5*, 166–187.

Bradshaw, J. L., Gates, A., & Nettleton, N. C. Bihemispheric involvement in lexical decisions: Handedness and a possible sex difference. *Neuropsychologia*, 1977, *15*, 277–286.

Bradshaw, J. L., Gates, A., & Patterson, K. Hemispheric differences in processing visual patterns. *Quarterly Journal of Experimental Psychology*, 1976, *26*, 667–681.

Bradshaw, J. L., & Nettleton, N. C. The nature of hemispheric specialization in man. *The Behavioral and Brain Sciences*, 1981, *4*, 51–92.

Bradshaw, J. L., & Taylor, M. J. A word-naming deficit in nonfamilial sinistrals? Laterality effects of vocal responses to tachistoscopically presented letter strings. *Neuropsychologia*, 1979, *17*, 21–32.

Brady, J. P., & Berson, J. Stuttering, dichotic listening and cerebral dominance. *Archives of General Psychiatry*, 1975, *32*, 1449–1452.

Breitmeyer, B. G., & Ganz, L. Implications of sustained and transient channels for theories of visual pattern masking, saccadic suppression and information processing. *Psychological Review*, 1976, *83*, 1–36.

Breitmeyer, B. G., Julesz, B., & Kropfl, W. Dynamic random-dot stereograms reveal an up–down anisotropy and left–right isotropy between cortical hemifields. *Science*, 1975, *187*, 269–270.

Briggs, G. G., & Nebes, R. D. The effects of handedness, family history and sex on the performance of a dichotic listening task. *Neuropsychologia*, 1976, *14*, 129–134.

Brinkman, J., & Kuypers, H. G. J. M. Splitbrain monkeys: Cerebral control of ipsilateral and contralateral arm, hand and finger movements. *Science*, 1972, *176*, 536–539.

Broadbent, D. E. The role of auditory localization in attention and memory span. *Journal of Experimental Psychology*, 1954, *47*, 191–196.

Broca, P. Nouvelle observation d'aphemie produite par une lesion de la moite posterieure des deuxieme et troisieme circonvolutions frontales. *Bulletin de la Society Anatomique de Paris*, 1861, *36*, 398–407.

Bryden, M. P. Order of report in dichotic listening. *Canadian Journal of Psychology*, 1962, *16*, 291–299.

Bryden, M. P. Ear preference in auditory perception. *Journal of Experimental Psychology*, 1963, *65*, 103–105.

Bryden, M. P. Tachistoscopic recognition, handedness, and cerebral dominance. *Neuropsychologia*, 1965, *3*, 1–8.

Bryden, M. P. Left–right differences in tachistoscopic recognition: Directional scanning or cerebral dominance? *Perceptual and Motor Skills*, 1966, *23*, 1127–1134.

Bryden, M. P. An evaluation of some models of laterality effects in dichotic listening. *Acta Oto-Laryngologica*, 1967, *63*, 595–604. (a)

Bryden, M. P. A model for the sequential organization of behaviour. *Canadian Journal of Psychology*, 1967, *21*, 36–56. (b)

Bryden, M. P. Binaural competition and division of attention as determinants of the laterality effect in dichotic listening. *Canadian Journal of Psychology*, 1969, *23*, 101–113.

Bryden, M. P. Laterality effects in dichotic listening: Relations with handedness and reading ability in children. *Neuropsychologia*, 1970, *8*, 433–450.

Bryden, M. P. Perceptual asymmetry in vision: Relation to handedness, eyedness, and speech lateralization. *Cortex*, 1973, *9*, 418–435.

Bryden, M. P. Speech lateralization in families: A preliminary study using dichotic listening. *Brain and Language*, 1975, *2*, 201–211.

Bryden, M. P. Response bias and hemispheric differences in dot localization. *Perception and Psychophysics*, 1976, *19*, 23–28. (a)

Bryden, M. P. *Sex differences in cerebral organization*. Paper presented at the Fourth Annual Meeting of the International Neuropsychology Society, Toronto, Canada, February 1976. (b)

Bryden, M. P. Measuring handedness with questionnaires. *Neuropsychologia*, 1977, *15*, 617–624.

Bryden, M. P. Strategy effects in the assessment of hemispheric asymmetry. In G. Underwood (Ed.), *Strategies of information processing*. London: Academic Press, 1978.

Bryden, M. P. Evidence for sex-related differences in cerebral organization. In M. Wittig & A. C. Petersen (Eds.), *Sex-related differences in cognitive functioning: Developmental issues*. New York: Academic Press, 1979. (a)

Bryden, M. P. *Patterns of cerebral asymmetry in sinistrals*. Paper presented at Body for Advancement of Brain, Behaviour and Language Enterprises (BABBLE), Niagara Falls, March 1979. (b)

Bryden, M. P. *Possible genetic mechanisms of handedness and laterality*. Paper presented in a symposium on the Origin and Development of Human Lateralization, at the annual meeting of the Canadian Psychological Association, Quebec City, June 1979. (c)

Bryden, M. P., & Allard, F. Visual hemifield differences depend on typeface. *Brain and Language*, 1976, *3*, 191–200.

Bryden, M. P., & Allard, F. Dichotic listening and the development of linguistic processes. In M. Kinsbourne (Ed.), *Asymmetrical functions of the brain*. Cambridge: Cambridge Univ. Press, 1978.

Bryden, M. P., & Allard, F. Do auditory perceptual asymmetries develop? *Cortex*, 1981, *17*, 313–318.

Bryden, M. P., Ley, R. G., & Sugarman, J. H. A left-ear advantage for identifying the emotional quality of tonal sequences. *Neuropsychologia*, 1982, *20*, 83–87.

Bryden, M. P., Munhall, K., & Allard, F. *Attentional biases and the right-ear effect in dichotic listening*. Paper presented at the annual meeting of the Canadian Psychological Association, Calgary, June 1980.

Bryden, M. P., & Sprott, D. A. Statistical determination of degree of laterality. *Neuropsychologia*, 1981, *19*, 571–581.

Bryden, M. P., & Zurif, E. B. Dichotic listening performance in a case of agenesis of the corpus callosum. *Neuropsychologia*, 1970, *8*, 371–377.

Buchsbaum, M., & Fedio, P. Visual information and evoked responses from the left and right hemispheres. *Electroencephalography and Clinical Neurophysiology*, 1969, *26*, 266–272.

Buchtel, H. A., Campari, F., DeRisio, C., & Rota, R. Hemispheric differences in discriminative reaction time to facial expressions. *Italian Journal of Psychology*, 1978, *5*, 159–169.

Buffery, A. W. H., & Gray, J. A. Sex differences in the development of spatial and linguistic skills. In C. Ounsted & D. C. Taylor (Eds.), *Gender differences: Their ontogeny and significance*. London: Churchill, 1972.

Butler, S. R., & Glass, A. Asymmetries in the electroencephalogram associated with cerebral dominance. *Electroencephalography and Clinical Neurophysiology*, 1974, *36*, 481–491.

Butler, S. R., & Glass, A. EEG correlates of cerebral dominance. In A. H. Riesen & R. F. Thompson (Eds.), *Advances in psychobiology* (Vol. 3). New York: Wiley, 1976.

Campbell, R. Asymmetries in interpreting and expressing a posed facial expression. *Cortex*, 1978, *14*, 327–342.

Caplan, P. J., & Kinsbourne, M. Baby drops the rattle: Asymmetry of duration of grasp by infants. *Child Development*, 1976, *47*, 532–534.

Carmon, A., & Bechtoldt, H. P. Dominance of the right cerebral hemisphere for stereopsis. *Neuropsychologia*, 1969, *7*, 29–39.

Carmon, A., & Benton, A. L. Tactile perception of direction and number in patients with unilateral cerebral disease. *Neurology*, 1969, *19*, 525–532.

Carmon, A., Bilstrom, D. E., & Benton, A. L. Thresholds for pressure and sharpness in the right and left hands. *Cortex*, 1969, *5*, 27–35.

Carmon, A., Lavy, S., Gordon, H., & Portnoy, Z. Hemispheric differences in rCBF during verbal and nonverbal tasks. In *Brain work: Alfred Benzon Symposium VIII.* Munksgaard, 1975.

Carmon, A., & Nachshon, I. Ear asymmetry in perception of emotional non-verbal stimuli. *Acta Psychologica*, 1973, *37*, 351–357.

Carmon, A., Nachshon, I., & Starinsky, R. Developmental aspects of visual hemifield differences in perception of verbal material. *Brain and Language*, 1976, *3*, 463–469.

Carr, B. M. Ear effect variables and order of report in dichotic listening. *Cortex*, 1969, *5*, 63–68.

Carter-Saltzman, L. Patterns of cognitive functioning in relation to handedness and sex related differences. In M. A. Wittig & A. C. Petersen (Eds.), *Sex-related differences in cognitive functioning: Developmental issues.* New York: Academic Press, 1979.

Carter-Saltzman, L., Scarr-Salapatek, S., Barker, W. B., & Katz, S. Left-handedness in twins: Incidence and patterns of performance in an adolescent sample. *Behavior Genetics*, 1976, *6*, 189–203.

Catlin, J., & Neville, H. The laterality effect in reaction time to speech stimuli. *Neuropsychologia*, 1976, *14*, 141–144.

Catlin, J., VanderVeer, N., & Teicher, R. Monaural right-ear advantage in target–identification task. *Brain and Language*, 1976, *4*, 471–481.

Chall, J. *Learning to read: The great debate.* New York: McGraw-Hill, 1967.

Chamberlain, H. D. The inheritance of left-handedness. *Journal of Heredity*, 1928, *19*, 557–559.

Chaney, R. E., & Webster, J. C. Information in certain multidimensional sounds. *Journal of the Acoustical Society of America*, 1966, *40*, 447–455.

Chapman, R. M., McCrary, J. W., Bragdon, H. R., & Chapman, J. A. Latent components of evoked potentials functionally related to information processing. In J. E. Desmedt (Ed.), *Progress in clinical neurophysiology* (Vol. 6): *Cognitive components in cerebral event-related potentials and selective attention.* Basel, Switzerland: Karger, 1979.

Charness, N., & Shea, J. *Enumeration and the hemispheres: Is counting right?* Paper presented at the annual meeting of the Canadian Psychological Association, Toronto, June 1981.

Cohen, G. Hemispheric differences in a letter classification task. *Perception and Psychophysics*, 1972, *11*, 139–142.

Cohen, G. Hemispheric differences in serial vs. parallel processing. *Journal of Experimental Psychology*, 1973, *97*, 349–356.

Cohen, G. Components of the laterality effect in letter recognition: Asymmetries in iconic storage. *Quarterly Journal of Experimental Psychology*, 1976, *28*, 105–114.

Cohen, G. Comment on "Information processing in the cerebral hemispheres: Selective activation and capacity limitations" by Hellige, Cox, and Litvac. *Journal of Experimental Psychology: General*, 1979, *108*, 309–315.

Collins, R. L. The sound of one paw clapping: An inquiry into the origin of left-handedness. In G. Lindzey & D. D. Thiessen (Eds.), *Contributions to behaviour–genetic analysis: The mouse as prototype*. New York: Appleton, 1970.

Collins, R. L. Toward an admissible genetic model for the inheritance of the degree and direction of asymmetry. In S. Harnad, R. W. Doty, L. Goldstein, J. Jaynes, & G. Krauthamer (Eds.), *Lateralization in the nervous system*. New York: Academic Press, 1977.

Corballis, M. C. The left–right problem in psychology. *Canadian Psychologist*, 1974, *15*, 16–33.

Corballis, M. C., & Beale, I. L. *The psychology of left and right*. Hillsdale, N.J.: Erlbaum, 1976.

Corballis, M. C., & Morgan, M. J. On the biological basis of human laterality: I. Evidence for a maturational left–right gradient. *The Behavioral and Brain Sciences*, 1978, *1*, 261–269.

Coren, S., & Kaplan, C. P. Patterns of ocular dominance. *American Journal of Optometry and Archives of American Academy of Optometry*, 1973, *50*, 283–292.

Coren, S., & Porac, C. Fifty centuries of right-handedness: The historical record. *Science*, 1977, *198*, 631–632.

Coren, S., & Porac, C. Birth factors and laterality: Effects of birth order, parental age, and birth stress on four indices of lateral preference. *Behavior Genetics*, 1980, *10*, 123–138. (a)

Coren, S., & Porac, C. Family patterns in four dimensions of lateral preference. *Behavior Genetics*, 1980, *10*, 333–348. (b)

Corkin, S. The role of different cerebral structures in somesthetic perception. In E. C. Carterette & M. P. Friedman (Eds.), *Handbook of perception* (Vol. 6). New York: Academic Press, 1978.

Cornil, L., & Gestaut, H. Etude électroencéphalographique de la dominance sensorielle d'un hémisphere cérébral. *Presse Medicale*, 1947, *37*, 421–422.

Corsi, P. M. *Human memory and the medial temporal region of the brain*. Unpublished doctoral dissertation, McGill University, 1972.

Cranney, J., & Ashton, R. Witelson's dichhaptic task as a measure of hemispheric asymmetry in deaf and hearing populations. *Neuropsychologia*, 1980, *18*, 95–98.

Crider, B. A battery of tests for the dominant eye. *Journal of General Psychology*, 1944, *31*, 179–190.

Critchley, M. *The parietal lobes*. London: Arnold, 1953.

Crovitz, H. F. Differential acuity of the two eyes and the problem of ocular dominance. *Science*, 1961, *134*, 614.

Crovitz, H. F., & Zener, K. A group-test for assessing hand and eye dominance. *American Journal of Psychology*, 1962, *75*, 271–276.

Cullen, J. K., Jr., Thompson, C. L., Hughes, L. F., Berlin, C. I., & Samson, D. S. The effects of varied acoustic parameters on performance in dichotic speech perception tasks. *Brain and Language*, 1974, *1*, 307–322.

Curry, F. K. W. A comparison of left-handed and right-handed subjects on verbal and non-verbal dichotic listening tasks. *Cortex*, 1967, *3*, 343–352.

Curry, F. K. W., & Rutherford, D. R. Recognition and recall of dichotically presented verbal stimuli by right- and left-handed persons. *Neuropsychologia*, 1967, *5*, 119–126.

Curtiss, S. *Genie: A psycholinguistic study of a modern-day "wild child."* New York: Academic Press, 1977.

Cutting, J. E. Two left-hemisphere mechanisms in speech perception. *Perception and Psychophysics*, 1974, *16*, 601–612.

Damasio, A. R., & Damasio, H. Musical faculty and cerebral dominance. In M. Critchley & R. A. Henson (Eds.), *Music and the brain: Studies in the neurology of music.* Springfield, Ill.: Thomas, 1977.

Darwin, C. J. Ear differences in the recall of fricatives and vowels. *Quarterly Journal of Experimental Psychology,* 1971, 23, 46–62.

Darwin, C. J., & Baddeley, A. D. Acoustic memory and the perception of speech. *Cognitive Psychology,* 1974, 6, 41–60.

Darwin, C. J., Howell, P., & Brady, S. A. Laterality and localization a "right ear advantage" for speech heard on the left. In J. Requin (Ed.), *Attention and performance VII.* Hillsdale, N.J.: Erlbaum, 1978.

Davidoff, J. Hemispheric sensitivity differences in the perception of colour. *Quarterly Journal of Experimental Psychology,* 1976, 28, 387–394.

Davidoff, J. B. Hemispheric differences in dot detection. *Cortex,* 1977, 13, 434–444.

Davies, S., & Bryden, M. P. *The relationship of lateral eye movement patterns to dichotic laterality effects and cognitive style.* Paper presented at the annual meeting of the Canadian Psychological Association, Calgary, June 1980.

Davis, A. E., & Wada, J. A. Hemispheric asymmetry: Frequency analysis of visual and auditory evoked responses to non-verbal stimuli. *Electroencephalography and Clinical Neurophysiology,* 1974, 37, 1–9.

Davis, A. E., & Wada, J. A. Hemispheric asymmetries of visual and auditory information processing. *Neuropsychologia,* 1977, 15, 799–806. (a)

Davis, A. E., & Wada, J. A. Spectral analysis of evoked potential asymmetries related to speech dominance. In J. E. Desmedt (Ed.), *Language and hemispheric specialization in man: Cerebral event-related potentials.* Basel: Karger, 1977. (b)

Davis, A. E., & Wada, J. A. Speech dominance and handedness in the normal human. *Brain and Language,* 1978, 5, 42–55.

Davis, R., & Schmit, V. Visual and verbal coding in the inter-hemispheric transfer of information. *Acta Psychologica,* 1973, 37, 229–240.

Dawson, J. L. M. B. Alaskan Eskimo hand, eye, auditory dominance and cognitive style. *Psychologia,* 1977, 20, 121–135.

Day, J. Right-hemisphere language processing in normal right-handers. *Journal of Experimental Psychology: Human Perception and Performance,* 1977, 3, 518–528.

Day, J. Visual half-field word recognition as a function of syntactic class and imageability. *Neuropsychologia,* 1979, 17, 515–520.

Day, M. E. An eye movement phenomenon relating to attention, thought and anxiety. *Perceptual and Motor Skills,* 1964, 19, 443–446.

Dax, M. Lésions de la moitié gauche de l'encéphale coincident avec l'oubli des signes de la pensée. *Gazette Bebdom,* 1865, 11, 259–260.

Dee, H. L. Auditory asymmetry and strength of manual preference. *Cortex,* 1971, 7, 236–245.

Dee, H. L., & Fontenot, D. J. Cerebral dominance and lateral differences in perception and memory. *Neuropsycholgia,* 1973, 11, 167–173.

Deglin, V. L. Clinical–experimental studies of unilateral electroconvulsive shock. *Journal of Neuropathology and Psychiatry,* 1973, 11, 1609–1621.

DeKosky, S. T., Heilman, K. M., Bowers, D., & Valenstein, E. Recognition and discrimination of emotional faces and pictures. *Brain and Language,* 1980, 9, 206–214.

Delacato, C. H. (Ed.). *Neurological organization and reading.* Springfield, Ill.: Thomas, 1966.

Demarest, L., & Demarest, J. *The interaction of handedness, familial sinistrality, and sex in determining cerebral dominance for verbal material.* Paper presented at the annual meeting of the Eastern Psychological Association, Philadelphia, April 1979.

Dennis, M., & Kohn, B. Comprehension of syntax in infantile hemiplegics after cerebral hemidecortication: Left-hemisphere superiority. *Brain and Language*, 1975, *2*, 472–482.

Dennis, M., & Whitaker, H. A. Hemispheric equipotentiality and language acquisition. In S. J. Segalowitz & F. A. Gruber (Eds.), *Language development and neurological theory*. New York: Academic Press, 1977.

DeRenzi, E., & Spinnler, H. Impaired performance on color tasks in patients with hemispheric damage. *Cortex*, 1967, *3*, 194–217.

Desmedt, J. E. (Ed.). *Language and hemispheric specialization in man: Cerebral event-related potentials*. Basel: Karger, 1977.

Diamond, R., & Carey, S. Developmental changes in the representation of faces. *Journal of Experimental Child Psychology*, 1977, *23*, 1–22.

Dimond, S. J., & Beaumont, J. G. Hemisphere function and color naming. *Journal of Experimental Psychology*, 1972, *96*, 87–91.

Dimond, S. J., & Blizard, D. A. (Eds.). Evolution and lateralization of the brain. *Annals of the New York Academy of Sciences*, 1977, *299*.

Divenyi, P. L., & Efron, R. Spectral versus temporal features in dichotic listening. *Brain and Language*, 1979, *7*, 375–386.

Dodds, A. G. Hemispheric differences in tactuo-spatial processing. *Neuropsychologia*, 1978, *16*, 247–254.

Donchin, E., Kutas, M., & McCarthy, G. Electrocortical indices of hemispheric utilization. In S. R. Harnad, R. W. Doty, L. Goldstein, J. Jaynes, & G. Krauthamer (Eds.), *Lateralization in the nervous system*. New York: Academic Press, 1977.

Donchin, E., McCarthy, G., & Kutas, M. Electroencephalographic investigations of hemispheric specialization. In J. E. Desmedt (Ed.), *Language and hemispheric specialization in man: Cerebral event-related potentials*. Basel: Karger, 1977.

Dorman, M. F., & Geffner, D. S. Hemispheric specialization for speech perception in six-year-old black and white children from low and middle socioeconomic classes. *Cortex*, 1974, *10*, 171–176.

Doyle, J. C., Ornstein, R., & Galin, D. Lateral specialization of cognitive mode: II. EEG frequency analysis. *Psychophysiology*, 1974, *11*, 567–578.

Drake, R. M. *Drake Musical Aptitude Test*. Chicago: Science Research Associates, 1954.

Durnford, M., & Kimura, D. Right hemisphere specialization for depth perception reflected in visual field differences. *Nature*, 1971, *231*, 394–395.

Ehrlichman, H. Field-dependence–independence and lateral eye movements following verbal and spatial questions. *Perceptual and Motor Skills*, 1977, *44*, 1229–1230.

Ehrlichman, H., & Weinberger, A. Lateral eye movements and hemispheric asymmetry: A critical review. *Psychological Bulletin*, 1978, *85*, 1080–1101.

Ehrlichman, H., Weiner, S. L., & Baker, A. H. Effects of verbal and spatial questions on initial gaze shifts. *Neuropsychologia*, 1974, *12*, 265–277.

Ellis, H. D., & Shepherd, J. W. Recognition of abstract and concrete words presented in left and right visual fields. *Journal of Experimental Psychology*, 1974, *103*, 1035–1036.

Entus, A. K. Hemispheric asymmetry in processing of dichotically presented speech and nonspeech stimuli by infants. In S. J. Segalowitz & F. A. Gruber (Eds.), *Language development and neurological theory*. New York: Academic Press, 1977.

Fairweather, H. Sex differences in cognition. *Cognition*, 1976, *4*, 231–280.

Fennell, E., Satz, P., VanDenAbell, T., Bowers, D., & Thomas, R. Visuospatial competency, handedness, and cerebral dominance. *Brain and Language*, 1978, *5*, 206–214.

Fennell, E., Satz, P., & Wise, R. Laterality differences in the perception of pressure. *The Journal of Neurology, Neurosurgery and Psychiatry*, 1967, *30*, 337–340.

Ferraro, J. A., & Minckler, J. The human lateral lemniscus and its nuclei. The human auditory pathways: A quantitative study. *Brain and Language*, 1977, *4*, 277–294.

Flor-Henry, P. Lateralized temporal-limbic dysfunction and psychopathology. *Annals of the New York Academy of Sciences*, 1976, *280*, 777–795.

Fontenot, D. J. Visual field differences in the recognition of verbal and nonverbal stimuli in man. *Journal of Comparative and Physiological Psychology*, 1973, *85*, 564–569.

Fontenot, D. J., & Benton, A. L. Tactile perception of direction in relation to hemispheric locus of lesion. *Neuropsychologia*, 1971, *9*, 83–88.

Forgays, D. G. The development of differential word recognition. *Journal of Experimental Psychology*, 1953, *45*, 165–168.

Frankfurter, A., & Honeck, R. Ear differences in the recall of monaurally presented sentences. *Quarterly Journal of Experimental Psychology*, 1973, *25*, 138–146.

Friedman, D., Simson, R., Ritter, W., & Rapin, I. Cortical evoked potentials elicited by real speech words and human sounds. *Electroencephalography and Clinical Neurophysiology*, 1975, *38*, 13–19.

Fromkin, V., Krashen, S., Curtiss, S., Rigler, D., & Rigler, M. The development of language in Genie: A case of language acquisition beyond the critical period. *Brain and Language*, 1974, *1*, 81–107.

Gaede, S. E., Parsons, O. A., & Bertera, J. H. Hemispheric differences in music perception: Aptitude vs. experience. *Neuropsychologia*, 1978, *16*, 369–374.

Gainotti, G. Reactions "catastrophiques" et manifestations d'indifference au cours des atteintes cérébrales. *Neuropsychologia*, 1969, *7*, 195–204.

Gainotti, G. Emotional behavior and hemispheric side of the lesion. *Cortex*, 1972, *8*, 41–55.

Galin, D. Implications for psychiatry of left and right cerebral specialization. *Archives of General Psychiatry*, 1974, *31*, 572–583.

Galin, D., Diamond, R., & Braff, D. Lateralization of conversion symptoms: More frequent on the left. *American Journal of Psychiatry*, 1977, *134*, 578–580.

Galin, D., & Ellis, R. R. Asymmetry in evoked potentials as an index of lateralized cognitive processes: Relation to EEG alpha asymmetry. *Neuropsychologia*, 1975, *13*, 45–50.

Galin, D., Johnstone, J., & Herron, J. Effects of task difficulty on EEG measures of cerebral engagement. *Neuropsychologia*, 1978, *16*, 461–472.

Galin, D., & Ornstein, R. Lateral specialization of cognitive mode: An EEG study. *Psychophysiology*, 1972, *9*, 412–418.

Galin, D., & Ornstein, R. Individual differences in cognitive style: I. Reflective eye movements. *Neuropsychologia*, 1974, *12*, 367–376.

Gardiner, M. F., & Walter, D. O. Evidence of hemispheric specialization from infant EEG. In S. Harnad, R. W. Doty, L. Goldstein, J. Jaynes, & G. Krauthamer (Eds.), *Lateralization in the nervous system*. New York: Academic Press, 1977.

Gardner, E. B., & Branski, D. M. Unilateral cerebral activation and perception of gaps: A signal detection analysis. *Neuropsychologia*, 1976, *14*, 43–53.

Gardner, E. B., English, A. G., Flannery, B. M., Hartnett, M. B., McCormick, J. K., & Wilhelmy, B. B. Shape-recognition accuracy and response latency in a bilateral tactile task. *Neuropsychologia*, 1977, *15*, 607–616.

Gardner, R. W., Holzman, P. S., Klein, G. S., Linton, H. B., & Spence, D. P. Cognitive control: A study of individual differences in cognitive behavior. *Psychological Issues*, 1959, *1*, No. 4.

Gates, A., & Bradshaw, J. L. Music perception and cerebral asymmetries. *Cortex*, 1977, *13*, 390–401. (a)

Gates, A., & Bradshaw, J. L. The role of the cerebral hemispheres in music. *Brain and Language*, 1977, *4*, 403–431. (b)

Gazzaniga, M. S. *The bisected brain.* New York: Appleton, 1970.

Gazzaniga, M. S., Bogen, J. E., & Sperry, R. W. Some functional effects of sectioning the cerebral commissures in man. *Proceedings of the National Academy of Sciences,* 1962, *48,* 1765.

Gazzaniga, M. S., Bogen, J. E., & Sperry, R. W. Laterality effects in somesthesis following cerebral commissurotomy in man. *Neuropsychologia,* 1963, *1,* 209–221.

Gazzaniga, M. S., Bogen, J. E., & Sperry, R. W. Observations in visual perception after disconnection of the cerebral hemispheres in man. *Brain,* 1965, *88,* 221–236.

Gazzaniga, M. S., & LeDoux, J. E. *The integrated mind.* New York: Plenum, 1978.

Geffen, G. Development of hemispheric specialization for speech perception. *Cortex,* 1976, *12,* 337–346.

Geffen, G. The development of the right ear advantage in dichotic listening with focused attention. *Cortex,* 1978, *14,* 169–177.

Geffen, G., Bradshaw, J. L., & Nettleton, N. C. Hemispheric asymmetry: Verbal and spatial coding of visual stimuli. *Journal of Experimental Psychology,* 1972, *95,* 25–31.

Geffen, G., Bradshaw, J. L., & Wallace, G. Interhemispheric effects on reaction time to verbal and nonverbal visual stimuli. *Journal of Experimental Psychology,* 1971, *87,* 415–422.

Geffen, G., & Caudrey, D. Reliability and validity of the dichotic monitoring test for language laterality. *Neuropsychologia,* 1981, *19,* 413–424.

Geffen, G., & Traub, E. The effects of duration of stimulation, preferred hand and familial sinistrality in dichotic monitoring. *Cortex,* 1980, *16,* 83–94.

Geffen, G., Traub, E., & Stierman, I. Language laterality assessed by unilateral ECT and dichotic monitoring. *Journal of Neurology, Neurosurgery, and Psychiatry,* 1978, *41,* 354–360.

Geffner, D. S., & Dorman, M. Hemispheric specialization for speech perception in four-year-old children from low and middle socioeconomic classes. *Cortex,* 1976, *12,* 71–73.

Geffner, D. S., & Hochberg, I. Ear laterality performance of children from low and middle socioeconomic levels on a verbal dichotic listening task. *Cortex,* 1971, *7,* 193–203.

Geschwind, N., & Levitsky, W. Human brain: Left–right asymmetries in temporal speech region. *Science,* 1968, *161,* 186–187.

Gesell, A., & Ames, L. B. The development of handedness. *Journal of Genetic Psychology,* 1947, *70,* 155–175.

Gevins, A. S., Zeitlin, G. M., Doyle, J. C., Schaffer, R. E., Yingling, C. D., Callaway, E., & Yeager, C. L. EEG correlates of higher cortical functions. *Science,* 1979, *203,* 665–668.

Ghent, L. Developmental changes in tactual thresholds on dominant and nondominant sides. *Journal of Comparative and Physiological Psychology,* 1961, *54,* 670–673.

Gibson, A. R., Dimond, S. J., & Gazzaniga, M. S. Left field superiority for word matching. *Neuropsychologia,* 1972, *10,* 463–466.

Gibson, C., & Bryden, M. P. *Cerebral lateralization in deaf children using a dichhaptic task.* Paper presented at the annual meeting of the International Neuropsychology Society, Pittsburgh, February 1982.

Glass, A., & Butler, S. R. Asymmetries in suppression of alpha rhythm possibly related to cerebral dominance. *Electroencephalography and Clinical Neurophysiology,* 1973, *34,* 729.

Godfrey, J. J. Perceptual difficulty and the right-ear advantage for vowels. *Brain and Language,* 1974, *1,* 323–336.

Goldstein, K. *The organism: A holistic approach to biology derived from pathological data in man.* New York: American Books, 1939.

Goodglass, H., & Barton, M. Handedness and differential perception of verbal stimuli in left and right visual fields. *Perceptual and Motor Skills,* 1963, *17,* 851–854.

Goodglass, H., & Calderon, M. Parallel processing of verbal and musical stimuli in right and left hemispheres. *Neuropsychologia,* 1977, *15,* 397–407.

Goodglass, H., & Quadfasel, F. A. Language laterality in left-handed aphasics. *Brain,* 1954, *77,* 521–548.

Goodglass, H., Shai, A., Rosen, M., & Oscar-Berman, M. *New observations on right–left differences in tachistoscopic recognition of verbal and non-verbal stimuli.* Paper presented at the annual meeting of the International Neuropsychological Society, Washington, D.C., September 1971.

Gordon, H. W. Hemispheric asymmetries in the perception of musical chords. *Cortex,* 1970, *6,* 387–398.

Gordon, H. W. Degree of ear asymmetries for perception of dichotic chords and for illusory chord localization in musicians of different levels of competence. *Journal of Experimental Psychology: Human Perception and Performance,* 1980, *6,* 516–527.

Gordon, H. W., & Bogen, J. E. Hemispheric lateralization of singing after intracarotid sodium amylobarbitone. *Journal of Neurology, Neurosurgery and Psychiatry,* 1974, *37,* 727.

Gottlieb, G., Doran, C., & Whitley, S. Cerebral dominance and speech acquisition in deaf children. *Journal of Abnormal and Social Psychology,* 1964, *69,* 182–189.

Graves, R., Landis, T., & Goodglass, H. Laterality and sex differences for visual recognition of emotional and nonemotional words. *Neuropsychologia,* 1981, *19,* 95–102.

Gronwall, D. M. A., & Sampson, H. Ocular dominance: A test of two hypotheses. *British Journal of Psychology,* 1971, *62,* 175–185.

Gross, K., Rothenberg, S., Schottenfeld, S., & Drake, K. Duration thresholds for letter identification in left and right visual fields for normal and reading-disabled children. *Neuropsychologia,* 1978, *16,* 709–715.

Gross, M. Hemispheric specialization for processing of visually-presented verbal and spatial stimuli. *Perception and Psychophysics,* 1972, *12,* 537–563.

Gross, Y., Franko, R., & Lewin, I. Effects of voluntary eye movements on hemispheric activity and choice of cognitive mode. *Neuropsychologia,* 1978, *16,* 653–657.

Gur, R. C., & Reivich, M. Cognitive task effects on hemispheric blood flow in humans: Evidence for individual differences in hemispheric activation. *Brain and Language,* 1980, *9,* 78–92.

Gur, R. E. Cognitive concomitants of hemispheric dysfunction in schizophrenia. *Archives of General Psychiatry,* 1979, *36,* 269–274.

Gur, R. E., & Gur, R. C. Defense mechanisms, psychosomatic symptomatology, and conjugate lateral eye movements. *Journal of Consulting and Clinical Psychology,* 1975, *43,* 416–420.

Gur, R. E., Gur, R. C., & Harris, L. J. Cerebral activation, as measured by subjects' lateral eye movements, is influenced by experimenter location. *Neuropsychologia,* 1975, *13,* 35–44.

Haaland, K. Y. The effect of dichotic, monaural and diotic verbal stimuli on auditory evoked potentials. *Neuropsychologia,* 1974, *12,* 339–345.

Haggard, M. P. Encoding and the REA for speech signals. *Quarterly Journal of Experimental Psychology,* 1971, *23,* 34–45.

Haggard, M. P., & Parkinson, A. M. Stimulus and task factors in the perceptual lateralization of speech signals. *Quarterly Journal of Experimental Psychology,* 1971, *23,* 168–177.

Halperin, Y., Nachshon, I., & Carmon, A. Shift of ear superiority in dichotic listening to temporally patterned nonverbal stimuli. *Journal of the Acoustical Society of America,* 1973, *53,* 46–50.

Halwes, T. G. Effects of dichotic fusion on the perception of speech. *Supplement to Status Report on Speech Research.* New Haven, Conn.: Haskins Laboratories, 1969.

Hamers, J. F., & Lambert, W. E. Visual field and cerebral hemisphere preferences in bilinguals. In S. J. Segalowitz & F. A. Gruber (Eds.), *Language development and neurological theory.* New York: Academic Press, 1977.

Hannay, H. J. Asymmetry in reception and retention of colors. *Brain and Language,* 1979, *8,* 191–201.

Hannay, H. J., & Boyer, C. L. Sex differences in hemispheric asymmetry revisited. *Perceptual and Motor Skills,* 1978, *47,* 315–321.

Hannay, H. J., & Malone, D. R. Visual field effects and short-term memory for verbal material. *Neuropsychologia,* 1976, *14,* 203–209.

Harcum, E. R., & Filion, R. D. L. Effects of stimulus reversals on lateral dominance in word recognition. *Perceptual and Motor Skills,* 1963, *17,* 779–794.

Hardyck, C., Goldman, R., & Petrinovitch, L. A note on the distribution of handedness in relation to sex, race, and age. *Human Biology,* 1975, *47,* 369–373.

Hardyck, C., & Petrinovitch, L. F. Left handedness. *Psychological Bulletin,* 1977, *84,* 385–404.

Hardyck, C., Petrinovitch, L. F., & Goldman, R. D. Left-handedness and cognitive deficit. *Cortex,* 1976, *12,* 266–280.

Harris, A. J. *Harris tests of lateral dominance* (3rd ed.). New York: The Psychological Corporation, 1958.

Harris, L. J. Left-handedness: Early theories, facts, and fancies. In J. Herron (Ed.), *Neuropsychology of left-handedness.* New York: Academic Press, 1980.

Harshman, R. A., & Remington, R. Sex, language, and the brain, Part I: A review of the literature on adult sex differences in lateralization. Unpublished manuscript, University of California, Los Angeles, 1975.

Harshman, R. A., Remington, R., & Krashen, S. D. Sex, language and the brain, Part II: Evidence from dichotic listening for adult sex differences in verbal lateralization. Unpublished manuscript, University of California, Los Angeles, 1975.

Hatta, T. The functional asymmetry of tactile pattern learning in normal subjects. *Psychologia,* 1978, *21,* 83–89. (a)

Hatta, T. Visual field differences in a mental transformation task. *Neuropsychologia,* 1978, *16,* 637–641. (b)

Hatta, T., & Nakatsuka, Z. Note on hand preference of Japanese people. *Perceptual and Motor Skills,* 1976, *42,* 530.

Haun, F. Functional dissociation of the hemispheres using foveal visual input. *Neuropsychologia,* 1978, *16,* 725–733.

Hayashi, R., & Hatta, T. Hemispheric differences in mental rotation task with Kanji stimuli. *Psychologia,* 1978, *21,* 210–215.

Hayashi, T., & Bryden, M. P. Ocular dominance and perceptual asymmetry. *Perceptual and Motor Skills,* 1967, *25,* 605–612.

Hayden, M. E., Kirstein, E., & Singh, S. Role of distinctive features in dichotic perception of 21 English consonants. *Journal of the Acoustical Society of America,* 1979, *65,* 1039–1046.

Hebb, D. O. *The organization of behavior.* New York: Wiley, 1949.

Hécaen, H. Clinical symptomatology in right and left hemispheric lesions. In V. B. Mountcastle (Ed.), *Interhemispheric relations and cerebral dominance.* Baltimore: Johns Hopkins Press, 1962.

Hécaen, H. Acquired aphasia in children and the ontogenesis of hemispheric functional specialization. *Brain and Language,* 1976, *3,* 114–134.

Hécaen, H. Personal communication, 1981.

Hécaen, H., & Ajuriaguerra, J. *Left-handedness: Manual superiority and cerebral dominance.* New York: Grune & Stratton, 1964.

Hécaen, H., Ajuriaguerra, J., & Angelergues, R. Apraxia and its various aspects. In L. Halpern (Ed.), *Problems of dynamic neurology.* Jerusalem: Hebrew University, 1963.

Hécaen, H., & Albert, M. L. *Human neuropsychology.* New York: Wiley, 1978.

Hécaen, H., & Angelergues, R. Agnosia for faces (prosopagnosia). *Archives of Neurology,* 1962, *7,* 92–100.

Hécaen, H., DeAgostini, M., & Monzon-Montes, A. Cerebral organization in left-handers. *Brain and Language,* 1981, *12,* 261–284.

Hécaen, H., & Sauguet, J. Cerebral dominance in left-handed subjects. *Cortex,* 1971, *7,* 19–48.

Heilman, K. M., & VanDenAbell, T. Right hemispheric dominance for mediating cerebral activation. *Neuropsychologia,* 1979, *17,* 315–322.

Hellige, J. B. Visual laterality patterns for pure- versus mixed-list presentation. *Journal of Experimental Psychology: Human Perception and Performance,* 1978, *4,* 121–131.

Hellige, J. B., & Cox, P. J. Effects of concurrent verbal memory on recognition of stimuli from the left and right visual fields. *Journal of Experimental Psychology: Human Perception and Performance,* 1976, *2,* 210–221.

Hellige, J. B., Cox, P. J., & Litvac, L. Information processing in the cerebral hemispheres: Selective hemispheric activation and capacity limitations. *Journal of Experimental Psychology: General,* 1979, *108,* 251–279.

Hellige, J. B., & Webster, R. Right hemisphere superiority for initial stages of letter processing. *Neuropsychologia,* 1979, *17,* 653–660.

Henry, R. G. J. Monaural studies eliciting hemispheric asymmetry: A bibliography. *Perceptual and Motor Skills,* 1979, *48,* 335–338.

Hermelin, B., & O'Connor, N. Functional asymmetry in the reading of Braille. *Neuropsychologia,* 1971, *9,* 431–435.

Heron, W. Perception as a function of retinal locus and attention. *American Journal of Psychology,* 1957, *70,* 38–48.

Herron, J. Two hands, two brains, two sexes. In J. Herron (Ed.), *Neuropsychology of left-handedness.* New York: Academic Press, 1980.

Higgenbottam, J. A. Relationships between sets of lateral and perceptual preference measures. *Cortex,* 1973, *9,* 402–409.

Hilliard, R. D. Hemispheric laterality effects on a facial recognition task in normal subjects. *Cortex,* 1973, *9,* 246–258.

Hines, D. Independent functioning of the two cerebral hemispheres for recognizing bilaterally presented tachistoscopic visual half-field stimuli. *Cortex,* 1975, *11,* 132–143.

Hines, D. Recognition of verbs, abstract nouns and concrete nouns from the left and right visual half-fields. *Neuropsychologia,* 1976, *14,* 211–216.

Hines, D. Differences in tachistoscopic recognition between abstract and concrete words as a function of visual half-field and frequency. *Cortex,* 1977, *13,* 66–73.

Hines, D., & Martindale, C. Induced lateral eye-movements and creative and intellectual performance. *Perceptual and Motor Skills,* 1974, *39,* 153–154.

Hines, D., & Satz, P. Superiority of right visual half fields in right handers for recall of digits presented at varying rates. *Neuropsychologia,* 1971, *9,* 21–26.

Hines, D., Satz, P., Schell, B., & Schmidlin, S. Differential recall of digits in the left and right visual half-fields under free and fixed order of report. *Neuropsychologia,* 1969, *7,* 13–22.

Hink, R. F., Hillyard, S. A., & Benson, P. J. Event-related brain potentials and selective attention to acoustic and phonetic cues. *Biological Psychology,* 1978, *6,* 1–16.

Hirata, K., & Bryden, M. P. Right visual field superiority for letter recognition with partial report. *Canadian Journal of Psychology,* 1976, *30,* 134–139.

Hiscock, M. Effects of examiner's location and subject's anxiety on gaze laterality. *Neuropsychologia*, 1977, *15*, 409–416. (a)

Hiscock, M. Eye-movement asymmetry and hemispheric function: An examination of individual differences. *Journal of Psychology*, 1977, *97*, 49–52. (b)

Hiscock, M., & Kinsbourne, M. Selective listening asymmetry in preschool children. *Developmental Psychology*, 1977, *13*, 217–224.

Honda, H. Shift of visual laterality difference by loading of auditory discrimination tasks. *Japanese Journal of Psychology*, 1978, *49*, 8–14.

Huang, M. Hemispheric differentiation and category width. *Cortex*, 1979, *15*, 531–540.

Hubel, D. H., & Wiesel, T. N. Receptive fields of cells in striate cortex of very young visually inexperienced kittens. *Journal of Neurophysiology*, 1963, *26*, 994–1002.

Hublet, C., Morais, J., & Bertelson, P. Spatial constraints on focused attention: Beyond the right-side advantage. *Perception*, 1976, *5*, 3–8.

Hudson, P. J. W. The genetics of handedness—a reply to Levy and Nagylaki. *Neuropsychologia*, 1975, *13*, 331–339.

Hulme, M. R. *Eye movements and egocentric direction.* Unpublished doctoral dissertation, University of Waterloo, 1979.

Humphrey, M. E., & Zangwill, O. L. Cessation of dreaming after brain injury. *Journal of Neurology, Neurosurgery, and Psychiatry*, 1951, *14*, 322–325.

Hunt, E., Lunneborg, C., & Lewis, J. What does it mean to be high verbal? *Cognitive Psychology*, 1975, *7*, 194–227.

Inglis, J. Dichotic stimulation, temporal-lobe damage, and the perception and storage of auditory stimuli—a note on Kimura's findings. *Canadian Journal of Psychology*, 1962, *16*, 11–17.

Inglis, J. Dichotic listening and cerebral dominance. *Acta Oto-laryngologica*, 1965, *60*, 231.

Inglis, J. Dichotic listening performance. *British Journal of Psychology*, 1968, *59*, 415–422.

Inglis, J., & Lawson, J. S. Sex differences in the effects of unilateral brain damage on intelligence. *Science*, 1981, *212*, 693–695.

Inglis, J., & Sykes, D. H. Some sources of variation in dichotic listening performance in children. *Journal of Experimental Child Psychology*, 1967, *5*, 480–488.

Ingram, D. Cerebral speech lateralization in young children. *Neuropsychologia*, 1975, *13*, 103–105. (a)

Ingram, D. Motor asymmetries in young children. *Neuropsychologia*, 1975, *13*, 95–102. (b)

Jackson, J. H. Clinical remarks on cases of defects of expression (by words, writing, signs, etc.) in diseases of the nervous system. *Lancet*, 1864, *2*, 604.

Jackson, J. H. On the nature of the duality of the brain. *Medical Press and Circular*, 1874, *1*, 19.

Jackson, J. H. On affections of speech from disease of the brain. *Brain*, 1878–1879, *1*, 304–330.

Jasper, H. H. The ten twenty electrode system. *Electroencephalography and Clinical Neurophysiology*, 1958, *10*, 371–375.

Johnstone, J., Galin, D., & Herron, J. Choice of handedness measures in studies of hemispheric specialization. *International Journal of Neuroscience*, 1979, *9*, 71–80.

Jones, R. K. Observations on stammering after localized cerebral injury. *Journal of Neurology, Neurosurgery, and Psychiatry*, 1966, *24*, 192–195.

Julesz, B., Breitmeyer, B., & Kropfl, W. Binocular-disparity-dependent upper–lower hemifield anisotropy and left–right hemifield isotropy as revealed by dynamic random-dot stereograms. *Perception*, 1976, *5*, 129–141.

Kail, R. V., & Siegel, A. W. Sex and hemispheric differences in the recall of verbal and spatial information. *Cortex*, 1978, *14*, 557–563.

Kallman, H. J. Can expectancy explain reaction time ear asymmetries? *Neuropsychologia,* 1978, *16,* 225–228.

Kallman, H. J., & Corballis, M. C. Ear asymmetry in reaction time to musical sounds. *Perception and Psychophysics,* 1975, *17,* 368–370.

Kaushall, P. Functional asymmetries of the human visual system as revealed by binocular rivalry and binocular brightness matching. *American Journal of Optometry and Physiological Optics,* 1975, *52,* 509–520.

Kelly, R. R., & Orton, K. D. Dichotic perception of word-pairs with mixed image values. *Neuropsychologia,* 1979, *17,* 363–372.

Kelly, R. R., & Tomlinson-Keasey, C. Hemispheric laterality of deaf children for processing words and pictures visually presented to the hemifields. *American Annals of the Deaf,* 1977, *122,* 525–533.

Kershner, J. R. Cerebral dominance in disabled readers, good readers, and gifted children: Search for a valid model. *Child Development,* 1977, *48,* 61–67.

Kershner, J. R., & Jeng, A. G. Dual functional hemispheric asymmetry in visual perception: Effects of ocular dominance and postexposural processes. *Neuropsychologia,* 1972, *10,* 437–445.

Kershner, J., Thomae, R., & Callaway, R. Nonverbal fixation control in young children induces a left-field advantage in digit recall. *Neuropsychologia,* 1977, *15,* 569–576.

Kimura, D. Cerebral dominance and the perception of verbal stimuli. *Canadian Journal of Psychology,* 1961, *15,* 166–171. (a)

Kimura, D. Some effects of temporal lobe damage on auditory perception. *Canadian Journal of Psychology,* 1961, *15,* 156–165. (b)

Kimura, D. Speech lateralization in young children as determined by an auditory test. *Journal of Comparative and Physiological Psychology,* 1963, *56,* 899–902.

Kimura, D. Left–right differences in the perception of melodies. *Quarterly Journal of Psychology,* 1964, *16,* 355–358.

Kimura, D. Dual functional asymmetry of the brain in visual perception. *Neuropsychologia,* 1966, *4,* 275–285.

Kimura, D. Functional asymmetry of the brain in dichotic listening. *Cortex,* 1967, *3,* 163–178.

Kimura, D. Spatial localization in left and right visual fields. *Canadian Journal of Psychology,* 1969, *23,* 445–448.

Kimura, D. Manual activity during speaking—I. Right-handers. *Neuropsychologia,* 1973, *11,* 45–50. (a)

Kimura, D. Manual activity during speaking—II. Left-handers. *Neuropsychologia,* 1973, *11,* 51–56. (b)

Kimura, D. The neural basis of language qua gesture. In H. Avakian-Whitaker & H. A. Whitaker (Eds.), *Current trends in neurolinguistics.* New York: Academic Press, 1976.

Kimura, D. Acquisition of a motor skill after left-hemisphere damage. *Brain,* 1977, *100,* 527–542.

Kimura, D. Neuromotor mechanisms in the evolution of human communication. In H. D. Steklis & M. J. Raleigh (Eds.), *Neurobiology of social communication in primates.* New York: Academic Press, 1979.

Kimura, D., & Archibald, Y. Motor functions of the left hemisphere. *Brain,* 1974, *97,* 337–350.

Kimura, D., & Durnford, M. Normal studies on the function of the right hemisphere in vision. In S. Dimond & J. Beaumont (Eds.), *Hemisphere function in the human brain.* New York: Wiley, 1974.

King, F. L., & Kimura, D. Left-ear superiority in dichotic perception of vocal nonverbal sounds. *Canadian Journal of Psychology,* 1972, *26,* 111–116.

Kinsbourne, M. The cerebral basis of lateral asymmetries in attention. *Acta Psychologica,* 1970, *33,* 193–201.

Kinsbourne, M. Eye and head turning indicates cerebral lateralization. *Science,* 1972, *176,* 539–541.

Kinsbourne, M. The control of attention by interaction between the cerebral hemispheres. In S. Kornblum (Ed.), *Attention and performance IV.* New York: Academic Press, 1973.

Kinsbourne, M. Direction of gaze and distribution of cerebral thought processes. *Neuropsychologia,* 1974, *12,* 279–281. (a)

Kinsbourne, M. Mechanisms of hemispheric interaction in man. In M. Kinsbourne & W. L. Smith (Eds.), *Hemispheric disconnection and cerebral function.* Springfield, Ill.: Thomas, 1974. (b)

Kinsbourne, M. The mechanism of hemispheric control of the lateral gradient of attention. In P. M. A. Rabbitt & S. Dornic (Eds.), *Attention and performance V.* New York: Academic Press, 1975. (a)

Kinsbourne, M. The ontogeny of cerebral dominance. In D. Aaronson & R. W. Rieber (Eds.), Developmental psycholinguistics and communication disorders. *Annals of the New York Academy of Sciences,* 1975, *263,* 244–250. (b)

Kinsbourne, M., & Cook, J. General and lateralized effects of concurrent verbalization on a unimanual skill. *Quarterly Journal of Experimental Psychology,* 1971, *23,* 341–345.

Kinsbourne, M., & Hicks, R. E. Functional cerebral space: A model for overflow, transfer and interference effects in human performance. In J. Requin (Ed.), *Attention and performance VII.* New York: Academic Press, 1978.

Kinsbourne, M., & Hiscock, M. Does cerebral dominance develop? In S. J. Segalowitz & F. A. Gruber (Eds.), *Language development and neurological theory.* New York: Academic Press, 1977.

Kinsbourne, M., & McMurray, J. The effect of cerebral dominance on time sharing between speaking and tapping by preschool children. *Child Development,* 1975, *46,* 240–242.

Kinsbourne, M., & Warrington, E. Developmental factors in reading and writing backwardness. *British Journal of Psychology,* 1963, *54,* 145–156.

Kirsner, K. Hemispheric differences in recognition memory for letters. *Bulletin of the Psychonomic Society,* 1979, *13,* 2–4.

Klatzky, R. L. Interhemispheric transfer of test stimulus representations in memory scanning. *Psychonomic Science,* 1970, *21,* 201–203.

Klatzky, R. L., & Atkinson, R. C. Specialization of the cerebral hemispheres in scanning for information in short-term memory. *Perception and Psychophysics,* 1971, *10,* 335–338.

Klisz, D. K., & Parsons, O. A. Ear asymmetry in reaction time tasks as a function of handedness. *Neuropsychology,* 1975, *13,* 323–330.

Knights, R. M., & Bakker, D. J. (Eds.), *The neuropsychology of learning disorders: Theoretical approaches.* Baltimore: Univ. Park Press, 1976.

Knopman, D. S., Rubens, A. B., Klassen, A. C., Meyer, M. W., & Niccum, N. Regional cerebral blood flow patterns during verbal and nonverbal auditory activation. *Brain and Language,* 1980, *9,* 93–112.

Knox, A. W., & Boone, D. R. Auditory laterality and tested handedness. *Cortex,* 1970, *6,* 164–173.

Knox, C., & Kimura, D. Cerebral processing of nonverbal sounds in boys and girls. *Neuropsychologia,* 1970, *8,* 227–237.

Kocel, D., Galin, D., Ornstein, R., & Merrin, E. L. Lateral eye movements and cognitive mode. *Psychonomic Science,* 1972, *27,* 223–224.

Kohn, B., & Dennis, M. Selective impairments of visuospatial abilities in infantile hemiplegics after right cerebral hemi-decortication. *Neuropsychologia,* 1974, *12,* 505–512. (a)

Kohn, B., & Dennis, M. Somatosensory functions after cerebral hemidecortication for infantile hemiplegia. *Neuropsychologia*, 1974, *12*, 119–130. (b)

Krashen, S. D. Lateralization, language learning, and the critical period: Some new evidence. *Language Learning*, 1973, *23*, 63–74.

Lachman, R., Lachman, J. L., & Butterfield, E. C. *Cognitive psychology and information processing: An introduction.* Hillsdale, N.J.: Erlbaum, 1979.

Lake, D. A., & Bryden, M. P. Handedness and sex differences in hemispheric asymmetry. *Brain and Language*, 1976, *3*, 266–282.

Landis, T., Assal, G., & Perret, E. Opposite cerebral hemispheric superiorities for visual associative processing of emotional facial expressions and objects. *Nature*, 1979, *278*, 739–740.

Lansdell, H. The effect of neurosurgery on a test of proverbs. *American Psychologist*, 1961, *16*, 448.

Lansdell, H. A sex difference in effect of temporal lobe neurosurgery on design preference. *Nature*, 1962, *194*, 852–854.

Lansdell, H. Effect of extent of temporal lobe ablations on two lateralized deficits. *Physiology and Behavior*, 1968, *3*, 271–273. (a)

Lansdell, H. The use of factor scores from the Wechsler–Bellevue Scale of Intelligence in assessing patients with temporal lobe removals. *Cortex*, 1968, *4*, 257–268. (b)

Lansdell, H. Effect of neurosurgery on the ability to identify popular word associations. *Journal of Abnormal Psychology*, 1973, *81*, 255–258.

Lansdell, H., & Urbach, N. Sex differences in personality measures related to size and side of temporal lobe ablations. *Proceedings of the 73rd Annual Convention of the American Psychological Association*, 1965, 113–114.

Lassonde, M. C., Lortie, J., & Ptito, M. Dichotic listening in children suffering from agenesis of the corpus callosum. *Society for Neuroscience Abstracts*, 1979, *5*, 24.

Ledlow, A., Swanson, J. M., & Kinsbourne, M. Reaction times and evoked potentials as indicators of hemispheric differences for laterally presented name and physical matches. *Journal of Experimental Psychology: Human Perception and Performance*, 1978, *4*, 440–454.

Lenneberg, E. *Biological foundations of language.* New York: Wiley, 1967.

Leong, C. K. Lateralization in severely disabled readers in relation to functional cerebral development and synthesis of information. In R.M. Knights & D. J. Bakker (Eds.), *The neuropsychology of learning disorders: Theoretical approaches.* Baltimore: University Park Press, 1976.

Levy, J. Possible basis for the evolution of lateral specialization of the human brain. *Nature*, 1969, *224*, 614–615.

Levy, J. Lateral specialization of the human brain: Behavioral manifestations and possible evolutionary basis. In J. A. Kiger (Ed.), *The biology of behavior.* Corvallis: Oregon State Univ. Press, 1972.

Levy, J. Psychological implications of bilateral asymmetry. In S. Dimond & J. G. Beaumont (Eds.), *Hemisphere function in the human brain.* London: Paul Elek, Ltd., 1974.

Levy, J. A review of evidence for a genetic component in handedness. *Behavior Genetics*, 1976, *6*, 429–453.

Levy, J. The origins of lateral asymmetry. In S. R. Harnad, R. W. Doty, L. Goldstein, J. Jaynes, & G. Krauthamer (Eds.), *Lateralization in the nervous system.* New York: Academic Press, 1977.

Levy, J., & Nagylaki, T. A model for the genetics of handedness. *Genetics*, 1972, *72*, 117–128.

Levy, J., & Reid, M. Variations in writing posture and cerebral organization. *Science*, 1976, *194*, 337–339.

Levy, J., & Reid, M. Variations in cerebral organization as a function of handedness, hand posture in writing, and sex. *Journal of Experimental Psychology: General*, 1978, *107*, 119–144.

Levy-Agresti, J., & Sperry, R. W. Differential perceptual capacities in major and minor hemispheres. *Proceedings of the National Academy of Sciences*, 1968, *61*, 1151.

Ley, R. G. *Asymmetry of hysterical conversion symptoms*. Paper presented at the annual meeting of the Canadian Psychological Association, Ottawa, June 1978.

Ley, R. G. An archival examination of an asymmetry of hysterical conversion symptoms. *Journal of Clinical Neuropsychology*, 1980, *2*, 1–9. (a)

Ley, R. G. *Emotion and the right hemisphere*. Unpublished doctoral dissertation, University of Waterloo, 1980. (b)

Ley, R. G., & Bryden, M. P. Hemispheric differences in recognizing faces and emotions. *Brain and Language*, 1979, *7*, 127–138. (a)

Ley, R. G., & Bryden, M. P. *Right hemisphere emotional effect for emotional, imagic words*. Paper presented at the annual meeting of the Psychonomic Society, Phoenix, November 1979. (b)

Ley, R. G., & Bryden, M. P. Consciousness, emotion, and the right hemisphere. In G. Underwood & R. Stevens (Eds.), *Aspects of consciousness* (Vol. 2). London: Academic Press, 1981.

Ley, R. G., & Bryden, M. P. A dissociation of right and left hemispheric effects for recognizing emotional tone and verbal content. *Brain and Cognition*, 1982, *1*, 3–9. (a)

Ley, R. G., & Bryden, M. P. Right hemispheric involvement in imagery and affect. In E. Perceman (Ed.), *Cognitive processing in the right hemisphere*. New York: Academic Press, forthcoming.

Liberman, A. M., Cooper, F. S., Shankweiler, D. P., & Studdert-Kennedy, M. Perception of the speech code. *Psychological Review*, 1967, *74*, 431–461.

Liberman, I. Y., Shankweiler, D., Orlando, C., Harris, K. S., & Berti, F. B. Letter confusion and reversals of sequence in the beginning reader: Implications for Orton's theory of developmental dyslexia. *Cortex*, 1971, *7*, 127–142.

Liederman, J., & Kinsbourne, M. Rightward motor bias in newborns depends upon parental right-handedness. *Neuropsychologia*, 1980, *18*, 579–584.

Lindsay, P. H., & Norman, D. A. *Human information processing: An introduction to psychology* (2nd ed.). New York: Academic Press, 1977.

Lindsley, D. B., & Wicke, J. D. The electroencephalogram: Autonomous electrical activity in man and animals. In R. F. Thompson & M. M. Patterson (Eds.), *Bioelectric recording techniques: Part B. Electroencephalography and human brain potentials*. New York: Academic Press, 1974.

Lomas, J. Competition within the left hemisphere between speaking and unimanual tasks performed without visual guidance. *Neuropsychologia*, 1980, *18*, 141–149.

Lomas, J., & Kimura, D. Intrahemispheric interaction between speaking and sequential manual activity. *Neuropsychologia*, 1976, *14*, 23–33.

Lowe, S. S., Cullen, J. K., Jr., Berlin, C. I., Thompson, C. L., & Willett, M. E. Perception of simultaneous dichotic and monotic monosyllables. *Journal of Speech and Hearing Research*, 1970, *13*, 812–822.

Luria, A. R. *The higher cortical functions in man*. New York: Basic Books, 1965.

Maccoby, E. E., & Jacklin, C. N. *The psychology of sex differences*. Stanford, Calif.: Stanford Univ. Press, 1974.

Mackavey, W., Curcio, F., & Rosen, J. Tachistoscopic word recognition performance under conditions of simultaneous bilateral presentation. *Neuropsychologia*, 1975, *13*, 27–33.

MacKinnon, G. E., Forde, J., & Piggins, D. J. Stabilized images, steadily fixated figures, and prolonged afterimages. *Canadian Journal of Psychology*, 1969, *23*, 184–195.

Majkowski, J., Bochenck, Z., Bochenck, W., Knapik-Fijalkowska, D., & Kopec, J. Latency of averaged evoked potentials to contralateral and ipsilateral auditory stimulation in normal subjects. *Brain Research,* 1971, *25,* 416–419.

Malone, D. R., & Hannay, H. J. Hemispheric dominance and normal color memory. *Neuropsychologia,* 1978, *16,* 51–59.

Manning, A., Goble, W., Markman, R., & La Breche, T. Lateral cerebral differences in the deaf in response to linguistic and nonlinguistic stimuli. *Brain and Language,* 1977, *4,* 309–321.

Marcel, T., Katz, L., & Smith, M. Laterality and reading proficiency. *Neuropsychologia,* 1974, *12,* 131–139.

Marcel, T., & Rajan, P. Lateral specialization for recognition of words and faces in good and poor readers. *Neuropsychologia,* 1975, *13,* 489–497.

Marsh, G. R. Asymmetry of electrophysiological phenomena and its relation to behavior in humans. In M. Kinsbourne (Ed.), *Asymmetrical function of the brain.* Cambridge: Cambridge Univ. Press, 1978.

Marshall, J. C., Caplan, D., & Holmes, J. M. The measure of laterality. *Neuropsychologia,* 1975, *13,* 315–322.

Martin, M. Hemispheric specialization for local and global processing. *Neuropsychologia,* 1979, *17,* 33–40.

Marzi, C. A., & Berlucchi, G. Right visual field superiority for accuracy of recognition of famous faces in normals. *Neuropsychologia,* 1977, *15,* 751–756.

Marzi, C. A., DiStefano, M., Tassinari, G., & Crea, F. Iconic storage in the two hemispheres. *Journal of Experimental Psychology: Human Perception and Performance,* 1979, *5,* 31–41.

Mateer, C., & Kimura, D. Impairment of nonverbal oral movements in aphasia. *Brain and Language,* 1977, *4,* 262–276.

Maynard Smith, J. Evolution and the theory of games. *American Scientist,* 1976, *64,* 41–45.

Mazzucchi, A., & Parma, M. Responses to dichotic listening tasks in temporal epileptics with or without clinically evident lesions. *Cortex,* 1978, *14,* 381–390.

McCall, G. N., & Cunningham, N. M. Two-point discrimination: Asymmetry in spatial discrimination on the two sides of the tongue, a preliminary report. *Perceptual and Motor Skills,* 1971, *32,* 368–370.

McFarland, K., McFarland, M. L., Bain, J. D., & Ashton, R. Ear differences of abstract and concrete word recognition. *Neuropsychologia,* 1978, *16,* 555–561.

McFie, J., & Piercy, M. F. Intellectual impairment with localized cerebral lesions. *Brain,* 1952, *75,* 292–311.

McFie, J., Piercy, M. F., & Zangwill, O. L. Visual-spatial agnosia associated with lesions of the right cerebral hemisphere. *Brain,* 1950, *73,* 167–190.

McGee, M. G. Human spatial abilities: Psychometric studies and environmental, genetic, hormonal, and neurological influences. *Psychological Bulletin,* 1979, *86,* 889–918.

McGlone, J. Sex differences in functional brain asymmetry. *Cortex,* 1978, *14,* 122–128.

McGlone, J. Sex differences in human brain organization: A critical survey. *The Behavioral and Brain Sciences,* 1980, *3,* 215–227.

McGlone, J., & Davidson, W. The relation between cerebral speech laterality and spatial ability with special reference to sex and hand preference. *Neuropsychologia,* 1973, *11,* 105–113.

McGlone, J., & Kertesz, A. Sex differences in cerebral processing of visuospatial tasks. *Cortex,* 1973, *9,* 313–320.

McKeever, W. F. Lateral word recognition: Effects of unilateral and bilateral presentation, asynchrony of bilateral presentation, and forced order of report. *Quarterly Journal of Experimental Psychology*, 1971, 23, 410–416.

McKeever, W. F. Does post-exposural directional scanning offer a sufficient explanation for lateral differences in tachistoscopic recognition? *Perceptual and Motor Skills*, 1974, 38, 43–50.

McKeever, W. F. Handwriting posture in left-handers: Sex, familial sinistrality and language laterality correlates.*Neuropsychologia*, 1979, 17, 429–444.

McKeever, W. F., & Gill, K. M. Interhemispheric transfer time for visual stimulus information varies as a function of the retinal locus of stimulation. *Psychonomic Science*, 1972, 26, 308–310.

McKeever, W. F., Hoemann, H. W., Florian, V. A., & VanDeventer, A. D. Evidence of minimal cerebral asymmetries for the processing of English words and American Sign Language in the congenitally deaf. *Neuropsychologia*, 1976, 14, 413–423.

McKeever, W. F., & Huling, M. D. Lateral dominance in tachistoscopic word recognition at two levels of ability. *Quarterly Journal of Experimental Psychology*, 1970, 22, 600–604.

McKeever, W. F., & Huling, M. D. Lateral dominance in tachistoscopic word recognition performance obtained with simultaneous bilateral input. *Neuropsychologia*, 1971, 9, 15–20.

McKeever, W. F., & Jackson, T. L. Cerebral dominance assessed by object- and color-naming latencies: Sex and familial sinistrality effects. *Brain and Language*, 1979, 7, 175–190.

McKeever, W. F., & VanDeventer, A. D. Dyslexic adolescents: Evidence of impaired visual and auditory language processing with normal lateralization and visual responsivity. *Cortex*, 1975, 11, 361–378.

McKeever, W. F., & VanDeventer, A. D. Familial sinistrality and degree of left-handedness. *British Journal of Psychology*, 1977, 68, 469–471. (a)

McKeever, W. F., & VanDeventer, A. D. Visual and auditory language processing asymmetries: Influences of handedness, familial sinistrality, and sex. *Cortex*, 1977, 13, 225–241. (b)

McKeever, W. F., VanDeventer, A. D., & Suberi, M. Avowed, assessed, and familial handedness and differential hemispheric processing of brief sequential and nonsequential visual stimuli. *Neuropsychologia*, 1973, 11, 235–238.

McNutt, J. C. Asymmetry in two-point discrimination on the tongues of adults and children. *Journal of Communication Disorders*, 1975, 8, 213–220.

Meadows, J. C. The anatomical basis of prosopagnosia. *Journal of Neurology, Neurosurgery and Psychiatry*, 1974, 37, 489–501. (a)

Meadows, J. C. Disturbed perception of colors associated with localized cerebral lesions. *Brain*, 1974, 97, 615–632. (b)

Mercure, R., & Warren, S. A. Inadequate and adequate readers' performance on a dichotic listening task. *Perceptual and Motor Skills*, 1978, 46, 709–710.

Meyer, G. E. Right hemispheric sensitivity for the McCollough effect. *Nature*, 1976, 264, 751–753.

Miglioli, M. D., Buchtel, H. A., Campanini, M. D., & DeRisio, C. Cerebral hemispheric lateralization of cognitive deficits due to alcoholism. *The Journal of Nervous and Mental Disease*, 1979, 167, 212–217.

Miles, W. R. Ocular dominance in human adults. *Journal of General Psychology*, 1930, 3, 412–420.

Miller, L. K., & Turner, S. Development of hemifield differences in word recognition. *Journal of Educational Psychology*, 1973, 65, 172–176.

Milner, B. Psychological defects produced by temporal lobe excision. *Research Publications of the Association for Nervous and Mental Diseases*, 1958, *36*, 244–257.

Milner, B. Hemispheric specialization: Scope and limits. In F. O. Schmitt & F. G. Worden (Eds.), *The neurosciences: Third study program*. Cambridge, Mass.: MIT Press, 1974.

Milner, B., Branch, C., & Rasmussen, T. Observations on cerebral dominance. In A. V. S. DeReuck & M. O'Connor (Eds.), *Disorders of language (CIBA Foundation Symposium)*. London: Churchill, 1964.

Milner, B., Taylor, L., & Sperry, R. W. Lateralized suppression of dichotically-presented digits after commissural section in man. *Science*, 1968, *161*, 184–186.

Mishkin, M., & Forgays, D. G. Word recognition as a function of retinal locus. *Journal of Experimental Psychology*, 1952, *43*, 43–48.

Molfese, D. Auditory evoked potentials in left and right hemispheres of infants. Paper presented at the Fourth Annual Meeting of the International Neuropsychology Society, Toronto, February 1976.

Molfese, D. L. Left and right hemisphere involvement in speech perception: Electrophysiological correlates. *Perception and Psychophysics*, 1978, *23*, 237–243. (a)

Molfese, D. L. Neuroelectrical correlates of categorical speech perception in adults. *Brain and Language*, 1978, *5*, 25–35. (b)

Molfese, D. L. Cortical involvement in the semantic processing of coarticulated speech cues. *Brain and Language*, 1979, *7*, 86–100.

Molfese, D. L. Hemispheric specialization for temporal information: Implications for the perception of voicing cues during speech perception. *Brain and Language*, 1980, *11*, 285–299.

Molfese, D. L., Freeman, R. B., Jr., & Palermo, D. S. The ontogeny of brain lateralization for speech and nonspeech stimuli. *Brain and Language*, 1975, *2*, 356–368.

Molfese, D. L., & Hess, T. M. Hemispheric specialization for VOT perception in the preschool child. *Journal of Experimental Child Psychology*, 1978, *26*, 71–84.

Molfese, D. L., & Molfese, V. J. Hemisphere and stimulus differences as reflected in the cortical responses of newborn infants to speech stimuli. *Developmental Psychology*, 1979, *15*, 505–511. (a)

Molfese, D. L., & Molfese, V. J. VOT distinctions in infants: Learned or innate? In H. A. Whitaker & H. Whitaker (Eds.), *Studies in neurolinguistics* (Vol. 4). New York: Academic Press, 1979. (b)

Molfese, D. L., & Molfese, V. J. Cortical responses of preterm infants to phonetic and nonphonetic speech stimuli. *Developmental Psychology*, 1980, *16*, 574–581.

Mononen, L. J., & Seitz, M. R. An AER analysis of contralateral advantage in the transmission of auditory information. *Neuropsychologia*, 1977, *15*, 165–173.

Morais, J., & Bertelson, P. Laterality effects in diotic listening. *Perception*, 1973, *2*, 107–111.

Morais, J., & Bertelson, P. Spatial position versus ear of entry as determinant of the auditory laterality effects: A stereophonic test. *Journal of Experimental Psychology: Human Perception and Performance*, 1975, *1*, 253–262.

Morgan, M. Embryology and inheritance of asymmetry. In S. Harnad, R. W. Doty, L. Goldstein, J. Jaynes, & G. Krauthamer (Eds.), *Lateralization in the nervous system*. New York: Academic Press, 1977.

Morgan, M. J., & Corballis, M. C. On the biological basis of human laterality: II. The mechanisms of inheritance. *The Behavioral and Brain Sciences*, 1978, *1*, 270–277.

Morrell, L. K., & Salamy, J. G. Hemispheric asymmetry of electrocortical response to speech stimuli. *Science*, 1971, *174*, 164–166.

Moscovitch, M. The development of lateralization of language functions and its relation to cognitive and linguistic development: A review and some theoretical speculatons. In

S. J. Segalowitz & F. A. Gruber (Eds.), *Language development and neurological theory*. New York: Academic Press, 1977.

Moscovitch, M. Information processing and the cerebral hemispheres. In M. S. Gazzaniga (Ed.), *Handbook of behavioral neurobiology* (Vol. 2, Neuropsychology). New York: Plenum, 1979.

Moscovitch, M., & Klein, D. Material-specific perceptual interference for visual words and faces: Implications for models of capacity limitations, attention and laterality. *Journal of Experimental Psychology: Human Perception and Performance*, 1980, 6, 590–604.

Moscovitch, M., & Olds, J. Asymmetries in spontaneous facial expressions and their possible relation to hemispheric specialization. *Neuropsychologia*, 1982, 20, 71–81.

Moscovitch, M., Scullion, D., & Christie, D. Early versus late stages of processing and their relation to functional hemispheric asymmetries in face recognition. *Journal of Experimental Psychology: Human Perception and Performance*, 1976, 2, 401–416.

Moscovitch, M., & Smith, L. Differences in neural organization between individuals with inverted and noninverted hand postures during writing. *Science*, 1979, 205, 710–712.

Murray, J. E., Brown, P. R., Saxby, L., Tapley, S. M., & Bryden, M. P. *Laterality effects for stops, nasals, and fricatives under conditions of controlled attention*. Paper presented at the annual meeting of the Canadian Psychological Association, Toronto, June 1981.

Nachshon, I. Handedness and dichotic listening to nonverbal features of speech. *Perceptual and Motor Skills*, 1978, 47, 1111–1114.

Nachshon, I., & Carmon, A. Hand preference in sequential and spatial discrimination tasks. *Cortex*, 1975, 11, 123–131.

Nagafuchi, M. Development of dichotic and monaural hearing abilities in young children. *Acta Oto-laryngologica*, 1970, 69, 409–415.

Naylor, H. Reading disability and lateral asymmetry: An information-processing analysis. *Psychological Bulletin*, 1980, 87, 531–545.

Nebes, R. D. Handedness and the perception of whole–part relationship. *Cortex*, 1971, 7, 350–356.

Netley, C. Dichotic listening performance of hemispherectomized patients. *Neuropsychologia*, 1972, 10, 223–240.

Newman, H. H. Studies of human twins. II. Asymmetry or mirror imaging in identical twins. *Biological Bulletin*, 1928, 55, 298–315.

Nielsen, H., & Sorensen, J. H. Hemispheric dominance, dichotic listening and lateral eye movement behavior. *Scandinavian Journal of Psychology*, 1976, 17, 129–132.

Norman, D. A., & Bobrow, D. G. On data-limited and resource-limited processes. *Cognitive Psychology*, 1975, 7, 44–64.

O'Connor, K. P., & Shaw, J. C. Field dependence, laterality and the EEG. *Biological Psychology*, 1978, 6, 93–109.

Ogle, K. Ocular dominance and binocular retinal rivalry. In H. Davson (Ed.), *The eye* (Vol. 4). New York: Academic Press, 1962.

Ojemann, G., & Mateer, C. Human language cortex: Localization of memory, syntax, and sequential motor-phoneme identification systems. *Science*, 1979, 205, 1401–1403.

Oldfield, R. C. The assessment and analysis of handedness: The Edinburgh Inventory. *Neuropsychologia*, 1971, 9, 97–113.

O'Neil, B. *Word attributes in dichotic recognition and memory*. Unpublished doctoral dissertation, University of Western Ontario, 1971.

Orbach, J. Differential recognition of Hebrew and English words in right and left visual fields as a function of cerebral dominance and reading habits. *Neuropsychologia*, 1967, 5, 127–134.

Ornstein, R. W. *The psychology of consciousness*. San Francisco: Freeman, 1972.

Ornstein, R., Johnstone, J., Herron, J., & Swencionis, C. Differential right hemisphere engagement in visuospatial tasks. *Neuropsychologia*, 1980, *18*, 49–64.

Orton, S. T. Specific reading disability–strephosymbolia. *Journal of American Medical Association*, 1928, *90*, 1095–1099.

Orton, S. *Reading, writing and speech problems in children*. New York: Norton, 1937.

Oscar-Berman, M., Rehbein, L., Porfert, A., & Goodglass, H. Dichhaptic hand-order effects with verbal and nonverbal tactile stimulation. *Brain and Language*, 1978, *6*, 323–333.

Oscar-Berman, M., Zurif, E. B., & Blumstein, S. Effects of unilateral brain damage on the processing of speech sounds. *Brain and Language*, 1975, *2*, 345–355.

Ounsted, C., & Taylor, D. C. (Eds.). *Gender differences: Their ontogeny and significance*. London: Churchill, 1972.

Overton, W., & Wiener, M. Visual field position and word-recognition threshold. *Journal of Experimental Psychology*, 1966, *71*, 249–253.

Oxbury, S., Oxbury, J., & Gardiner, J. Laterality effects in dichotic listening. *Nature*, 1967, *214*, 742–743.

Paivio, A. Mental imagery in associative learning and thought. *Psychological Review*, 1969, *76*, 241–263.

Paivio, A. *Imagery and verbal processes*. New York: Holt, 1971.

Paivio, A. The relationship between verbal and perceptual codes. In E. C. Carterette & M. P. Friedman (Eds.), *Handbook of perception* (Vol. 13). *Perceptual coding*. New York: Academic Press, 1978.

Palmer, R. D. Development of a differentiated handedness. *Psychological Bulletin*, 1964, *62*, 257–272.

Papanicolaou, A. C. Cerebral excitation profiles in language processing: The photic probe paradigm. *Brain and Language*, 1980, *9*, 269–280.

Papcun, G., Krashen, S., Terbeek, D., Remington, R., & Harshman, R. Is the left hemisphere specialized for speech, language and/or something else? *Journal of the Acoustical Society of America*, 1974, *55*, 319–327.

Paradowski, W., Brucker, B., Zaretsky, H., & Alba, A. The effect of unilateral brain damage on the appearance of question-induced CLEM reactions. *Cortex*, 1978, *14*, 420–430.

Patterson, K., & Bradshaw, J. L. Differential hemispheric mediation of nonverbal visual stimuli. *Journal of Experimental Psychology: Human Perception and Performance*, 1975, *1*, 246–252.

Penfield, W., & Jasper, H. H. *Epilepsy and the functional anatomy of the human brain*. New York: Little, Brown, 1954.

Penfield, W., & Rasmussen, T. *The cerebral cortex of man*. New York: MacMillan, 1950.

Penfield, W., & Roberts, L. *Speech and brain mechanisms*. Princeton, N.J.: Princeton Univ. Press, 1959.

Pennal, B. E. Human cerebral asymmetry in color discrimination. *Neuropsychologia*, 1977, *15*, 563–568.

Peters, M., & Durding, B. Handedness as continuous variable. *Canadian Journal of Psychology*, 1978, *32*, 257–261.

Pettigrew, T. F. The measurement and correlates of category width as a cognitive variable. *Journal of Personality*, 1958, *26*, 532–544.

Pettit, J. M., & Helms, S. B. Hemispheric language dominance of language-disordered, articulation-disordered, and normal children. *Journal of Learning Disabilities*, 1979, *12*, 12–17.

Pettit, J. M., & Noll, J. D. Cerebral dominance in aphasia recovery. *Brain and Language,* 1979, 7, 191–200.

Phippard, D. Hemifield differences in visual perception in deaf and hearing subjects. *Neuropsychologia,* 1977, 15, 555–562.

Piazza, D. M. The influence of sex and handedness in the hemispheric specialization of verbal and nonverbal tasks. *Neuropsychologia,* 1980, 18, 163–176.

Pirot, M., Pulton, T. W., & Sutker, L. W. Hemispheric asymmetry in reaction time to color stimuli. *Perceptual and Motor Skills,* 1977, 45, 1151–1155.

Pirozzolo, F. J. *The neuropsychology of developmental reading disorders.* New York: Praeger, 1979.

Pirozzolo, F. J., & Rayner, K. Cerebral organization and reading disability. *Neuropsychologia,* 1979, 17, 485–491.

Pirozzolo, F. J., & Wittrock, M. C. (Eds.). *Neuropsychological and cognitive processes in reading.* New York: Academic Press, 1981.

Pitblado, C. B. Cerebral asymmetries in random-dot stereopsis: Reversal of direction with changes in dot size. *Perception,* 1979, 8, 683–690.

Pizzamiglio, L. Handedness, ear-preference, and field-dependence. *Perceptual and Motor Skills,* 1974, 38, 700–702.

Pohl, W., Butters, N., & Goodglass, H. Spatial discrimination system and cerebral lateralization. *Cortex,* 1972, 8, 305–314.

Poon, L. W., Thompson, L. W., & Marsh, G. R. Average evoked potential changes as a function of processing complexity. *Psychophysiology,* 1976, 13, 43–49.

Porac, C., & Coren, S. Is eye dominance a part of generalized laterality? *Perceptual and Motor Skills,* 1975, 40, 763–769.

Porac, C., & Coren, S. The dominant eye. *Psychological Bulletin,* 1976, 83, 880–897.

Porac, C., & Coren, S. Individual and familial patterns in four dimensions of lateral preference. *Neuropsychologia,* 1979, 17, 543–548.

Porter, R. J., Jr., & Whittaker, R. G. Dichotic and monotic masking of CV's by CV second formants with different transition starting values. *Journal of the Acoustical Society of America,* 1980, 67, 1772–1780.

Posner, M. I., Boies, S. J., Eichelman, W. H., & Taylor, R. L. Retention of visual and name codes of single letters. *Journal of Experimental Psychology,* 1969, 79, 1–16.

Posner, M., & Keele, S. Decay of visual information from a single letter. *Science,* 1967, 158, 137–139.

Posner, M. I., & Mitchell, R. F. Chronometric analysis of classification. *Psychological Review,* 1967, 74, 392–409.

Pritchard, R. M., Heron, W., & Hebb, D. O. Visual perception approached by the method of stabilized images. *Canadian Journal of Psychology,* 1960, 14, 66–77.

Provins, K. A., & Cunliffe, P. The reliability of some motor performance tests of handedness. *Neuropsychologia,* 1972, 10, 199–206.

Provins, K. A., & Jeeves, M. A. Hemisphere differences in response time to simple auditory stimuli. *Neuropsychologia,* 1975, 13, 207–211.

Raczkowski, D., Kalat, J. W., & Nebes, R. Reliability and validity of some handedness questionnaire items. *Neuropsychologia,* 1974, 12, 43–47.

Raney, E. T. Brain potentials and lateral dominance in identical twins. *Journal of Experimental Psychology,* 1939, 24, 21–39.

Rasmussen, T., & Milner, B. The role of early left-brain injury in determining lateralization of cerebral speech functions. *Annals of the New York Academy of Sciences,* 1977, 299, 355–369.

Rasmussen, T., & Penfield, W. Further studies of the sensory and motor cerebral cortex of man. *Federation Proceedings, Federation of American Societies for Experimental Biology,* 1947, *6,* 452–460.

Ratcliff, G. Spatial thought, mental rotation and the right cerebral hemisphere. *Neuropsychologia,* 1979, *17,* 49–54.

Reitsma, P. Visual asymmetry in children. In *Lateralization of brain functions.* Boerhaave Committee for Postgraduate Education. The Netherlands: Univ. of Leiden Press, 1975.

Repp, B. H. Measuring laterality effects in dichotic listening. *Journal of the Acoustical Society of America,* 1977, *62,* 720–737.

Repp, B. H. Stimulus dominance and ear dominance in the perception of dichotic voicing contrasts. *Brain and Language,* 1978, *5,* 310–330.

Reuter-Lorenz, P., & Davidson, R. J. Differential contributions of the two cerebral hemispheres to the perception of happy and sad faces. *Neuropsychologia,* 1981, *19,* 609–614.

Rife, D. C. Handedness, with special reference to twins. *Genetics,* 1940, *25,* 178–186.

Risberg, J. Regional cerebral blood flow measurements by ^{133}Xe-Inhalation: Methodology and applications in neuropsychology and psychiatry. *Brain and Language,* 1980, *9,* 9–34.

Rizzolatti, G., & Buchtel, H. A. Hemispheric superiority in reaction time to faces: A sex difference. *Cortex,* 1977, *13,* 300–305.

Rizzolatti, G., Umilta, C., & Berlucchi, G. Opposite superiorities of the right and left cerebral hemispheres in discriminative reaction time to physiognomical and alphabetical material. *Brain,* 1971, *94,* 431–442.

Roberts, L. In P. J. Vinken & G. W. Bruyn (Eds.), *Handbook of clinical neurology* (Vol. 4). Amsterdam: Elsevier, 1968.

Robertshaw, S., & Sheldon, M. Laterality effects in judgment of the identity and position of letters: A signal detection analysis. *Quarterly Journal of Experimental Psychology,* 1976, *28,* 115–121.

Robertson, A. D., & Inglis, J. The effects of electroconvulsive therapy on human learning and memory. *Canadian Psychological Review,* 1977, *18,* 285–307.

Robinson, G. M., & Solomon, D. J. Rhythm is processed by the speech hemisphere. *Journal of Experimental Psychology,* 1974, *102,* 508–511.

Rodney, M. L. *Motor sequencing and hemispheric specialization.* Unpublished doctoral dissertation, University of Waterloo, 1980.

Rosenfield, D. B., & Goodglass, H. Dichotic testing of cerebral dominance in stutterers. *Brain and Language,* 1980, *11,* 170–180.

Rosenzweig, M. R. Representations of the two ears at the auditory cortex. *American Journal of Physiology,* 1951, *167,* 147–214.

Ross, E. D., & Mesulam, M. Dominant language functions of the right hemisphere? *Archives of Neurology,* 1979, *36,* 144–148.

Rossi, G. F., & Rosadini, G. Experimental analysis of cerebral dominance in man. In F. L. Darley (Ed.), *Brain mechanisms underlying speech and language.* New York: Grune & Stratton, 1967.

Rotter, J. B. *Social learning and clinical psychology.* Englewood Cliffs, N.J.: Prentice-Hall, 1954.

Rubens, A. B. Anatomical asymmetries of human cerebral cortex. In S. Harnad, R. W. Doty, L. Goldstein, J. Jaynes, & G. Krauthamer (Eds.), *Lateralization in the nervous system.* New York: Academic Press, 1977.

Rudel, R. G., Denckla, M. B., & Hirsch, S. The development of left-hand superiority for discriminating Braille configurations. *Neurology,* 1977, *27,* 160–164.

Rugg, M. D., & Beaumont, J. G. Interhemispheric asymmetries in the visual evoked response: Effects of stimulus lateralization and task. *Biological Psychology*, 1978, *6*, 283–292. (a)

Rugg, M. D., & Beaumont, J. G. Visual evoked responses to visual-spatial and verbal stimuli: Evidence of differences in cerebral processing. *Physiological Psychology*, 1978, *6*, 501–504. (b)

Rutter, M. Prevalence and types of dyslexia. In A. L. Benton & D. Pearl (Eds.), *Dyslexia: An appraisal of current knowledge.* New York: Oxford Univ. Press, 1978.

Ryan, W. J., & McNeil, M. Listener reliability for a dichotic task. *Journal of the Acoustical Society of America*, 1974, *56*, 1922–1923.

Sackheim, H. A., Gur, R. C., & Saucy, M. C. Emotions are expressed more intensely on the left side of the face. *Annals of the New York Academy of Sciences*, 1978, *202*, 424–435.

Safer, M. A. Sex and hemisphere differences in access to codes for processing emotional expressions and faces. *Journal of Experimental Psychology: General*, 1981, *110*, 86–100.

Safer, M., & Leventhal, H. Ear differences in evaluating emotional tones of voice and verbal content. *Journal of Experimental Psychology: Human Perception and Performance*, 1977, *3*, 75–82.

St. John, R. C. Lateral asymmetry in face perception. *Canadian Journal of Pyshcology*, 1981, *35*, 213–223.

Satz, P. Pathological left-handedness: An explanatory model. *Cortex*, 1972, *8*, 121–135.

Satz, P. Left-handedness and early brain insult: An explanation. *Neuropsychologia*, 1973, *11*, 115–117.

Satz, P. Cerebral dominance and reading disability: An old problem revisited. In R. M. Knights & D. J. Bakker (Eds.), *The neuropsychology of learning disorders: Theoretical approaches.* Baltimore: University Park Press, 1976.

Satz, P. Incidence of aphasia in left-handers: A test of some hypothetical models of cerebral speech organization. In J. Herron (Ed.), *Neuropsychology of left-handedness.* New York: Academic Press, 1980.

Satz, P., Achenbach, K., & Fennell, E. Correlations between assessed manual laterality and predicted speech laterality in a normal population. *Neuropsychologia*, 1967, *5*, 295–310.

Satz, P., Achenbach, K., Pattishall, E., & Fennell, E. Order of report, ear asymmetry and handedness in dichotic listening. *Cortex*, 1965, *1*, 377–396.

Satz, P., Bakker, D. J., Teunissen, J., Goebel, R., & Van der Vlugt, H. Developmental parameters of the ear asymmetry: A multivariate approach. *Brain and Language*, 1975, *2*, 171–185.

Satz, P., Baymur, L., & Van der Vlugt, H. Pathological left-handedness: Cross-cultural tests of a model. *Neuropsychologia*, 1979, *17*, 77–82.

Satz, P., & Sparrow, S. Specific developmental dyslexia: A theoretical formulation. In D. Bakker & P. Satz (Eds.), *Specific reading disability.* Rotterdam: Rotterdam Univ. Press, 1970.

Schmuller, J., & Goodman, R. Bilateral tachistoscopic perception, handedness and laterality. *Brain and Language*, 1979, *8*, 81–91.

Schmuller, J., & Goodman, R. Bilateral tachistostopic perception, handedness, and laterality. II. Nonverbal stimuli. *Brain and Language*, 1980, *11*, 12–18.

Schulhoff, C., & Goodglass, H. Dichotic listening, side of brain injury and cerebral dominance. *Neuropsychologia*, 1969, *7*, 149–160.

Schulman-Galambos, C. Dichotic listening performance in elementary and college students. *Neuropsychologia*, 1977, *15*, 577–584.

Schwartz, M. *Competition in dichotic listening.* Unpublished doctoral dissertation, University of Waterloo, 1970.

Schwartz, M. Left-handedness and high-risk pregnancy. *Neuropsychologia*, 1977, *15*, 341–344.

Schwartz, M. *Familial laterality and cerebral dominance.* Paper presented at the annual meeting of the Canadian Psychological Association, Quebec City, June 1979.

Schwartz, N. H., & Dean, R. S. Laterality preference patterns of learning disabled children. *Perceptual and Motor Skills*, 1978, *47*, 869–870.

Scotti, G., & Spinnler, H. Colour imperception in unilateral hemisphere damaged patients. *Journal of Neurology, Neurosurgery and Psychiatry*, 1970, *33*, 22–28.

Seamon, J. G., & Gazzaniga, M. S. Coding strategies and cerebral laterality effects. *Cognitive Psychology*, 1973, *5*, 249–256.

Segalowitz, S. J., & Bryden, M. P. Individual differences in hemispheric representation of language. In S. J. Segalowitz (Ed.), *Language functions and brain organization.* New York: Academic Press, forthcoming.

Segalowitz, S. J., & Stewart, C. Left and right lateralization for letter matching: Strategy and sex differences. *Neuropsychologia*, 1979, *17*, 521–525.

Semmes, J. Hemispheric specialization: A possible clue to mechanism. *Neuropsychologia*, 1968, *6*, 11–26.

Semmes, J. Protopathic and epicritic sensation: A reappraisal. In A. L. Benton (Ed.), *Contributions to clinical neuropsychology.* Chicago: Aldine, 1969.

Semmes, J., Weinstein, S., Ghent, L., & Teuber, H.-L. *Somatosensory changes after penetrating brain wounds in man.* Cambridge, Mass.: Harvard University Press, 1960.

Sergent, J., & Bindra, D. Differential hemispheric processing of faces: Methodological considerations and reinterpretation. *Psychological Bulletin*, 1981, *89*, 541–554.

Seth, G. Eye-hand co-ordination and 'handedness': A developmental study of visuo-motor behaviour in infancy. *British Journal of Educational Psychology*, 1973, *43*, 35–49.

Shankweiler, D. Effects of temporal lobe damage on perception of dichotically presented melodies. *Journal of Comparative and Physiological Psychology*, 1966, *62*, 115–119.

Shankweiler, D., & Studdert-Kennedy, M. A continuum of lateralization for speech perception? *Brain and Language*, 1975, *2*, 212–225.

Shepard, R., & Metzler, J. Mental rotation of three-dimensional objects. *Science*, 1971, *171*, 701–703.

Sherman, J. A. *Sex-related cognitive differences: An essay on theory and evidence.* Springfield, Ill.: Thomas, 1978.

Shucard, D. W., Shucard, J. L., & Thomas, D. G. Auditory evoked potentials as probes of hemispheric differences in cognitive processing. *Science*, 1977, *197*, 1295–1297.

Sidtis, J. J., & Bryden, M. P. Asymmetrical perception of language and music: Evidence for independent processing strategies. *Neuropsychologia*, 1978, *16*, 627–632.

Silva, D. A., & Satz, P. Pathological left-handedness: Evaluation of a model. *Brain and Language*, 1979, *7*, 8–16.

Silverberg, R., Bentin, S., Gaziel, T., Obler, L. K., & Albert, M. L. Shift of visual field preference for English words in native Hebrew speakers. *Brain and Language*, 1979, *8*, 184–190.

Smith, M. O., Chu, J., & Edmonston, W. E. Cerebral lateralization of haptic perception: Interaction of responses to Braille and music reveals a functional basis. *Science*, 1977, *197*, 689–690.

Spellacy, F. Lateral preferences in the identification of patterned stimuli. *Journal of the Acoustical Society of America*, 1970, *47*, 574–578.

Spellacy, F., & Blumstein, S. The influence of language set on ear preference in phoneme recognition. *Cortex*, 1970, *6*, 430–439.

Sperling, G. The information available in brief visual presentation. *Psychological Monographs*, 1960, *74*(Whole No. 498).

Spreen, O., Spellacy, F. J., & Reid, J. R. The effect of interstimulus interval and intensity on ear asymmetry for nonverbal stimuli in dichotic listening. *Neuropsychologia,* 1970, *8,* 245–250.

Springer, S. P. Hemispheric specialization for speech opposed by contralateral noise. *Perception and Psychophysics,* 1973, *13,* 391–393.

Springer, S. P., & Eisenson, J. Hemispheric specialization for speech in language-disordered children. *Neuropsychologia,* 1977, *15,* 287–293.

Springer, S. P., & Searleman, A. The ontogeny of hemispheric specialization: Evidence from dichotic listening in twins. *Neuropsychologia,* 1978, *16,* 269–281.

Sprott, D. A., & Bryden, M. P. Measurement of laterality effects. In J. B. Hellige (Ed.), *Cerebral hemisphere asymmetry: Method, theory, and application.* New York: Praeger Scientific, forthcoming.

Stern, D. Handedness and the lateral distribution of conversion reactions. *Journal of Nervous and Mental Disease,* 1977, *164,* 122–128.

Strauss, E., & Moscovitch, M. Perception of facial expressions. *Brain and Language,* 1981, *13,* 308–332.

Stroop, J. Studies of interference in serial verbal reactions. *Journal of Experimental Psychology,* 1935, *18,* 643–662.

Studdert-Kennedy, M., & Shankweiler, D. Hemispheric specialization for speech perception. *Journal of the Acoustical Society of America,* 1970, *48,* 579–594.

Studdert-Kennedy, M., Shankweiler, D., & Schulman, S. Opposed effects of a delayed channel on perception of dichotically and monotonically presented CV syllables. *Journal of the Acoustical Society of America,* 1970, *48,* 599–602.

Suberi, M., & McKeever, W. F. Differential right hemispheric memory storage of emotional and non-emotional faces. *Neuropsychologia,* 1977, *5,* 757–768.

Summers, J. J., & Sharp, C. A. Bilateral effects of concurrent verbal and spatial rehearsal on complex motor sequencing. *Neuropsychologia,* 1979, *17,* 331–344.

Sussman, H. The laterality effect in lingual-auditory tracking. *Journal of the Acoustical Society of America* 1971, *49,* 1874–1880.

Sussman, H. M. Evidence for left hemisphere superiority in processing movement-related tonal signals. *Journal of Speech and Hearing Research,* 1979, *22,* 224–235.

Sussman, H., & MacNeilage, P. F. Studies of hemispheric specialization for speech production. *Brain and Language,* 1975, *2,* 131–151.

Sussman, H. M., & Westbury, J. R. A laterality effect in isometric and isotonic labial tracking. *Journal of Speech and Hearing Research,* 1978, *21,* 563–579.

Swanson, J., Ledlow, A., & Kinsbourne, M. Lateral asymmetries revealed by simple reaction time. In M. Kinsbourne (Ed.), *Asymmetrical function of the brain.* London: Cambridge Univ. Press, 1978.

Tanguay, P. E., Taub, J. M., Doubleday, C., & Clarkson, D. An interhemispheric comparison of auditory evoked responses to consonant–vowel stimuli. *Neuropsychologia,* 1977, *15,* 123–131.

Tapley, S. M., & Bryden, M. P. *A group test to assess hand performance.* Poster session at the annual meeting of the Canadian Psychological Association, Calgary, June 1980.

Templer, D. I., Goldstein, R., & Penick, S. B. Stability and inter-rater reliability of lateral eye movement. *Perceptual and Motor Skills,* 1972, *34,* 469–470.

Teng, E. L. Dichotic ear difference is a poor index for the functional asymmetry between the cerebral hemispheres. *Neuropsychologia,* 1981, *19,* 235–240.

Teng, E. L., Lee, P. H., Yang, K., & Chang, P. C. Handedness in a Chinese population: Biological, social, and pathological factors. *Science,* 1976, *193,* 1148–1150.

Terzian, H. Behavioral and EEG effects of intracarotid sodium amytal injections. *Acta Neurochirugia,* 1964, *12,* 230–240.

Thomson, M. E. A comparison of laterality effects in dyslexics and controls using verbal dichotic listening tasks. *Neuropsychologia*, 1976, *14*, 243–246.

Todor, J. I., & Doane, T. Handedness classification: Preference versus proficiency. *Perceptual and Motor Skills*, 1977, *45*, 1041–1042.

Tomlinson-Keasey, C., Kelly, R. R., & Burton, J. K. Hemispheric changes in information processing during development. *Developmental Psychology*, 1978, *14*, 214–223.

Trankell, A. Aspects of genetics in psychology. *American Journal of Human Genetics*, 1955, *7*, 264–276.

Treisman, A., & Geffen, G. Selective attention and cerebral dominance in perceiving and responding to speech messages. *Quarterly Journal of Experimental Psychology*, 1968, *20*, 139–150.

Tucker, D. M. Lateral brain function, emotion, and conceptualization. *Psychological Bulletin*, 1981, *89*, 19–46.

Tucker, G. H., & Suib, M. R. Conjugate lateral eye movement (CLEM) direction and its relationship to performance on verbal and visuospatial tasks. *Neuropsychologia*, 1978, *16*, 251–254.

Turkewitz, G. The development of lateral differences in the human infant. In S. Harnad, R. W. Doty, L. Goldstein, J. Jaynes, & G. Krauthamer (Eds.), *Lateralization in the nervous system*. New York: Academic Press, 1977.

Turkewitz, G., Gordon, E. W., & Birch, H. G. Head turning in the human neonate: Effect of prandial condition and lateral preference. *Journal of Comparative and Physiological Psychology*, 1965, *59*, 189–192. (a)

Turkewitz, G., Gordon, E. W., & Birch, H. G. Head turning in the human neonate: Spontaneous patterns. *Journal of Genetic Psychology*, 1965, *107*, 143–158. (b)

Turkewitz, G., Moreau, T., & Birch, H. Relation between birth condition and neurobehavioral organization in the neonate. *Pediatric Research*, 1968, *2*, 243–249.

Turvey, M. T., Pisoni, D. B., & Croog, J. F. A right-ear advantage in the retention of words presented monaurally. *Haskins Laboratories Status Report on Speech Research*, 1972, SR-31/32, 67–74.

Umilta, C., Rizzolatti, G., Marzi, C. A., Zamboni, G., Franzini, C., Carmada, R., & Berlucchi, G. Hemispheric differences in the discrimination of line orientation. *Neuropsychologia*, 1974, *12*, 165–174.

Uttal, W. R. *The psychobiology of sensory coding*. New York: Harper, 1973.

Vaid, J., & Genesee, F. Neuropsychological approaches to bilingualism: A critical review. *Canadian Journal of Psychology*, 1980, *34*, 417–445.

Vandenberg, S. G., & Kuse, A. R. Mental rotations: A group test of three-dimensional spatial visualization. *Perceptual and Motor Skills*, 1978, *47*, 599–604.

Vanderplas, J. M., & Garvin, E. A. The association of random shapes. *Journal of Experimental Psychology*, 1959, *57*, 147–154.

Van Lancker, D., & Fromkin, V. A. Hemispheric specialization for pitch and "tone": Evidence from Thai. *Journal of Phonetics*, 1973, *1*, 101–109.

Vargha-Khadem, F., & Corballis, M. C. Cerebral asymmetry in infants. *Brain and Language*, 1979, *8*, 1–9.

Varney, N. R., & Benton, A. L. Tactile perception of direction in relation to handedness and familial handedness. *Neuropsychologia*, 1975, *13*, 449–454.

Viviani, J., Turkewitz, G., & Karp, E. A relationship between laterality of functioning at 2 days and at 7 years of age. *Bulletin of the Psychonomic Society*, 1978, *12*, 189–192.

Wada, J. A. *Cerebral anatomical asymmetry in infant brains*. Paper presented at the Fourth Annual Meeting of the International Neuropsychology Society, Toronto, February 1976.

Wada, J. A., Clark, R., & Hamm, A. Cerebral hemispheric asymmetry in humans. *Archives of Neurology*, 1975, *32*, 239–246.

Wada, J. A., & Rasmussen, T. Intracarotid injection of sodium amytal for the lateralization of cerebral speech dominance. *Journal of Neurosurgery*, 1960, *17*, 266–282.

Wall, P. D. The somatosensory system. In M. S. Gazzaniga & C. Blakemore (Eds.), *Handbook of psychobiology*. New York: Academic Press, 1975.

Walter, J. L., Bryden, M. P., & Allard, F. *Hemispheric differences for nonverbal visual material*. Paper presented at the Annual Meeting of the Canadian Psychological Association, Toronto, June 1976.

Walters, J., & Zatorre, R. J. Laterality differences for word identification in bilinguals. *Brain and Language*, 1978, *6*, 158–167.

Warrington, E. K., & James, M. Tachistoscopic number estimation in patients with unilateral cerebral lesions. *Journal of Neurology, Neurosurgery and Psychiatry*, 1967, *30*, 468–474.

Warrington, E. K., & Pratt, R. T. C. Language laterality in left handers assessed by unilateral ECT. *Neuropsychologia*, 1973, *11*, 423–428.

Weinstein, E. A., & Kahn, R. L. *Denial of illness: Symbolic and physiological aspects*. Springfield, Ill.: Thomas, 1955.

Weinstein, S. Tactile sensitivity of the phalanges. *Perceptual and Motor Skills*, 1962, *14*, 351–354.

Weinstein, S. The relationship of laterality and cutaneous area to breast sensitivity in sinistrals and dextrals. *American Journal of Psychology*, 1963, *76*, 475–479.

Weinstein, S. Intensive and extensive aspects of tactile sensitivity as a function of body part, sex, and laterality. In D. R. Kenshalo (Ed.), *The skin senses*. Springfield, Ill.: Thomas, 1968.

Weinstein, S., & Sersen, E. A. Tactual sensitivity as a function of handedness and laterality. *Journal of Comparative and Physiological Psychology*, 1961, *54*, 665–669.

Weisenberg, T., & McBride, K. E. *Aphasia: A clinical and psychological study*. New York: Commonwealth Fund, 1935.

Weiss, M. S., & House, A. S. Perception of dichotically presented vowels. *Journal of the Acoustical Society of America*, 1973, *53*, 51–58.

Wertheim, N. Is there an anatomical localization for musical faculties? In M. Critchley & R. A. Henson (Eds.), *Music and the brain: Studies in the neurology of music*. Springfield, Ill.: Thomas, 1977.

White, K., & Ashton, R. Handedness assessment inventory. *Neuropsychologia*, 1976, *14*, 261–264.

White, M. J. Visual hemifield differences in the perception of letters and contour orientations. *Canadian Journal of Psychology*, 1971, *25*, 207–212.

White, M. J. Hemispheric asymmetries in tachistoscopic information processing. *British Journal of Psychology*, 1972, *63*, 497–508.

White, M. J. Does cerebral dominance offer a sufficient explanation for laterality differences in tachistoscopic recognition? *Perceptual and Motor Skills*, 1973, *36*, 479–485.

Wigan, A. L. *The duality of the mind*. London: Longman, 1844.

Wilkins, A., & Stewart, A. The time course of lateral asymmetries in visual perception of letters. *Journal of Experimental Psychology*, 1974, *102*, 905–908.

Wilson, R., Dirks, D., & Carterette, E. C. The effects of ear preference and order bias on the perception of verbal materials. *Journal of Speech and Hearing Research*, 1968, *11*, 502–522.

Witelson, S. F. Hemispheric specialization for linguistic and nonlinguistic tactual perception using a dichotomous stimulation technique. *Cortex*, 1974, *10*, 3–17.

Witelson, S. F. Abnormal right hemisphere specialization in developmental dyslexia. In R. M. Knights & D. J. Bakker (Eds.), *The neuropsychology of learning disorders: Theoretical approaches.* Baltimore: University Park Press, 1976. (a)

Witelson, S. F. Sex and the single hemisphere: Specialization of the right hemisphere for spatial processing. *Science,* 1976, *193,* 425–427. (b)

Witelson, S. F. Early hemisphere specialization and interhemispheric plasticity: An empirical and theoretical review. In S. J. Segalowitz & F. A. Gruber (Eds.), *Language development and neurological theory.* New York: Academic Press, 1977.

Witelson, S. F. Neuroanatomical asymmetry in left-handers: A review and implications for functional asymmetry. In J. Herron (Ed.), *Neuropsychology of left-handedness.* New York: Academic Press, 1980.

Witelson, S. F., & Pallie, W. Left hemisphere specialization for language in the newborn: Neuroanatomical evidence of asymmetry. *Brain,* 1973, *96,* 641–646.

Witelson, S., & Rabinovitch, M. S. Children's recall strategies in dichotic listening. *Journal of Experimental Child Psychology,* 1971, *12,* 106–113.

Witelson, S., & Rabinovitch, S. Hemispheric speech lateralization with auditory-linguistic deficits. *Cortex,* 1972, *8,* 413–426.

Witkin, H. A., Dyk, R. B., Faterson, H. F., Goodenough, D. R., & Karp, S. A. *Psychological differentiation.* New York: Wiley, 1962.

Wittig, M., & Petersen, A. C. (Eds.). *Sex-related differences in cognitive functioning: Developmental issues.* New York: Academic Press, 1979.

Woo, T. L., & Pearson, K. Dextrality and sinistrality. *Biometrika,* 1927, *19,* 192–198.

Wood, C. C., Goff, W. R., & Day, R. S. Auditory evoked potentials during speech perception. *Science,* 1971, *173,* 1248–1251.

Wood, F. Theoretical, methodological, and statistical implications of the inhalation rCBF technique for the study of brain-behavior relationships. *Brain and Language,* 1980, *9,* 1–8.

Woodworth, R. S. *Experimental psychology.* New York: Holt, 1938.

Wyke, M. Postural arm drift associated with brain lesions in man. *Archives of Neurology,* 1966, *15,* 329–334.

Wyke, M. Effect of brain lesions on the rapidity of arm movement. *Neurology,* 1967, *17,* 1113–1120.

Wyke, M. Effect of brain lesions in the performance of an arm–hand precision task. *Neuropsychologia,* 1968, *6,* 125–134.

Wyke, M. Influence of direction on the rapidity of bilateral arm movements. *Neuropsychologia,* 1969, *7,* 189–194.

Wyke, M. The effects of brain lesions on the learning performance of a bimanual coordination task. *Cortex,* 1971, *7,* 59–72. (a)

Wyke, M. The effects of brain lesions on the performance of bilateral arm movements. *Neuropsychologia,* 1971, *9,* 33–42. (b)

Yeni-Komshian, G. H., & Gordon, J. F. The effect of memory load on the right ear advantage in dichotic listening. *Brain and Language,* 1974, *1,* 375–381.

Yeni-Komshian, G. H., Isenberg, D., & Goldberg, H. Cerebral dominance and reading disability: Left visual field deficit in poor readers. *Neuropsychologia,* 1975, *13,* 83–94.

Yin, R. Face recognition by brain injured patients: A dissociable ability? *Neuropsychologia,* 1970, *8,* 395–402.

Young, A. W., & Bion, P. J. Hemispheric laterality effects in the enumeration of visually presented collections of dots by children. *Neuropsychologia,* 1979, *17,* 99–102.

Young, A. W., & Ellis, A. W. Perception of numerical stimuli felt by fingers of the left and right hands. *Quarterly Journal of Experimental Psychology,* 1979, *31,* 263–272.

Young, A. W., & Ellis, A. W. Asymmetry of cerebral hemispheric function in normal and poor readers. *Psychological Bulletin,* 1981, *89,* 183–190.

Zaidel, E. Language, dichotic listening, and the disconnected hemispheres. In D. O. Walter, L. Rogers, & J. M. Finzi-Fried (Eds.), *Conference on human brain function.* Los Angeles: Brain Information Service (Report No. 42), 1976.

Zajonc, R. B. Feeling and thinking: Preferences need no inferences. *American Psychologist,* 1980, *35,* 151–175.

Zangwill, O. L. *Cerebral dominance and its relation to psychological function.* Edinburgh: Oliver & Boyd, 1960.

Zoccolotti, P., & Oltman, P. K. Field dependence and lateralization of verbal and configurational processing. *Cortex,* 1978, *14,* 155–163.

Zurif, E. B., & Bryden, M. P. Familial handedness and left–right differences in auditory and visual perception. *Neuropsychologia,* 1969, *7,* 179–187.

Index

PERSPECTIVES IN
NEUROLINGUISTICS, NEUROPSYCHOLOGY, AND
PSYCHOLINGUISTICS: A Series of Monographs and Treatises

Harry A. Whitaker, Series Editor
DEPARTMENT OF HEARING AND SPEECH SCIENCES
UNIVERSITY OF MARYLAND
COLLEGE PARK, MARYLAND 20742

HAIGANOOSH WHITAKER and HARRY A. WHITAKER (Eds.).
Studies in Neurolinguistics, Volumes 1, 2, 3, and 4

NORMAN J. LASS (Ed.). Contemporary Issues in Experimental Phonetics

JASON W. BROWN. Mind, Brain, and Consciousness: The Neuropsychology of Cognition

SIDNEY J. SEGALOWITZ and FREDERIC A. GRUBER (Eds.). Language Development and Neurological Theory

SUSAN CURTISS. Genie: A Psycholinguistic Study of a Modern-Day "Wild Child"

JOHN MACNAMARA (Ed.). Language Learning and Thought

I. M. SCHLESINGER and LILA NAMIR (Eds.). Sign Language of the Deaf: Psychological, Linguistic, and Sociological Perspectives

WILLIAM C. RITCHIE (Ed.). Second Language Acquisition Research: Issues and Implications

PATRICIA SIPLE (Ed.). Understanding Language through Sign Language Research

MARTIN L. ALBERT and LORAINE K. OBLER. The Bilingual Brain: Neuropsychological and Neurolinguistic Aspects of Bilingualism

TALMY GIVÓN. On Understanding Grammar

CHARLES J. FILLMORE, DANIEL KEMPLER, and WILLIAM S-Y. WANG (Eds.). Individual Differences in Language Ability and Language Behavior

JEANNINE HERRON (Ed.). Neuropsychology of Left-Handedness

FRANÇOIS BOLLER and MAUREEN DENNIS (Eds.). Auditory Comprehension: Clinical and Experimental Studies with the Token Test

R. W. RIEBER (Ed.). Language Development and Aphasia in Children: New Essays and a Translation of "Kindersprache und Aphasie" by Emil Fröschels

GRACE H. YENI-KOMSHIAN, JAMES F. KAVANAGH, and CHARLES A. FERGUSON (Eds.). Child Phonology, Volume 1: Production and Volume 2: Perception